Serono Symposia USA
Norwell, Massachusetts

Springer Science+Business Media, LLC

PROCEEDINGS IN THE SERONO SYMPOSIA USA SERIES

MALE STERILITY AND MOTILITY DISORDERS:
Etiological Factors and Treatment: A Serono Symposia S.A. Publication
Edited by Samir Hamamah, Roger Mieusset, François Olivennes, and René Frydman

NUTRITIONAL ASPECTS OF OSTEOPOROSIS: A Serono Symposia S.A. Publication
Edited by Peter Burckhardt, Bess Dawson-Hughes, and Robert P. Heaney

GERM CELL DEVELOPMENT, DIVISION, DISRUPTION AND DEATH
Edited by Barry R. Zirkin

CELL DEATH IN REPRODUCTIVE PHYSIOLOGY
Edited by Jonathan L. Tilly, Jerome F. Strauss III, and Martin Tenniswood

INHIBIN, ACTIVIN AND FOLLISTATIN: Regulatory Functions
in System and Cell Biology: A Serono Symposia S.A. Publication
Edited by Toshihiro Aono, Hiromu Sugino, and Wylie W. Vale

PERIMENOPAUSE
Edited by Rogerio A. Lobo

GROWTH FACTORS AND WOUND HEALING: Basic Science and
Potential Clinical Applications
Edited by Thomas R. Ziegler, Glenn F. Pierce, and David N. Herndon

POLYCYSTIC OVARY SYNDROME
Edited by R. Jeffrey Chang

IDEA TO PRODUCT: The Process
Edited by Nancy J. Alexander and Anne Colston Wentz

BOVINE SPONGIFORM ENCEPHALOPATHY: The BSE Dilemma
Edited by Clarence J. Gibbs, Jr.

GROWTH HORMONE SECRETAGOGUES
Edited by Barry B. Bercu and Richard F. Walker

CELLULAR AND MOLECULAR REGULATION OF TESTICULAR CELLS
Edited by Claude Desjardins

GENETIC MODELS OF IMMUNE AND INFLAMMATORY DISEASES
Edited by Abul K. Abbas and Richard A. Flavell

MOLECULAR AND CELLULAR ASPECTS OF PERIIMPLANTATION PROCESSES
Edited by S.K. Dey

THE SOMATOTROPHIC AXIS AND THE REPRODUCTIVE PROCESS IN HEALTH
AND DISEASE
Edited by Eli Y. Adashi and Michael O. Thorner

GHRH, GH, AND IGF-I: Basic and Clinical Advances
Edited by Marc R. Blackman, S. Mitchell Harman, Jesse Roth, and Jay R. Shapiro

Continued after Index

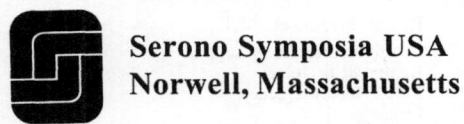

Serono Symposia USA
Norwell, Massachusetts

Samir Hamamah   Roger Mieusset
François Olivennes   René Frydman
Editors

Male Sterility and Motility Disorders

Etiological Factors and Treatment

A Serono Symposia S.A. Publication

Foreword by R.G. Edwards

With 26 Figures

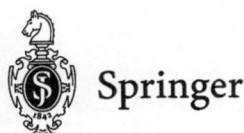
Springer

Samir Hamamah, Ph.D.

Service de FIV
Hôpital A. Béclère
92141 Clamart cedex
France

François Olivennes, M.D., Ph.D.

Service de Gynéco-Obstétrique
Hôpital A. Béclère
157, rue de la Porte-de-Trivaux
92141 Clamart cedex
France

Roger Mieusset, M.D.

Centre de Stérilité Masculine
Hôpital de la Grave
31052 Toulouse cedex
France

René Frydman. Ph.D.

Service de Gynéco-Obstétrique
Hôpital A. Béclère
157, rue de la Porte-de-Trivaux
92141 Clamart cedex
France

Proceedings of the International Symposium on Male Sterility for Motility Disorders, sponsored by Serono Symposia S.A., held January 30 to 31, 1998, in Paris, France.

For information on previous volumes, contact Serono Symposia USA, Inc.

Library of Congress Cataloging-in-Publication Data
Male sterility and motility disorders: etiological factors and
   treatment / Samir Hamamah [et al.].
      p.   cm.
   "Serono Symposia USA."
   "Proceedings of the International Symposium on Male Sterility for
Motility Disorders, sponsored by Serono Symposia S.A., held
January 30–31, 1998, in Paris, France"—T.p. verso.
   Includes bibliographical references and index.
   ISBN 978-1-4612-7177-2   ISBN 978-1-4612-1522-6 (eBook)
   DOI 10.1007/978-1-4612-1522-6
   1. Spermatozoa—Motility—Disorders—Congresses.   I. Hamamah, S.
II. Serono Symposia S.A.   III. International Symposium on Male
Sterility for Motility Disorders (1998 : Paris, France.)
   [DNLM: 1. Infertility, Male—etiology congresses.   2. Infertility,
Male—therapy congresses.   3. Sperm Motility—physiology congresses.
4. Spermatozoa—physiology congresses.   WJ 709 M2457 1999]
RC889.2.M34   1999
616.6'92—dc21   98-33322

Printed on acid-free paper.

© 1999 Springer Science+Business Media New York
Originally published by Springer-Verlag New York, Inc. in 1999
Softcover reprint of the hardcover 1st edition 1991

Production coordinated by Chernow Editorial Services, Inc., and managed by Francine McNeill; manufacturing supervised by Joe Quatela.
Typeset by KP Company, Brooklyn, NY.

9 8 7 6 5 4 3 2 1

ISBN 978-1-4612-7177-2

SYMPOSIUM ON MALE STERILITY FOR MOTILITY DISORDERS

Scientific Committee

Mohamed Benahmed, M.D.
INSERM U 407
Laboratoire de Recherche sur les Communications Cellulaires
   en Biologie de la Reproduction
Centre Hospitalier Lyon-Sud
69 495 Pierre-Bénite cedex, France

René Frydman, Ph.D.
Service de Gynéco-Obstétrique
Hôpital A. Béclère
157, rue de la Porte-de-Trivaux
92141 Clamart cedex, France

Samir Hamamah, Ph.D.
Service de FIV
Hôpital A. Béclère
92141 Clamart cedex, France

Roger Mieusset, M.D.
Centre de Stérilité Masculine
Hôpital de la Grave
31052 Toulouse cedex, France

Yigal Soffer, M.D.
Infertility and IVF Unit
Assaf Harofeh Medical Center
Zerifin 70300, Israel

Herman Tournaye, M.D.
Centre for Reproductive Medicine
University Hospital, Dutch-Speaking Brussels Free University
Laarbeeklaan 101, B-1090 Brussels, Belgium

Organizing Secretary

Maria Grazia Calì
Serono Symposia S.A.
15 bis Chemin des Mines
CH-1202 Geneva, Switzerland

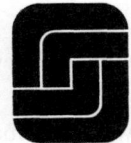

Foreword

This conference, dedicated to the etiology and treatment of motility disorders in spermatozoa and male sterility, attracted some of the finest investigators in the field. Standards were immensely high throughout, and discussions were meaningful and detailed. Analyses on disorders in sperm motility demand a broad-based approach, involving cytologists, geneticists, andrologists, and embryologists, because the topic has many clinical and scientific overtones. Human spermatozoa are at the mercy of so many factors as they form and mature in the testis and epididymis. Their survival and fundamental characteristics are essential for fertilization, and the male genome imposes its influence on the embryo as it becomes active in male pronuclei very soon after sperm entry into the oocyte.

All of these fundamental aspects of sperm biology demanded a broad breadth of topics in the symposium. The opening session quickly got down to fundamentals with contributions from J.-L. Gatti, J.G. Alvarez, C. Gagnon, and H. Breitbart. They discussed the mechanism and regulation of motility, the metabolic strategy of human spermatozoa, the effects of exogenous factors such as antibodies, infections, and toxins, and finally the role of intracellular calcium on sperm motility. To these topics, the postcoffee session on the first morning described the genetics of motility disorders and the etiology and management of necrozoospermia. The excellent presentation provided the background detail of the symposium and opened the way for the discussion of various clinical aspects of the topic.

Therapy was covered by three speakers. P. Jouannet evaluated the assessment of flagellar dyskinesia, medial therapy was analyzed by R. Mieusset, and in vitro therapy by S. Hamamah. These French contributions outlined both the opportunities and limitations of present-day methods, preparatory to a debate on the value of ICSI in cases of immotile spermatozoa. ICSI clearly remains the best hope at present, as shown in the minisymposium devoted to it. The use of HOST or supravital staining to identify live immotile spermatozoa—evidently an important aspect of establishing pregnancies with ICSI—

was described by J. Cohen. The necessary conditions for choosing and injecting immotile spermatozoa were covered by S. Fishel, including means of
selection, breakages in sperm tails, and the use of different media.
R. Ron-El analyzed the use of thawed immotile spermatozoa in ICSI, and
H. Tournaye complemented this paper by assessing the wider clinical factors
involved in the use of immotile spermatozoa. Several short reports by seven
investigators were devoted to the value of ICSI in difficult cases. Several
excellent posters were also discussed during this session, selected from a
larger number of carefully designed and presented posters on display at the
meeting.

The second day of the conference opened with analyses on the physiology
and pathology of testicular spermatozoa. Fundamental studies on testis cells
including spermatozoa emerged once again. Testis function was analyzed by
M. Benahmed in a discussion on growth factors, L.D. Russell, who analyzed
apopotosis in testicular tissues, and an analyses of gene expression in the
regulation of apopotosis by D. de Rooij. This session ended with a description from A. Ogura and R. Yanagimachi of fundamental molecular controls in
immature sperm cells, which are essential for fertilization. These papers continued the very high quality apparent in the first day and introduced two final
clinical sessions.

The first of these, testicular sperm retrieval and its value for ICSI, was
covered initially by G. Tritto, A. Ditmar, and G. Arvis, on the value of
microcaptors and testicular sperm extraction before the use of ICSI. S. Silber
described the methods and means for identifying the ideal testicular site for
sperm retrieval, P. Schlegel was concerned with possible pathological risks
after multiple biopsies for TESE, and V. Izard, D. Marmor, A. Benoit, and
A. Jardin dealt with peroperative cytology of the population of germinal cells
in relation to the strategy of sperm retrieval. This session concluded with the
discussion of four abstracts on the genetics and cell biology of the spermatozoon. Once again, large amounts of material were presented and discussed by
each author. A similar theme continued in the final session, with the presentation of studies on genetic aspects of male sterility, including work on the
AZFa, b, and c deletions by P. Vogt, the quality of conceptuses derived from
testicular spermatozoa by H. Hazout, and, finally, the genetic problems of
ICSI children, presented by M. Bonduelle and L. Liebars.

This book should prove to be of immense value to scientists and clinicians
involved in scientific studies or patient care. The problem of male infertility
is a huge one, and the introduction of ICSI has opened one approach to its
alleviation. This conference will be valuable to many readers for having analyzed the basic and applied aspects of the field in great detail. No stone has
been left unturned, and the symposium will doubtless have a prominent place
in the libraries of most investigators concerned with male infertility and sperm
motility.

R.G. EDWARDS

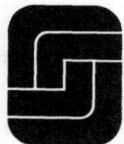

Contents

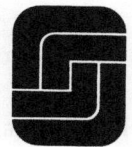

Contributors

MOHAMED A. ABOULGHAR, The Egyptian IVF-ET Center, Maadi, Cairo, Egypt.

JUAN G. ALVAREZ, Department of Obstetrics and Gynecology, Beth Israel Deaconess Medical Center, Harvard Medical School, Boston, Massachusetts, USA.

YAHIA M. AMIN, The Egyptian IVF-ET Center, Maadi, Cairo, Egypt.

GABRIEL ARVIS, Service of Uro-Andrology, Tenon Hospital, Paris, France.

AYSE AYTOZ, Centre for Medical Genetics, Dutch-Speaking Brussels Free University, Brussels, Belgium.

CLAIRE BARTHELEMY, Reproductive Unit, Obstetrics and Gynecology Department, Centre Hospitalier Universitaire Bretonneau, Tours, France.

MOHAMED BENAHMED, Laboratoire de Recherche sur les Communications Cellulairés, INSERM, Centre Hospitalier Lyon-Sud, 69 495 Pierre-Bénite cedex, France.

GÉRARD BENOÎT, Department of Urology, Hôpital Bicêtre, Le Kremlin Bicêtre, France.

ORNA BERN, IVF and Infertility Unit, Assaf Harofeh Medical Center, Tel-Aviv University, Zerifin, Israel.

TIM L. BEUMER, Department of Cell Biology, Utrecht University Medical School, Utrecht, The Netherlands.

MARYSE BONDUELLE, Centre for Medical Genetics, Dutch-Speaking Brussels Free University, Brussels, Belgium.

HAIM BREITBART, Life Sciences, Bar-Ilan University, Ramat-Gan, Israel.

ANDREA BUYSSE, Centre for Medical Genetics, Dutch-Speaking Brussels Free University, Brussels, Belgium.

NICOLE CARLON, Laboratoire d'Embryologie, Faculté de Médicine, Marseilles, France.

PAUL COHEN-BACRIE, IVF Unit, Laboratoire Déylau, Paris, France.

HÉLÈNE CORDONIER, Laboratoire de Biologie de la Reproduction, Hôpital Edouard Herriot, Lyon, France.

JAMES M. CUMMINS, Division of Veterinary and Biomedical Sciences, Murdoch University, Murdoch, Western Australia, Australia.

EVE DE LAMIRANDE, Urology Research Laboratory, Royal Victoria Hospital and Faculty of Medicine, McGill University, Quebec, Canada.

DIRK G. DE ROOIJ, Department of Cell Biology, Utrecht University Medical School, Utrecht, The Netherlands.

PAUL DEVROEY, Centre for Medical Genetics, Dutch-Speaking Brussels Free University, Brussels, Belgium.

ANDRÉ DITTMAR, INSA Lyon, CNRS LPM, Lyon, France.

KENNETH DOWELL, Centres for Assisted Reproduction, Nottingham, UK.

MARTINE DUMONT-HASSAN, IVF Unit, Laboratoire Déylau, Paris, France.

ALAIN FIGNON, Departement de Gynécologie-Obstétrique, CHU Bretonneau, 37044 Tours cedex, France.

SIMON FISHEL, Centres for Assisted Reproduction, Nottingham, UK.

SHEVACH FRIEDLER, IVF and Infertility Unit, Assaf Harofeh Medical Center, Tel-Aviv University, Zerifin, Israel.

CLAUDE GAGNON, Urology Research Laboratory, Royal Victoria Hospital and Faculty of Medicine, McGill University, Quebec, Canada.

LOUISE GARRATT, Centres for Assisted Reproduction, Nottingham, UK.

JEAN-LUC GATTI, Chargé Recherche Thèse d'Université en Science de la Vie, Laboratoire de Physiologie de la Reproduction, INRA Nouzilly, France.

STEVEN GREEN, Centres for Assisted Reproduction, Nottingham, UK.

GENEVIÈVE GRIZARD, Laboratoire de la Reproduction, Hôtel Dieu, Clermont-Ferrand, France.

JEAN-FRANÇOIS GUÉRIN, Laboratoire de Biologie de la Reproduction, Hôpital Edouard Herriot, Lyon, France.

SAMIR HAMAMAH, Service de FIV, Hôpital A. Béclère, 92141 Clamart cedex, France.

ANDRE HAZOUT, 15, rue Faraday, Paris, France.

ALISON HUNTER-CAMPBELL, Centres for Assisted Reproduction, Nottingham, UK.

VINCENT IZARD, Department of Urology, Hôpital Bicêtre, Le Kremlin Bicêtre, France.

ALAIN JARDIN, Department of Urology, Hôpital Bicêtre, Le Kremlin Bicêtre, France.

AHMED KAMAL, The Egyptian IVF-ET Center, Maadi, Cairo, Egypt.

ESTI KASTERSTEIN, IVF and Infertility Unit, Assaf Harofeh Medical Center, Tel-Aviv University, Zerifin, Israel.

DAPHNA KOMAROVSKI, IVF and Infertility Unit, Assaf Harofeh Medical Center, Tel-Aviv University, Zerifin, Israel.

PIERRE J. LECOMTE, Department of Endocrinology, Centre Hospitalier Universitaire Bretonneau, Tours, France.

RACHEL LEVY, Laboratoire de Biologie de la Reproduction, Hôpital Edouard Herriot, Lyon, France.

PHILIP SHIHUA LI, Department of Urology, James Buchanan Brady Foundation, The New York Hospital—Cornell Medical Center, New York, New York, USA.

INGE LIEBAERS, Centre for Medical Genetics, Dutch-Speaking Brussels Free University, Brussels, Belgium.

JACQUELINE LORNAGE, Laboratoire de Biologie de la Reproduction, Hôpital Edouard Herriot, Lyon, France.

RAGAA T. MANSOUR, The Egyptian IVF-ET Center, Maadi, Cairo, Egypt.

DOMINIQUE MARMOR, Reproductive Biology Unit, Hôpital Bicêtre, Le Kremlin Bicêtre, France.

CLAIRE MAUDUIT, Laboratoire de Recherche sur les Communications Cellulairés, INSERM, Centre Hospitalier Lyon-Sud, 69 495 Pierre Bénite cedex, France.

HELEN MCDERMOTT, Centres for Assisted Reproduction, Nottingham, UK.

GEORGES MERCIER, Laboratoire d'Embryologie, Faculté de Médicine, Marseilles, France.

ROGER MIEUSSET, Centre de Stérilité Masculine, Hôpital de la Grave, 31052 Toulouse cedex, France.

DAVID MORTIMER, Sydney I.V.F., and Department of Obstetrics and Gynaecology, University of Sydney, New South Wales, Australia.

SHARON T. MORTIMER, Department of Animal Science, University of Sydney, New South Wales, Australia.

ZVI NAOR, Biochemistry, Tel-Aviv University, Tel-Aviv, Israel.

LEONARD NDUWAYO, Department of Endocrinology, Centre Hospitalier Universitaire Bretonneau, Tours, France.

MARIE-ODILE NORTH, International Center of Andrology of Roma, Rome, Italy.

ATSUO OGURA, Department of Veterinary Science, National Institute of Infectious Diseases, Tokyo, Japan.

VALÉRIE PARADIS, Department of Pathology, Hôpital Bicêtre, Le Kremlin Bicêtre, France.

ANNE PERON, Laboratoire of Biological Andrology, Hôpital Bicêtre, Le Kremlin Bicêtre, France.

MARIE-CLAUDE PINATEL, Laboratoire de Biologie de la Reproduction, Hôpital Edouard Herriot, Lyon, France.

ARIE RAZIEL, IVF and Infertility Unit, Assaf Harofeh Medical Center, Tel-Aviv University, Zerifin, Israel.

RAPHAEL RON-EL, IVF and Infertility Unit, Assaf Harofeh Medical Center, Tel-Aviv University, Zerifin, Israel.

LONNIE D. RUSSELL, Department of Physiology, Southern Illinois University School of Medicine, Carbondale, Illinois, USA.

MORY SCHACHTER, IVF and Infertility Unit, Assaf Harofeh Medical Center, Tel-Aviv University, Zerifin, Israel.

PETER N. SCHLEGEL, Department of Urology, James Buchanan Brady Foundation, The New York Hospital–Cornell Medical Center, New York, New York, USA.

GAMAL I. SEROUR, The Egyptian IVF-ET Center, Maadi, Cairo, Egypt.

FRANCOISE SHENFIELD, Reproductive Medicine Unit, University College Hospital, London, UK.

SHERMAN J. SILBER, Infertility Center of St. Louis, St. Luke's Hospital, St. Louis, Missouri, USA.

YIGAL SOFFER, Male Infertility and IVF Unit, Assaf Harofeh Medical Center, Tel-Aviv University, Zerifin, Israel.

JEAN-CLAUDE SOUFIR, Laboratoire of Biological Andrology, Hôpital Bicêtre, Le Kremlin Bicêtre, France.

DEBORAH STRASSBURGER, IVF and Infertility Unit, Assaf Harofeh Medical Center, Tel-Aviv University, Zerifin, Israel.

LI-MING SU, Department of Urology, James Buchanan Brady Foundation, The New York Hospital–Cornell Medical Center, New York, New York, USA.

NEVIN A. TAWAB, The Egyptian IVF-ET Center, Maadi, Cairo, Egypt.

SIMON THORNTON, Centres for Assisted Reproduction, Nottingham, UK.

HERMAN TOURNAYE, Centre for Reproductive Medicine, University Hospital, Dutch-Speaking Brussels Free University, B-1090 Brussels, Belgium.

JOSEPH TRITTO, Service of Urology, Saint Louis Hospital and Service of Uro-Andrology, Tenon Hospital, Paris, France.

ELVIRE VAN ASSCHE, Centre for Medical Genetics, Dutch-Speaking Brussels Free University, Brussels, Belgium.

ANDRE VAN STEIRTEGHEM, Centre for Medical Genetics, Dutch-Speaking Brussels Free University, Brussels, Belgium.

PETER H. VOGT, Reproduction Genetics, Institute of Human Genetics, Heidelberg, Germany.

JOHN WEBSTER, Centres for Assisted Reproduction, Nottingham, UK.

ANN WILIKENS, Centre for Medical Genetics, Dutch-Speaking Brussels Free University, Brussels, Belgium.

RYUZO YANAGIMACHI, Department of Anatomy and Reproductive Biology, University of Hawaii School of Medicine, Honolulu, Hawaii, USA.

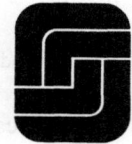

Introduction

The field of clinical andrology was to all intents and purposes declared extinct by leading reproductive specialists 5 years ago after an overwhelming series of events in male infertility treatment by assisted fertilization, principally the ICSI procedure. Although sweeping general statements such as this are often made after medical breakthroughs, they are, in fact, generally inspired by the moment, and they rarely survive intact for more than a few years. Even though the importance of ICSI led to a lessening of basic interest in spermatology, it has nevertheless opened avenues that previously were impossible to study. This book presents the proceedings of a meeting held in Paris in 1998 on the narrow but crucial topic of clinical andrology, describing the etiological factors and treatments of male sterility following disorders of sperm motility. Overall agreement between the many gifted scientific authors gathered for this meeting would have been nearly impossible to achieve were it not for the growing realization that ICSI by no means explains fertilization failure for subfertile men, nor does it shed any light on the causes of idiopathic hypokinesia.

A synopsis of the ultrastructure and metabolic strategy of human spermatozoa for motility support provides the background for an update on the mechanisms and regulation of sperm motility. Likely etiologies of nonmotile human sperm are addressed here in superb detail, as are the potential effects on sperm motility of both intracellular calcium and various extrinsic–intrinsic and cellular factors. It is being increasingly observed that motility disorders can be associated with genetic problems.

Early clinical assessment of flagellar dyskinesia is important because it lowers chances of normal fertilization and obviously suggests performing ICSI as the next step. For other motility disorders, various laboratory tools are presented here, but without any conclusive answers. We find that migration, selective washing techniques, and caffeine or pentoxifylline addition can improve motility, but such treatments are not always associated with positive outcome.

Identification of live immotile sperm is a prerequisite for selection of the cell to be injected into the oocyte. When a few individual sperm cells are frozen for use through ICSI, specific techniques of sperm cryopreservation are required, and it is important to minimize any motility loss. For injection of immotile sperm, various factors have to be taken into account, such as sperm selection, tail breakage, and the medium used for maturation and culture. Whatever procedure is used, however, the fertilizing capacity of thawed immotile sperm is rather low in terms of viable pregnancies. ICSI with ejaculated immotile sperm is mainly associated with fertilization failure, and some authors suggested a move to testicular sperm in cases of necrozoospermia. ICSI is also used in recognized "difficult" cases, such as Klinefelter, nonobstructive azoospermia (low success rates, embryonic development), immotile sperm (multiple structural sperm anomalies), and severe teratozoospermia. Whatever the specific details are, success rates in "difficult" ICSI cases are rather low.

Several growth factors that support testis development and function are described here as well. It has become increasingly evident that testicular cells may undergo apoptosis, or cell loss during spermatogenesis, in which a transcription factor seems to be important in initiating an apoptotic pathway, at least in animal models, but the debate between apoptosis or necrosis as the primary process involved is still open.

Another important problem concerns the possible negative consequences certain diagnostic and therapeutic testicular extraction procedures may have on testicular function. Repeated surgical procedures are not only costly and invasive, but in the case of testicular sperm extraction, can cause transient and even permanent adverse physiologic effects. Many questions such as methods, modalities, and ideal sites for sperm retrieval are being addressed, as well as the potential pathological risks following multiple biopsies.

Finally, considerations about the health of the conceptus obtained through ICSI from ejaculated as well as testicular sperm are covered here with special concern because many medical and ethical questions have arisen since its introduction.

JACQUES COHEN

Part I

The Immotile Sperm: Etiology

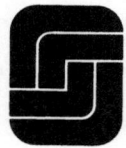

1

Motility Update

JEAN-LUC GATTI

Introduction

Although evolution has put strong selective pressure on ensuring that individuals have healthy, functioning gametes, at least 15% of human couples have fertility problems. The infertility can be due to either partner, but fecondation failure in the male partner occurs in one third of the cases (1). A large number of different causes can lead to this male infertility, but the most striking ones are those that affect the mobility of the sperm because the main function of this cell is to deliver the male nuclear package to the ovocyte. These cases of infertility can be treated by subzonal insemination or intracytoplasmic injection (2–4), with the risk that the genetic defect will be transmitted to the offspring.

To achieve their function, sperm have a highly specialized device for their displacement: the flagellum. In cases of motility problems, the normal beating of this flagellum may be decreased, abnormal, or totally absent, depending on the flagellar ultrastructural defects. The sperm flagellum has an internal complex structure composed of a central core that is common to almost all cilia and flagella: the axoneme (see Fig. 1.1). This axoneme is composed of an external ring formed by nine outer doublets of microtubules with two single microtubules at its center forming a central pair (the 9 + 2 structure). The assembly of this axoneme requires more than 200 different proteins. The axonemal structure is the active part of the flagellum and is responsible for the formation and the propagation of coordinated bending waves, which results in sperm displacement. In mammals, this axoneme is surrounded by large columnar structures formed by the outer dense fibers enclosed either with the ribbon formed by the mitochondria along the intermediate piece, or by the fibrous sheath along the principal piece (Fig. 1.1).

Several reviews have been published on axonemal structure and its composition [5–8; see also the series of papers published in *Cell Motility and Cytoskeleton* 1995; 32(2)] as well as on the different models that explain the motility mechanism and regulation (9–12). Readers are invited to refer to

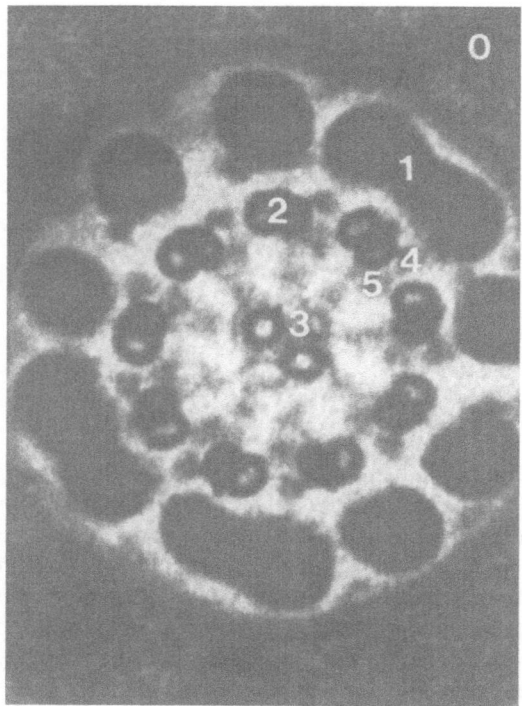

FIGURE 1.1. Transverse section of the intermediate piece of a mammalian sperm flagellum. Flagellum from boar sperm: 0, mitochondria surrounding the dense fibers and the axoneme; 1, outer dense fibers; 2, external doublet of microtubule; 3, central doublet of microtubule; 4, outer arm dynein attached to the A tubule; 5, inner arm dynein attached to the A tubule. The nine peripheral doublets and the two singlets form the 9 + 2 structure of the axoneme (about 250 nm in diameter).

these different papers for an excellent overview of the exploding fields of both axonemal motility and its cytoplasmic counterpart (13,14).

This chapter will focus on the new results as well as the questions raised by different molecular biology analyses of the flagellar components. Some of the data highlight the difficulties in reaching definitive conclusions on the role of certain axonemal components in sperm motility.

Building the Axoneme

Centriolar Structure

At the center of the axoneme is the centriole, a structure that is composed of nine triplets of microtubules. Several components of the pericentriolar material have been shown to be unique and necessary for nucleating microtubules. This is particularly the case for the gamma tubulin that self-assembles to form the ring complexes on which the microtubules are built (15,16). Indirect results have suggested that these gamma-tubulin elements could be present at the base of the microtubule that forms the axonemes (17).

Another protein described in the sperm centrosome is a zinc finger protein called basonuclin (18). This protein is found associated with the distal centriole at the base of the elongating flagellum during spermatozoan formation as well as within the nucleus and the acrosome, which suggests a role in the nucleation of the microtubular network involved in sperm shaping.

These different findings are interesting as defects in the sperm centriole result in an abnormal axoneme (19). Male centrioles also play a role in the formation of the sperm aster after fecondation and possible links exist between centrosomal defects and a failure in the assembly of the microtubule network that is necessary for the pronuclei fusion (20).

The Tubulins

The main part of the axoneme is chiefly comprised of the alpha- and beta-tubulins forming the $9 + 2$ microtubules and the nine triplets of the centriole. The idea has arisen that certain tubulin isotypes participate in particular functions in specialized cells (multitubulin hypothesis; 21). This hypothesis is supported by the fact that a specific beta-tubulin isoform is required for a functional assembly of the Drosophila sperm axoneme (see Ref. 21). It is not yet known whether the equivalent of this specific isoform exists in other organisms. Meanwhile, it has been demonstrated that tubulins in the axonemes are posttranslationally modified and thus exist as many different variants (for a review, see Ref. 22). Alpha-tubulin can be acetylated, and both alpha- and beta-tubulin are modified by polyglycylation and polyglutamylation (22). Alpha-tubulin can also be truncated at the carboxyl terminal amino acid (delta 2 alpha-tubulin), hence it will not allow the cyclic detyrozilation that can occur on the alpha-tubulin. All these different variants of the tubulins are involved in the stability of the microtubules within the axoneme, and it has been demonstrated that these variants are apparently not distributed at random and play a certain role in sperm motility. The A and B microtubules that form the outer doublet in the sea urchin axoneme differ in the composition of their tubulin variants (23). The A tubule is formed mainly by alpha- and beta-tubulin that has been tyrozinated, whereas the B tubule contains more than half of its alpha-tubulin in the detyrozinated form and about half of its beta-tubulin in the polyglycylated form. This is interesting because both microtubules have different functions: The A tubule supports the dynein arms and the radial spokes, and the B tubule is the site of ATP-sensitive attachment of the dynein-ATPases. Meanwhile, motility inhibition of reactivated flagella by specific antibodies shows that dynein-ATPases bind to both alpha- and beta-tubulin in an ATP-dependent manner (24), particularly to the C-terminal domain of tubulins.

This is not surprising because the C-terminal domain of the tubulins is very important, both for microtubule formation and for interactions with microtubule-associated proteins. This is also the site where a number of post-translational modifications occur, such as the glutamylation of the alpha chain (22), and Gagnon et al. (25) have shown that an antibody against the glutamylated alpha-tubulin was also able to inhibit the movement of demembranated sea urchin and *Oxyrrhis marina* flagellum. In addition, it was shown that kinesin, another molecular motor, binds specifically to polyglutamylated tubulins by its ATP site. In a similar experiment, Cosson et al. (26) showed that using a monoclonal antibody directed at a beta-tubulin variant strongly decreased the beat frequency of reactivated axonemes from different species without impairing the dynein–tubulin interactions. The precise epitope of the tubulin recognized by the antibody was not described. These different effects of the tubulin antibodies are reminiscent of some of the motility defaults observed in certain dynein-deficient mutants in *Chlamydomonas* and suggest that different dynein-ATPases (inner and outer) do not bind to the same type of tubulins in the B tubule. The preferential distribution of the tubulin variants in the different microtubules suggests the possibility that the tubulin variants are involved in the mechanical cycle of different heads of dynein and may play a role in the mechanism of motility. If the ATP-binding domain of different dynein heavy chains was obtained in vitro, it would certainly allow this hypothesis to be analyzed further (27,28).

Structural studies have also been conducted to determine the precise surface lattice of the microtubule (17). All four types of microtubules (A, B, and the two central singlets) have been shown to have the same building structure: a B lattice in which alpha- and beta-tubulin form a stacking of successive coiled rings. This type of lattice implies that a microtubule is not a closed tube, but that a discontinuity exists. Knowledge of the tubulin lattice could help in the understanding of how the dynein-ATPases interact and displace the adjacent microtubule in three dimensions (29), as well as how this could influence the beating pattern (30).

Assembly of the Axoneme

Kinesins

Kinesins are a family of molecular motors involved in cytoplasmic transport. Kinesin isoforms have been found in the ciliary axoneme of *Chlamydomonas* and also of the sea urchin embryo (31–33). In *Chlamydomonas,* the isoforms are at different levels: (1) near the plasma membrane with a definite association with the external doublets of microtubule and (2) between the central doublet and definitely linked to one of the microtubules. Several reports indicate that kinesin is involved in the assembly of the axoneme by delivering cargoes to the tip of the growing end (plus end) of the axoneme. For example, in *Chlamydomonas*, inner arm mutants cannot be rescued by mutants missing one of the kinesin isoforms (Fla10), but outer-arm mutants can be, which suggests that this kinesin is necessary in inner-arm assembly (34). The microinjection of monoclonal antibody against anti–kinesin II (another kinesin isoform) into sea urchin eggs profoundly affects the ciliogenesis of the blastula: Only short immotile cilia lacking the central pair of microtubules are observed (32). Thus, different kinesin isoforms could be involved in axonemal assembly. The results also confirm that dynein complexes, inner arms, and, certainly, also outer arms, are preassembled in the cell's cytoplasm before being transported and attached on the axoneme (35). The presence of kinesin has been demonstrated in the sea urchin sperm axoneme (36), but not, as yet, in the mammalian sperm flagellum. The role of this motor protein in the sperm flagellar assembly during spermiogenesis remains to be studied. Meanwhile, short-tailed sperm, which are associated with an absence of inner arms in the cilia axoneme, are described in some cases of male infertility.

Hsp70

In the axonemal structure of *Chlamydomonas,* a 70 kDa flagellar protein that is a chaperone of the heat shock protein (hsp) family has also been suggested to have a role in normal axonemal assembly (37). This hsp70 is associated with the 9 + 2 structure and is mainly concentrated at the plus end side of the axoneme, perhaps associated with the end-capping structure of the axoneme. Several hsp70 proteins are expressed in mammalian germ cells during gametogenesis, and the knockout of some of these proteins in mice produces sterility in males by affecting gametogenesis (38,39). One of the hsp70 proteins is expressed specifically in round and elongated spermatids (hsc70t). It is also observed in mature spermatozoa; thus, it is possible that this particular hsp70 protein also plays a role in the mammalian sperm axonemal assembly.

Accessory Proteins in the Microtubules

The Dynein Regulatory Complex

At least 10 proteins form a structure located on the microtubule close to the inner arms. This structure has been shown to participate in the regulation of axonemal beating and is thus called the dynein regulatory complex (drc). The drc plays a role in transferring information between the dynein of the inner and outer arms as well as between the radial spokes and the inner arms (for a review, see Ref. 5). Mutations in the protein of the drc allow paralyzed *Chlamydomonas* with a missing central pair or radial spokes to regain movement, although this is different from normal beating. A fine analysis using reactivation of isolated axonemes from central pair and radial spokes mutants showed that with a low ATP concentration, the axonemes of certain of these mutants exhibited movements similar to those of the wild-type axoneme (40). These results indirectly suggest that the proteins of the drc may be involved in the sensitivity of the dynein toward ATP, and that the correct microtubule sliding in central pair or radial spokes mutants could be inhibited by physiological concentrations of ATP.

The Docking Structure

It was shown by using *Chlamydomonas* motility mutants obtained by insertional mutagenesis that absence of the outer arm in the axoneme could also result in the disappearance of a supplementary structure involved in the outer arm binding to the microtubule (41,42). This "docking structure" is part of microtubule A and is formed by the association of three proteins of 105, 62, and 25 kDa. The 105 kDa protein was cloned and its sequence revealed no clear homology with other proteins. The cDNA of the protein suggested that the molecular weight of this chain should be about 85 kDa. The difference observed may be due to phosphorylations (42).

Other components of the microtubule include a 66 kDa protein with WD repeats. Some of the immotile *Chlamydomonas* mutants that were defective in the central pair of microtubules and their accessory structures can be rescued (i.e., they can regain flagellar beating) by the insertion of the gene of a protein of 66 kDa with five WD repeats, which is a sequence motif involved in interactions between proteins that is also found in dynein intermediate chains (for further details, see Ref. 43). The presence of the 66 kDa protein allows formation of the normal central pair in the deficient mutant. Immunological study shows that the protein is normally situated all along one of the internal microtubules as well as in the bridge that connects the central pair together. This suggests that the 66 kDa protein is required for the nucleation of the central pair and also for their stability in vivo. Thus, the lack of one protein is sufficient to destabilize the central pair structure and inhibit flagellar movement.

The Motors: The Dynein-ATPases

Dynein-ATPases are macromolecular complexes that act as microtubule-based translocators during the beating cycle of the axoneme in cilia and flagella. This class of enzyme is also involved in cytoplasmic transport, chromosome movement, and organelle sorting.

Knowledge of the molecular composition of dynein-ATPases as well as understanding of their architecture and organization are based mainly on studies of the outer arm dyneins from cilia and flagella of protists and invertebrates (*Chlamydomonas, Tetrahymena*, sea urchin, oyster, and mussels) or lower vertebrates such as fishes [trout and rockcod (44)]. In the axoneme, dynein-ATPases are found in the outer and inner arms of the outer doublet of microtubules. Outer-arm dynein can be solubilized by a high salt extraction of isolated axonemes, but inner-arm dynein needs a different treatment such as low ionic strength dialysis of axonemes. As general features, dynein-

ATPases are large complexes of more than 1 MDa formed by the association of one or two subunits (depending on species origin). Each subunit contains one, two, or three high-molecular weight polypeptide chains (HCs; molecular weight > 400 kDa) with an ATP hydrolytic site and, in general, intermediates (ICs) and lower molecular weight (LCs) polypeptides (for reviews, see Refs. 5–7). All of these protein chains form particles viewed by scanning transmission electron microscopy as globular heads joined by a stem, with a mass at the root of the stem. The number of heads corresponds to the number of heavy chains.

The dynein-ATPase complex comprising the outer arm of the axoneme appears to be homogenous all along the flagellum. This means that the complex has the same composition from base to tip. In contrast, studies of *Chlamydomonas* and the sea urchin show that inner-arm dynein is heterogeneous. At least seven different complexes can be observed in *Chlamydomonas*: One (inner arm 1; I1) is formed by a two-headed particle, but the others (I2 and I3) by one single head. These different complexes involved at least eight distinct HCs and several different ICs and LCs (45).

Molecular biology studies have been carried out over a 3-year period to decipher the different proteins involved in the formation of these dynein complexes in different organisms.

Outer-Arm Dynein (OAD)

The Low Molecular Weight Chains (LCs)

Dynein-ATPase associated LCs vary in number depending on the species. In trout sperm axonemes, six LCs were observed (46,47) and with two-dimensional gel electrophoresis the light chain LC 5 showed a faint component that was more basic (see Fig. 1.2). In *Chlamydomonas,* there are at least 10 different LCs associated with the outer arm complex. Six of these LCs with masses of 8, 11, 14, 16, 18, and 19 kDa have been sequenced (48–50). The 8 and 11 kDa light chains present a high percentage of homology (about 40%). Only one gene exists for each of these chains and their structure prediction suggests that they have an alpha-helix motif that is involved in protein–protein interactions (48). This is in agreement with results that show that these light chains are situated at the base of the dynein arms and interact with the intermediate chains. This IC–LC complex is part of the ATP-independent dynein anchor that is bound to the tubulins (see Ref. 5). The 8 kDa light chain is also found associated with the brain cytoplasmic dynein IC complex (51), and its absence in Drosophila leads to severe deficiencies during development (52). This 8 kDa protein is highly conserved through the different organisms with 92% homology found between the nematode and the human protein. The low molecular compound has been found to be associated with myosin and to inhibit the nitric oxide synthase (53). This study also shows that the 8 kDa chain forms a homodimer that has some importance in the nitric oxide synthase inhibition as well as in the binding of the protein to myosin and dynein. In addition, the LC has certain other binding sites in the axoneme that remain

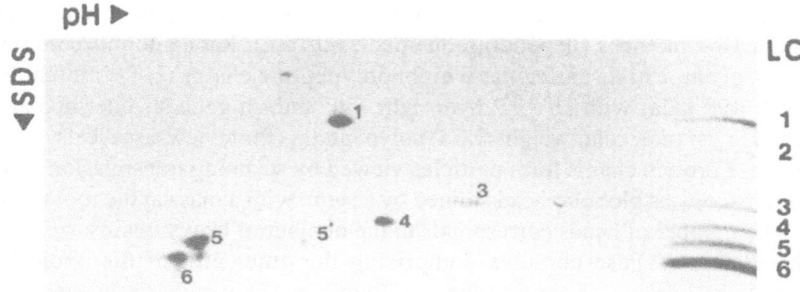

FIGURE 1.2. Two-dimensional gel electrophoresis of the trout sperm OAD light chains. The OAD LCs were separated by two-dimensional gel electrophoresis. The six LCs are visible on the control lane (right). LCs 1, 3, 4, 6 show only one spot while LC 5 has two spots, one important (5) and the other less visible (5'). LC2 was not found on the gel. (acidic side at left).

to be determined (53). From these data, it could be speculated that this highly conserved LC is present in the mammalian axoneme.

A second pair of ICs that have been sequenced are the 14 and 16 kDa proteins (50). These authors found that the two chains were homologous, both belong to the family of thioredoxin proteins, and both have one functional enzymatic active site. The thioredoxin are involved in controlling the redox state of important thiol groups in proteins, and they particularly avoid their destruction to maintain the quaternary structure. Thiol groups are involved in dynein-ATPase activity as shown by activation or inhibition (depending on the dose) with N-ethylmaleimide. Furthermore, the 16 kDa LC contains the P-loop motif for ATP binding that is also found on the dynein heavy chains, but this site is apparently not functional.

The 18 kDa LC has homology with the calmodulin calcium-binding protein family (49). This protein has at least one functional calcium-binding site and could be involved in the transition from asymmetric to symmetric beating that occurs in *Chlamydomonas* during the photo response (49).

The *Chlamydomonas* 19 kDa protein is tightly bound to the beta heavy chain. The chain sequence matches the sequence of the murine protein Tctex-2 as well as the rp3 protein found in humans, which is a cytoplasmic dynein LC (54). Another related Tctex product, Tctex-1, is also a cytoplasmic dynein LC expressed in the testis (55). It is interesting that the Tctex products are encoded by the *t* complex of the mouse chromosome 17. The complex is involved in spermatogenesis. Mice bearing a defective form of this region (*t* haplotype) present sperm with impaired motility (56). Whether the sperm motility defect is due to outer arm misassembly and/or cytoplasmic dynein dysfunction is not yet known, but the results do indicate that a defect in dynein LCs could be involved in infertility.

The Intermediate Molecular Weight Chains (ICs)

Outer-arm dyneins contain from two to six different intermediate chains, depending on the species. In *Chlamydomonas* two ICs are part of the OAD complex: IC69 and IC78. One, IC78, is essential for the correct binding of the outer arm to the *A* tubule because this protein binds directly to the tubulin (57,58). The other, IC69, is also involved in the interaction, but it apparently does not bind to tubulin (57, see also Ref. 5). Antibodies against these different ICs cross-reacted with ICs of several other species, such as sea urchin and trout sperm (47), which suggests that they share common epitopes. The sequence of these two *Chlamydomonas* chains, as well as the sequence of the three intermediate chains of the sea urchin sperm axoneme OAD and of the cytoplasmic dynein, are now known (58,59). Comparison of sequence and immunological data suggests that there are three different families of intermediate chains. In the first family, the intermediate chains contain five WD repeats in their C-terminal half (58,59). The WD is a sequence motif known to be involved in protein–protein interactions. Both IC69 and IC78 from *Chlamydomonas*, the IC2 and IC3 from sea urchin sperm OAD, and the IC74 from the cytoplasmic dynein fall in this family. From immunological data, the trout sperm IC1 and IC2 as well as two ICs from *Mytillus* sperm OAD (about 90 kDa) and two ICs from ascidian sperm OAD (85 and 96 kDa) could also be part of this family (46,47,59). The second family has only one member: the IC1 of sea urchin sperm OAD. This protein presents a hybrid sequence that contains both a thioredoxin-related part and a repeated homologous sequence to the nucleoside diphosphate kinase (NDPkinase; 59). Indirect results suggest that the thioredoxin part of this protein is functional and a homology of this chain with the light chains 14 and 16 kDa has been found (see earlier discussion). The role of these thioredoxins in vivo has to be clarified. The NDPkinase activity was not detected within the IC1, which suggests that this part of the protein is not functional (59).

The third family is suggested by immunological results showing that ICs from different species cross-reacted with antibody against the NDPkinase region of the sea urchin IC1 but not with its thioredoxin region (59).

Knowledge of the sequence of the intermediate chains in different species will be necessary to classify the different IC forms. It is also interesting to note that an antibody against IC1 was able to inhibit the motility of the axoneme in different species including human sperm (60). This suggests that a protein sharing some sequence with the IC1 chain could exist in the mammalian sperm axoneme and be involved in the regulation of motility.

Inner Arm Dynein (IAD)

In *Chlamydomonas,* the inner arm I1 has the same composition along the axoneme: It is composed of two HC (named 1-alpha and 1-beta) and two ICs of 140 and 110 kDa. The composition of I2 and I3 varies along the axoneme

(61; see also Ref. 5): Several heavy chains are involved (2A, 2B, 2', 3, 3'), as are several light chains, with the largest at 86 kDa, one at 43 kDa which is actin (62), one at about 28 kDa (named p28), and the lighter at 19 kDa, which is closely related to the calcium-binding protein caltractin/centrin (61). A similar structure was also observed within the inner arms from the sea urchin sperm and from the rockcod fish sperm.

Light Chains (LCs)

Actin, which is a 43 kDa protein widely found in cells, was demonstrated to be one of the LCs associated with almost all of the *Chlamydomonas* inner arms—only one inner arm dynein species was found to have no actin (61). When the single actin gene is mutated, the beating of the flagellar is altered and the cell displacement is slower. In the axoneme, the normal actin is apparently replaced by a novel protein that is closely related to actin. This new actin can substitute for a part of the activity of the normal form, but not completely because several of the dynein inner arms are missing in this mutant (62). This suggests that actin plays a role in mediating the binding of the inner arms on the *A* tubule.

The LC p28 is associated with the inner arm I2 and I3 in *Chlamydomonas*. The sequence of this protein has been obtained (63). The chain is an unknown protein that presents a large alpha-helical domain. An antisera against this protein shows that it is distributed all along the axoneme and immunoprecipitation studies indicate that it is linked with inner arm HC 2'. The same study shows that the centrin LC is associated with the 3 and 3', whereas the 2 could bind both of the LCs. The same authors have also shown that mutation in the p28 chain results in the absence in the inner arms of the dynein HCs normally linked with this protein (64).

Two different approaches have also shown that the p28 protein is present in other species and could be involved in sperm movement. A monoclonal antibody generated against axonemal proteins from sea urchin sperm was found to inhibit the motility of the demembranated-reactivated model (65). The protein of 33 kDa recognized by the antibody was further purified, sequenced, and its cDNA isolated. The nucleotidic sequence showed that this protein presents more than 60% homology with the *Chlamydomonas* p28. Thus, the p28 protein is also found in sperm axonemes from invertebrates and plays a role in movement. The human homologous p28 mRNA has been isolated (66) by using a probe design on the sequence of the *Chlamydomonas* p28. The mRNA was expressed mainly in the testis, but it was also found in several other tissues. The gene encoding the protein was localized on chromosome 1. This study also showed that homologous sequences are presented in different mammal species as well as in chicken and yeast. It is not yet known whether the protein is linked with the inner arms in the axoneme.

The Dynein Heavy Chains (HCs)

Because the sea urchin ciliary axonemal dynein beta HCs were sequenced (67,68), the number of HCs reported in different species has increased greatly every year. The three HCs (alpha, beta, and gamma) that constitute the *Chlamydomonas* OAD have also been completely sequenced (69–71). Analysis has shown that the *Chlamydomonas* alpha and beta chains are more closely related and homologous to the sea urchin cilia beta HC than they are to the gamma HC from *Chlamydomonas*. All of the sequences of the dynein HC present a central part that contains four consensus regions for the ATP-binding site (*p*-loop), but the N- and C-terminals consist of alpha helixes that form coiled-coil regions. Only one ATPase site (the first from the N-terminal) is functional, and the other sites are able to bind ATP but not split it (72). Although the role of the other binding sites is not yet known, it has been suggested that the binding of nucleotides to the HC could modulate ATPase activity (40).

From the initial sequence data, the region of the first ATP hydrolytic site appeared highly conserved (8). This region, therefore, was used to screen, with rt-PCR or hybridization (73), mRNA libraries from diverse sources including human tissues. A large number of HC mRNAs have been found and partially sequenced using this technique: At this time, 13 HCs have been reported in the sea urchin embryo (8), at least 12 in *Paramecium* (73), 12 dynein HCs have been found in *Chlamydomonas* (45), 14 in mouse (74,75), and 11 in human (75,76). These partial sequences have been used to generate phylogenetic trees (8,45,76). Three branches have been found, two of which are rapidly divergent and separate the axonemal and cytoplasmic dynein HCs (77). The axonemal dynein HC branch then splits into two: one group is formed by outer arm dynein HCs, and the second is suggested to be the inner arm HCs. Most of the dynein HCs reported from partial sequencing are classified using this approach. Meanwhile, it is not yet known in higher organisms if the HCs that form the inner or outer arms in axonemal cilia are the same as those in spermatozoa. It has also been suggested that only one HC exists in each organism for the cytoplasmic dynein and that this chain forms a functional homodimer. This idea is challenged by the finding that there are two different cytoplasmic dynein HCs: one distributed in all tissues and the other present only in ciliated tissue. The cellular distribution of these two cytoplasmic dyneins suggests that they have different functions: one might be to help in the building of the axoneme by transporting vesicles (78,79).

Mammalian Sperm Dynein Heavy Chains

Attempts have been made to analyze the mammalian sperm outer arm dynein. High salt extraction or an overnight low salt dialysis of sperm in the presence of low concentrations of protease inhibitors have been employed (80,81). These conditions appeared to be deleterious for the HCs because a partial proteolysis occurred during the extraction phase that was certainly due to proteases released from the acrosome (82). This alteration could be the origin for the discrepancies in the number of dynein subunits and HCs found in the different studies. It is surprising that the mammalian sperm outer arm dynein heavy chains cannot be extracted by high salt levels in the presence of high concentrations of protease inhibitors (80,82). In contrast, in the presence of low concentrations of protease inhibitors, and after a proteolysis has occurred, a part of the OAD is solubilized by the high salt treatment. Because the extraction was found to be better at the end of the flagellum than at the base where supplementary structures (like the mitochondrial and fibrous sheaths and the coarse fibers) are more important, it has been suggested that structures that surround the mammalian axoneme need to be partially destroyed before the dynein can diffuse out into the media. On the other hand, one could propose that the link between the OAD and the *A* tubule is particular to mammals. Study by electron microscopy of the 19S dynein particle obtained from bull sperm showed a bouquet with two globular heads (83), in agreement with different results which indicate that mammalian sperm OAD has two main heavy chains.

These HCs show, in situ and after extraction, molecular weight and photolytic properties close to those of the heavy chains from lower vertebrate and invertebrate species (8,47,82). Immunological similarities also exist between mammalian sperm heavy chains and certain heavy chains from invertebrates and lower vertebrates (83,84). Using an affinity purified antibody directed against the beta HC from trout sperm a cross-reactivity was found with the sea urchin beta but not alpha HC (84). A cross-reaction was also observed with one of the axonemal HCs from the boar and ram (see Fig. 1.3). These data and the results obtained with other vertebrate sperm (46,47,51) suggest that the mammalian sperm axonemal OAD should contain only two HCs. Meanwhile, from the 11 HCs that have been cloned from humans, nine are putative axonemal dynein and at least three are closely related to OAD HCs (76). Thus, by using available cross-reacting antibodies against the OAD HCs or by obtaining antibodies against particular specific peptides derived from the sequence of these chains, it should be possible to exactly define their position in the axoneme. These tools will certainly also be of great help in understanding human dynein pathology (see further).

Mammalian Sperm Accessory Structures

Mammalian sperm flagella possess a characteristic ultrastructural complex of nine outer dense fibers (ODFs) that surrounds the 9 + 2 axoneme, making the 9 + 9 + 2 pattern seen in cross-section by electron microscopy (85,86; see Fig. 1.1). At the base of the flagellum, these nine ODFs are joined to form a part of the connecting piece. In the intermediate piece of the flagellum, this 9 + 9 + 2 structure is surrounded by the mitochondrial sheath, after which the mitochondria are replaced along the principal piece by a tapered cylinder, the fibrous sheath (FS). In addition, in the principal piece the ODFs close to

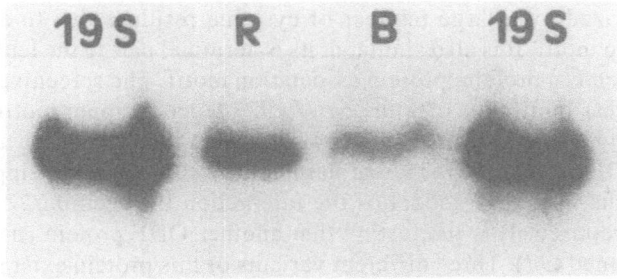

FIGURE 1.3. Cross-reactivity between dynein HCs. The HCs of the ram (R) and boar (B) sperm SDS extracts were probed with a trout affinity purified (see Ref. 84). One single heavy chain in boar and in ram reacted with the antibody suggesting sequence similarity with the trout beta HC. The 19S trout sperm OAD was used as positive control.

doublet 3 and 8 fuse with the FS to make two columnar structures. All of these supplementary structures are supposed to add stiffness to the flagellum to protect it from breaking, particularly during the ejaculation process. A role in increasing the force of the beating of the sperm flagella is also suggested from results obtained by computer simulation based on the geometrical clutch hypothesis (87). This idea is also supported by earlier results that show that a defect in the length of the ODFs impaired the motility of the human sperm by decreasing the wave amplitude (88,89).

In rats, the ODFs are composed of at least six major polypeptides of 84, 71, 40, 27, 20, and 14 kDa and some less abundant compounds. These proteins are highly phosphorylated on serine residues. It has also been reported that the rat FS has major proteins of 80, 67, 24, 11, and 5 kDa (85). Similar results have been obtained with human and rabbit ODFs (90). In humans, a 97 kDa protein has been observed in the FS that colocalized with actin (91), which indicates that actin could be a possible component of the FS as in the ODFs (92).

Outer Dense Fibers (ODFs)

The ODF and FS were suggested to be keratinlike structures because of their insolubility. One of the proteins of the ODF is effectively a keratinlike protein of 57 kDa (named sak57) that has also been observed in the manchette during sperm elongation. This protein is able to bind to the cytoplasmic beta-tubulin in vivo, and is found exclusively at the ODF level in mature sperm (93). This finding strongly suggests that the protein could be involved in the association of the ODF with the external doublet of microtubules, as indicated by functional observations (94; see also Ref. 87). Different groups have cloned the 27 kDa ODF protein (95). Transcript of this protein is found in several mammals, including humans. The protein, also named *odf1* or *odf27*, is characterized by a large number of cysteine residues due to a repetitive Cys-Gly-Pro motif. It is also similar at its N-terminal part to the leucine zipper region, which is a protein–protein association motif. The screening of a testis cDNA expression library with the *odf1/odf27* leucine zipper motif led to the detection and characterization of a 84 kDa protein (*odf84*), which also proved to be an ODF protein (96). This protein contains two leucine zipper motifs. Based on this finding, a model of the interaction between *odf27* and *odf84* has been proposed. It is interesting that another ODF protein (named *odf2*) has been cloned (97). Three different variants of this protein exist in the ODF (ranging between 65 and 70 kDa) derived from the same gene. The proteins have a large overall alpha-helical structure and also contain two identical leucine zipper regions. It could therefore be suggested that this motif is highly involved in the formation of the ODF, and also that sequence homologies between the different ODF proteins exist, which could indicate earlier gene duplication.

Fibrous Sheath (FS)

An FS protein of 85 kDa has been purified, characterized, and its cDNA cloned (98,99). This protein has a functional sequence domain that is able to bind the inhibitory regulatory domain (RII beta, a 55 kDa protein; 100) of protein kinase A. This kinase was demonstrated to be in the cytoplasm and also associated with the FS and the mitochondrial sheath (101). The protein kinase A is composed of two regulatory and two catalytic subunits, and the binding of cAMP to the enzyme results in dissociation of the subunits and an increase in the kinase activity. cAMP and sperm protein phosphorylations are implicated in the control of motility during different stages of sperm maturation as well as during its capacitation and hyperactivation (102). The 85 kDa protein is itself a target for tyrosine-phosphorylation by a calcium-calmodulin dependent mechanism (103). Moreover, a protein of 55 kDa (different from RII) in the sperm cytoplasm is phosphorylated by the PKA and its level of phosphorylation is correlated with sperm motility acquisition (104), [i.e., when PKA is inhibited from binding to its regulatory protein an inhibition of sperm motility occurs (105)]. Cross-talk between cAMP, cAMP-dependent protein kinases, and the protein phosphatases is certainly part of motility control, and it has been demonstrated that a cAMP-dependent protein kinase inhibits dynein-driven sliding of micotubules (106,107). The 85 kDa FS protein could thus participate in this activation cascade by its role in sequestering the PKA complex and then lowering the cell cytoplasm PKA activity.

As previously stated, the ODFs are composed of phosphoproteins. These proteins could be the target for phosphorylations/dephosphorylations, which may then result in changes in stiffness of the ODFs, and hence be one of the regulators of sperm flagellar beat under different conditions (see Ref. 87 and refs therein).

Protein kinase A is not the sole protein to bind to the FS. The glyceraldehyde 3 phosphate dehydrogenase is also found to be associated with the FS in mammalian sperm (108). These authors suggest that the ATP production pathway could be different in the intermediate piece, where there are the mitochondria and therefore oxidative phosphorylation, and the principal piece where glycolytic enzymes are bound to the FS and directly provide the energy substrate.

Conclusion and Relation with the Human Pathology

Most of the proteins described in this chapter have been found because their mutation in *Chlamydomonas* produces immobility or abnormal mobility in this biflagellated green alguae. From studies of this simple organism, great insights into the axonemal puzzle have been gained, enabling a better understanding of the interaction of these proteins to generate microtubule sliding. These studies have also shown that a large number of components are vital to gaining a fully motile axoneme. Some of the mutations produce the disruption of part or all of the axoneme, but others impair enzymatic function.

The diverse ultrastructural defects reported here have also been observed in human sperm with motility disorders (109; for review, see Ref. 110). In some cases, the sperm is filagellum abnormal, and defects have been observed in the axoneme of cilia from different tissues. This suggests two main classes of defect: First, problems are restricted to the sperm; second, the axonemal structure is affected throughout the body. This second group includes individuals affected by the immotile-cilia syndrome or Kartagener's syndrome (ICS; see Ref. 110). This pathology has also been found to be associated with situs inversus (i.e. visceral asymmetry), and it has been shown that a dynein HC related to the axonemal dynein could be involved in this left–right asymmetry (111). In mice carrying the mutation *inversus viscerum*, 50% of their descendants have situs inversus. A dynein HC gene (named left–right dynein: *lrd*) was found to be at the chromosomal location of the mutation. The HC bears a point mutation in the highly conserved *p*-loops region, and this provides the molecular basis for the left–right inversion. Meanwhile, the transcript of this chain is expressed at a low level in the testis, but is found in ciliated cells and is actively transcribed in nonciliated cells during embryogenesis. Thus, although this protein is related to the axonemal HC it could be an HC of an unknown cytoplasmic dynein, and it may be involved in the transport of materials during ciliogenesis. On the other hand, a dynein HC could have different functions at different times in the organism, or with alternative splicing give a different protein that could have different functions (76). The function of this dynein could also be directed by the accessory proteins bound to the HC, which could vary during development (14).

In rats, 14 dynein HC genes have been found and at least seven are involved in ciliogenesis (75,112). In humans, at least 11 heavy chain genes have been reported, but it is not known if one of these chains is equivalent to the *lrd* in rats (76). These 11 HCs are dispatched on several chromosomes and some of them on locations involved in genetic defects in cellular transport or axonemal function (75,76). It should be noted that in Drosophila one dynein gene was found within the *Y* chromosome (113), and deletions in the *Y* chromosome in humans are responsible for diverse forms of male sterility. Moreover, mutations in the sperm chromosomes are more likely to occur than they are in oocyte chromosomes because a sperm cell, in its formation, needs six times more cell divisions than does an ovocyte (114).

In conclusion, studies in invertebrates have opened up a large field of research on which the analysis of human pathologies can be based. It could be a long time, however, before all sperm axonemal problems have been mapped. For example, in *Chlamydomonas* (which has a simple axoneme) at least 75 different genetic loci are involved in motility, although some of these are certainly related to the specific function of the cell. Nevertheless, we shall see more and more reports on what constitutes the human sperm and ciliary axonemes and we will be able to classify some of the different types of diseases. This should also provide tools for detecting the defects and offer more possibilities to couples in cases of intracytoplasmic injection of immotile sperm.

References

1. Bourgereon T, Barbeaux S, McElreavy K, Fellous M. La genetique de la sterilite masculine. Med Sci 1996;11: I–VIII.
2. Wolf JP, Feneux D, Escalier D, Rodrigues D, Frydman R, Jouannet P. Pregnancy after subzonal insemination with spermatozoa lacking outer dynein arms. J Reprod Fertil 1993;97:487–92.
3. Vandervorst M, Tournaye H, Camus M, Nagy ZP, Van Steirteghem A, Devroey P. Patient with absolutely immotile and intracytoplasmic sperm injection. Hum Reprod 1997;12:2429–33.
4. Papadimas J, Tarlatzis BC, Bili H, et al. Therapeutic approach of immotile cilia syndrome by intracytoplasmic sperm injection: a case report. Fertil Steril 1997;67:562–65.
5. Witman GB, Wilkerson CG, King SM. The biochemistry, genetic and molecular biology of flagellar dynein. In: Hyam JS, Lloyd CW, editors. Microtubules. New York: Wiley-Liss, 1994:229–49.
6. Dutcher SK. Flagellar assembly in two hundred and fifty easy to follow steps. Trends Genet 1995;11:398–404.
7. Gatti JL, Dacheux JL. Molecular basis of axonemal movement. Front Endocrinol (Serono Symposia) 1995;11:53–72.
8. Gibbons IR. The role of dynein in microtubule based motility. Cell Struct Funct 1996;21:331–42.
9. Brokaw CJ. Control of flagellar bending: a new agenda based on dynein diversity. Cell Motil Cytoskeleton 1994;28:199–204.
10. Cosson J. A moving image of flagella: news and views on the mechanisms involved in axonemal beating. Cell Biol Int 1996;20:83–94.
11. Lindemann CB, Kanous KS. A model for flagellar motility. Int Rev Cytol 1997;173:1–72.

12. Brokaw CJ. Transient disruptions of the axonemal structure and microtubule sliding during bend propagation by ciona sperm flagella. Cell Motil 1997;37:346–62.
13. Allan V. Motor proteins: a dynamic duo. Curr Biol 1996;6:630–33.
14. Vallee RB, Sheetz MP. Targeting of motor proteins. Science 1996;271:1539–44.
15. Zheng Y, Wong ML, Alberts B, Mitchinson T. Nucleation of microtubule assembly by a gamma-tubulin-containing ring complex. Nature 1995;378:578–83.
16. Morritz M, Braunfield MB, Sedat JW, Alberts B, Agard DA. Microtubule nucleation by gamma-tubulin-containing rings in the centrosome. Nature 1995; 378:638–40.
17. Song YH, Mandelkow E. The anatomy of flagellar microtubules: polarity, seam, junctions, and lattice. J Cell Biol 1995;128:81–94.
18. Yang ZH, Gallicano GI, Yu QC, Fuchs E. An unexpected localization of basonuclin in the centrosome, mitochondria and acrosome of developing spermatids. J Cell Biol 1997;137:657–69.
19. Hrudka F, Betsch JM, Kenney RM. Anomalies of centriolar derivatives manifest in spermatic flagella and respiratory cilia of the stallion. Arch Androl 1991;27:161–75.
20. Navara SC, Simerly C, Zoran S, Schatten G. The sperm centrosomùe during fertilization in mammals: implication for fertility and reproduction. Reprod Fertil Dev 1995;7:747–54.
21. Wilson PG, Borisy GG. Evolution of the multitubulin hypothesis. BioEssays 1997;19:451–54.
22. Plessman U, Weber K. Mammalian sperm tubulin: an exceptionally large number of variants based on several post-translational modifications. J Protein Chem 1997;16:385–90.
23. Multigner L, Pignot-Paintrand I, Saoudi Y, et al. The A and B tubules of the outer doublets of sea urchin sperm axonemes are composed of different tubulin variants. Biochemistry 1996;35:10862–71.
24. Goldsmith M, Yarbrough L, Van der Kooy D. Mechanics of motility: distinct dynein-binding domains on alpha and beta tubulin. Biochem Cell Biol 1995; 73:665–71.
25. Gagnon C, White D, Cosson J, et al. The polyglutamylated lateral chain of alpha-tubulin plays a key role in flagellar motility. J Cell Sci 1996;109:1545–53.
26. Cosson J, White D, Huitorel P, et al. Inhibition of flagellar beat frequency by a new anti-beta-tubulin antibody. Cell Motil 1996;35:100–12.
27. Mazumdar M, Mikami A, Gee MA, Vallee RB. In vitro motility from recombinant dynein heavy chain. Proc Natl Acad Sci USA 1996;93:6552–56.
28. Koonce MP. Identification of a microtubule binding domain in a cytoplasmic dynein heavy chain. J Biol Chem 1997;272:19714–18.
29. Holwill ME, Foster GF, Hamasaki T, Satir P. Biophysical aspects and modelling of ciliary motility. Cell Motil Cytoskeleton 1995;32:114–20.
30. Takada S, Kamiya R. Beat frequency difference between the two flagella of Chlamydomonas depends on the attachment site of outer dynein arms on the outer doublet microtubules. Cell Motil Cytoskeleton 1997;36:68–75.
31. Kozminsky KG, Beech PL, Rosenbaum JL. The Chlamydomonas kinesin-like Fla10 is involved in motility associated with the flagellar membrane. J Cell Biol 1995;131:1517–27.
32. Morris RL, Scholley JM. Heterotrimeric Kinesin II is required for the assembly of motile 9 + 2 ciliary axonemes on sea urchin embryos. J Cell Biol 1997;138:1009–22.

33. Fox LA, Sawin KE, Sale WS. Kinesin related proteins in eukaryotic flagella. J Cell Sci 1994;107:1545–50.

34. Piperno G, Mead K, Henderson S. Inner dynein arms but not outer dynein arms require the activity of kinesin homologue protein KHP1(FLA10) to reach the distal part of flagella in *Chlamydomonas*. J Cell Biol 1996;133:371–79.

35. Piperno G, Mead K. Transport of a novel complex in the cytoplasmic matrix of *Chlamydomonas* flagella. Proc Natl Acad Sci USA 1997;94:4457–62.

36. Henson JH, Cole DG, Roesener CD, Capuano S, Mendola RJ, Scholey JM. The heterotrimeric motor protein kinesin-II localizes to the midpiece and the flagellum of sea urchin and sand dollar sperm. Cell Motil 1997;38:29–37. Stephens RE. Ciliogenesis in sea urchin embryos a subroutine in the program of development. Bioessays 1995;17:331–40.

37. Bloch MA, Johnson KA. Identification of a molecular chaperone in the eukaryotic flagellum and its localisation to the site of microtubule assembly. J Cell Sci 1995;108:3541–45.

38. Eddy EM. Chauvinist genes of male germ cells. Reprod Fertil Dev 1995;7:695–704.

39. Dix DJ. Hsp 70 expression and function during spermatogenesis. Cell Stress Chaperones 1997;2:73–77.

40. Frey E, Brokaw CJ, Omoto CK. Reactivation at low ATP distinguishes among classes of paralyzed flagella mutants. Cell Motil 1997;38:91–97.

41. Takada S, Kamiya R. Functional reconstitution of *Chlamydomonas* outer dynein arms from alpha beta and gamma subunits: requirement of a third factor. J Cell Biol 1994;126:737–45.

42. Koutoulis A, Pazour GJ, Wilkerson CG, et al. The *Chlamydomonas reinhardtii* ODA3 gene encodes a protein of the outer dynein arm docking complex. J Cell Biol 1997;137:1069–80.

43. Smith EF, Lefebvre PA. PF20 gene product contains WD repeats and localizes to the intermicrotubule bridges in *Chlamydomonas* flagella. Mol Biol Cell 1997;8:455–67.

44. King SM, Marchese Ragona SP, Parker SK, Detrich HW, 3rd. Inner and outer arm axonemal dyneins from the Antarctic rockcod Notothenia coriiceps. Biochemistry 1997;36:1306–14.

45. Porter ME, Knott JA, Myster SH, Farlow SJ. The dynein gene family in *Chlamydomonas reinhardtii*. Genetics 1996;144:569–85.

46. Gatti J-L, King SM, Moss AG, Witman GB. Outer arm dynein from trout spermatozoa. Purification, polypeptide composition and enzymatic properties. J Biol Chem 1989;264:11450–57.

47. King SM, Gatti J-L, Moss AG, Witman GB. Outer arm dynein from trout spermatozoa: substructural organization. Cell Motil 1990;16:266–78.

48. King SM, Patel-King RS. Identification of a Ca(2+) binding light chain within *Chlamydomonas* outer arm dynein. J Cell Sci 1995;108:3757–64.

49. King SM, Patel-King RS. The M(r) = 8,000 and 11,000 outer dynein light chains from *Chlamydomonas* flagella have cytoplasmic homologues. J Biol Chem 1995;270:11445–52.

50. Patel-King RS, Benashaki SE, Harrison A, King SM. Two functional thioredoxins containing redox sensitive vicinal dithiols from the *Chlamydomonas* outer dynein arm. J Biol Chem 1996;271:6283–91.

51. King SM, Barbarese E, Dillman JF III, Patel King RS, Carson JH, Pfister KK. Brain cytoplasmic and flagellar outer arm dyneins share a highly conserved Mr 8,000 light chain. J Biol Chem 1996;271:19358–66.

52. Phillis R, Statton D, Caruccio P, Murphey RK. Mutations in the 8 kDa dynein light chain gene disrupt sensory axon projections in the Drosophila imaginal CNS. Development 1996;122:2955–63.
53. Benashski SE, Harrison A, Patel-King RS, King SM. Dimerization of the highly conserved light chain shared by dynein and myosin V. J Biol Chem 1997;272: 20929–35.
54. Patel-King RS, Benashski SE, Harrison A, King SM. A *Chlamydomonas* homologue of the putative murine *t* complex distorder Tctex 2 is an outer arm dynein light chain. J Cell Biol 1997;137:1081–90.
55. King SM, Dillman JF, 3rd, Benashski SE, Lye RJ, Patel King RS, Pfister KK. The mouse *t* complex encoded protein Tctex 1 is a light chain of brain cytoplasmic dynein. J Biol Chem 1996;271:32281–87.
56. Olds-Clarke P. Models for male infertility: the *t* haplotypes. Rev Reprod 1997; 2:157–64.
57. King SM, Patel-King RS, Wilkerson CG, Witman GB. The 78,000 M(r) intermediate chain of *Chlamydomonas* outer arm dynein is a microtubule binding protein. J Cell Biol 1995;131:399–409.
58. Wilkerson CG, King SM, Koutoulis A, Pazour GJ, Witman GB. The 78,000 M(r) intermediate chain of *Chlamydomonas* outer arm dynein is a WD repeat protein required for arm assembly. J Cell Biol 1995;129:169–78.
59. Ogawa K, Kamiya R, Wilkerson CG, Witman GB. Interspecies conservation of outer arm dynein intermediate chain sequences defines two intermediate chain subclasses. Mol Biol Cell 1995;6:685–96.
60. Gagnon C, White D, Huitorel P, Cosson J. A monoclonal antibody against the dynein IC1 peptide of sea urchin spermatozoa inhibits the motility of sea urchin, dinoflagellate, and human flagellar axonemes. Mol Biol Cell 1994;5:1051–63.
61. Piperno G. Regulation of dynein activity within *Chlamydomonas* flagella. Cell Motil 1995;32:103–5.
62. Kato-Minoura T, Hirono M, Kamiya R. *Chlamydomonas* inner arm dynein mutant, ida5, has a mutation in an actin encoding gene. J Cell Biol 1997;137:649–56.
63. Piperno G, Luck DJ. An actin like protein is a component of axonemes from *Chlamydomonas* flagella. J Biol Chem 1979;254:2187–90.
64. LeDizet M, Piperno G. ida4-1, ida4-2, and ida4-3 are intron splicing mutations affecting the locus encoding p28, a light chain of *Chlamydomonas* axonemal inner dynein arms. Mol Biol Cell 1995;6:713–23.
65. Gingras D, White D, Garin J, et al. Purification, cloning, and sequence analysis of a Mr = 30,000 protein from sea urchin axonemes that is important for sperm motility. Relationship of the protein to a dynein light chain. J Biol Chem 1996;271:12807–13.
65. LeDizet M, Piperno G. The light chain p28 associates with a subset of inner dynein arm heavy chains in *Chlamydomonas* axonemes. Mol Biol Cell 1995;6:697–711.
66. Kastury K, Taylor WE, Shen R, et al. Complementary deoxyribonucleic acid cloning and characterization of a putative human axonemal dynein light chain gene. J Clin Endocrinol Metab 1997; 82:3047–53.
67. Gibbons IR, Gibbons BH, Mocz G, Asai DJ. Multiple nucleotide-binding sites in the sequence of dynein beta heavy chain. Nature 1991;352:640–43.
68. Ogawa K. Four ATP-binding sites in the midregion of the beta heavy chain of dynein. Nature 1991;352:643–45.
69. Wilkerson CG, King SM, Witman GB. Molecular analysis of the gamma heavy chain of *Chlamydomonas* flagellar outer arm dynein. J Cell Sci 1994;107:497–506.

70. Mitchell DR, Brown KS. Sequence analysis of the *Chlamydomonas* alpha and beta dynein heavy chain genes. J Cell Sci 1994;107: 635–44.

71. Mitchell DR, Brown KS. Sequence analysis of the *Chlamydomonas reinhardtii* flagellar alpha dynein gene. Cell Motil 1997;37:120–26.

72. Mocz G, Gibbons IR. Phase partition analysis of nucleotide binding to axonemal dynein. Biochemistry 1996;35:9204–11.

73. Asai DJ, Criswell PG. Identification of new dynein heavy chain genes by RNA directed polymerase chain reaction. Methods Cell Biol 1995;47:579–85.

74. Tanaka Y, Zhang Z, Hirokawa N. Identification and evolution of new dynein-like protein sequence in rat brain. J Cell Sci 1995;108:1883–93.

75. Vaughan KT, Mikami A, Paschal BM, et al. Multiple mouse chromosomal loci for dynein based motility. Genomics 1996;36:29–38.

76. Chapelin C, Duriez B, Magnino F, Goossens M, Escudier E, Amselem S. Isolation of several human axonemal dynein heavy chain genes: genomic structure of the catalytic site, phylogenetic analysis and chromosomal assignment. FEBS Lett 1997;412:325–30.

77. Mikami A, Paschal BM, Mazumdar M, Vallee RB. Molecular cloning of the retrograde transport motor cytoplasmic dynein (MAP1C). Neuron 1993;10:787–96.

78. Criswell PS, Ostrowski LE, Asai DJ. A novel cytoplasmic dynein heavy chain: expression of DHC1b in mammalian ciliated epithelial cells. J Cell Sci 1996;109:1891–98.

79. Vaisberg EA, Grissom PM, McIntosh JR. Mammalian cells express three distinct dynein heavy chains that are localized to different cytoplasmic organelles. J Cell Biol 1996;133:831–42.

80. Gagnon C. Extraction and properties of dynein from bull spermatozoa. Methods Enzymol 1986;134:318–24.

81. Baccetti B, Burrini AG, Colodel G, et al. Comparative observations on mammalian dyneins. In: Baccetti B, editor. Comparative spermatology 20 years after. New York: Raven Press, 1992:321–32.

82. Gatti JL, Nicolle JC, Dacheux JL. Characterisation of boar sperm dynein heavy chains by UV vanadate dependent photocleavage. Biol Cell 1994;82:203–10.

83. Marchese Ragona SP, Gagnon C, White D, Belles-Iles M, Johnson KA. Structure and mass analysis of 12 S and 19 S dynein obtained from bull sperm. Cell Motil 1987;8:366–74.

83. Yoshida T, Katsuta K, Takanari H, Izutsu K. Analysis of mammalian dynein using antibodies against A polypeptides of sea urchin flagellar dynein. Exp Cell Res 1989;184:440–48.

84. Gatti JL, Dacheux JL. Immunological cross reaction between sperm dynein heavy chains from different species. Reprod Nutr Dev 1996;36:213–20.

85. Vera JC, Brito M, Zuvic T, Burzio LO. Polypeptide composition of rat sperm outer dense fibers. J Biol Chem 1984;259:5970–77.

86. Fouquet JP, Kann ML. The cytoskeleton of mammalian spermatozoa. Biol Cell 1994;81:89–93.

87. Lindemann CB. Functional significance of the outer dense fibers of mammalian sperm examined by computer simulations with the geometric clutch model. Cell Motil 1996;34:258–70.

88. Feneux D, Serres C, Jouannet P. Sliding spermatozoa: a dyskinesia responsible for human infertility? Fertil Steril 1985;44:508–11.

89. Serres C, Feneux D, Jouanet P. Abnormal distribution of the periaxonemal structures in a human sperm flagellar dyskinesia. Cell Motil 1986;6:68–76.

90. Kim YH, de-Kretser DM, Temple-Smith PD, Hearn MT, McFarlane JR. Isolation and characterization of human and rabbit sperm tail fibrous sheath. Mol Hum Reprod 1997;3:307–13.
91. Escalier D, Gallo JM, Schrevel J. Immunochemical characterization of a human sperm fibrous sheath protein, its developmental expression pattern, and morphogenetic relationships with actin. J Histochem Cytochem 1997;45:909–22.
92. Paranko J, Yagi A, Kuusisto M. Immunocytochemical detection of actin and 53 kDa polypeptide in the epididymal spermatozoa of rat and mouse. Anat Rec 1994;240:516–27.
93. Tres LL, Kierszenbaum AL. Sak57, an acidic keratin initially present in the spermatid manchette before becoming a component of paraaxonemal structures of the developing tail. Mol Reprod Dev 1996;44:395–407.
94. Si Y, Okuno M. The sliding of the fibrous sheath through the axoneme proximally together with microtubule extrusion. Exp Cell Res 1993;208:170–74.
95. Burmester S, Hoyer-Fender S. Transcription and translation of the outer dense fiber gene (Odf1) during spermiogenesis in the rat. A study by in situ analyses and polysome fractionation. Mol Reprod Dev 1996;45:10–20.
96. Shao X, Tarnasky HA, Schalles U, Oko R, van der Hoorn FA. Interactional cloning of the 84-kDa major outer dense fiber protein Odf84. Leucine zippers mediate associations of Odf84 and Odf27. J Biol Chem 1997;272:6105–13.
97. Brohmann H, Pinnecke-S, Hoyer Fender S. Identification and characterization of new cDNAs encoding outer dense fiber proteins of rat sperm. J Biol Chem 1997;272:10327–32.
98. Carrera A, Gerton GL, Moss SB. The major fibrous sheath polypeptide of mouse sperm: structural and functional similarities to the A-kinase anchoring proteins. Dev Biol 1994;165:272–84.
99. Mei X, Singh IS, Erlichman M, Orr GA. Cloning and characterization of a testis specific, developmentally regulated A-kinase-anchoring protein (TAKAP-80) present on the fibrous sheath of rat sperm. Eur J Biochem 1997;246:425–32.
100. Pariset-C, Weinman S. Differential localization of two isoforms of the regulatory subunit RII alpha of cAMP-dependent protein kinase in human sperm: biochemical and cytochemical study. Mol Reprod Dev 1994;39:415–22.
101. MacLeod J, Mei X, Erlichman J, Orr GA. Association of the regulatory subunit of a type II cAMP-dependent protein kinase and its binding proteins with the fibrous sheath of rat sperm flagellum. Eur J Biochem 1994;225:107–14.
102. Leclerc P, de Lamirande E, Gagnon C. cAMP-dependent regulation of protein tyrosine phosphorylation in relation to human sperm capacitation and motility. Biol Reprod 1996;55:684–92.
103. Carrera A, Moos J, Ning XP, et al. Regulation of protein tyrosine phosphorylation in human sperm by a calcium/calmodulin-dependent mechanism: identification of A kinase anchor proteins as major substrates for tyrosine phosphorylation. Dev Biol 1996;180:284–96.
104. Vijarayaghavan S, Trautman KD, Goueli SA, Carr DW. A tyrosine-phosphorylated 55-kDa motility associated bovine sperm protein is regulated by cAMP and calcium. Biol Reprod 1997;56:1450–57.
105. Vijarayaghavan S, Goueli SA, Davey MP, Carr DW. Protein kinase A-anchoring inhibitor peptides arrest mammalian sperm motility. J Biol Chem 1997;272:4747–52.
106. Hamasaki T, Barkalow K, Satir P. Regulation of ciliary beat frequency by a dynein light chain. Cell Motil Cytoskeleton 1995;32:121–24.

107. Howard DR, Habermacher G, Glass DB, Smith EF, Sale WS. Regulation of *Chlamydomonas* flagellar dynein by an axonemal proteine kinase. J Cell Biol 1994;127:1683–92.

108. Westhoff D, Kamp G. Glyceraldehyde 3-phosphate dehydrogenase is bound to the fibrous sheath of mammalian spermatozoa. J Cell Sci 1997;110:1821–29.

109. Escalier D, David G. Pathology of the cytoskeleton of the human sperm flagellum: axonemal and peri-axonemal anomalies. Biol Cell 1984;50:37–52.

110. Afzelius BA. Situs inversus and ciliary abnormalities. What is the connection? Int J Dev Biol 1995;39:839–44.

111. Supp DM, Witte DP, Potter SS, Brueckner M. Mutation of an axonemal dynein affects left-right asymmetry in inversus viscerum mice. Nature 1997;389:963–66.

112. Andrews KL, Nettesheim P, Asai DJ, Ostrowski LE. Identification of seven rat axonemal dynein heavy chain genes: expression during ciliated cell differentiation. Mol Biol Cell 1996;7:71–79.

113. Gepner J, Hays TS. A fertility region on the Y chromosome of Drosophila melanogaster encodes a dynein microtubule motor. Proc Natl Acad Sci USA 1993;90:11132–36.

114. King SJ, Dutcher SK. Phosphoregulation of an inner dynein arm complex in *Chlamydomonas* is altered in phototactic mutant strains. J Cell Biol 1997;136:177–91.

2

Metabolic Strategy in Human Spermatozoa: Its Impact on Sperm Motility

JUAN G. ALVAREZ

Metabolic Strategy of Spermatozoa

Introduction

The mammalian spermatozoon must reach the site of fertilization in the oviduct to exert its ultimate biological role of delivering the male haploid DNA complement to the oocyte, thereby producing a pronucleate embryo and a subsequent pregnancy. In order to reach the oviduct in vivo, the sperm cell must be capable both of acquiring its characteristic motility pattern during maturation in the testes and of maintaining this motility pattern during its migration through the female reproductive tract. The capability of the sperm cell to display motion in vitro and in vivo is highly dependent on its ability to generate ATP, which, in turn, is used as the dynein ATPase substrate to transduce chemical energy into mechanical work by the contractile proteins of the flagellum. The ability of the spermatozoon to maintain its motility pattern in vitro and in vivo, therefore, is going to depend both on the normal function of the contractile proteins of the flagellum and its ability to generate ATP but also on the availability of metabolic substrate in the female reproductive tract to produce ATP.

Spermatozoa are subject to rather marked changes in environment as they move from the male reproductive tract to the site of fertilization in the oviduct. Ejaculation exposes epididymal sperm to the seminal plasma, which initiates motility and sharply increases sperm energy metabolism. Further environmental changes occur in the female reproductive tract as semen is diluted with uterine fluids. Under such conditions, sperm survival critically depends on the efficient utilization and control of the metabolism of nutrients from the surrounding medium.

The purpose of this review is to examine the metabolic strategy of mammalian and, in particular, human spermatozoa with specific reference to oxidative metabolism and glycolysis and the impact of this metabolic strategy on sperm motility.

Glycolysis

Much of the energy needed for motility and survival in human sperm, like that in most mammalian species, is generated by glycolysis, which is highly active under both aerobic and anaerobic conditions. Peterson and Freund reported the effects of substrate, substrate concentration, and changes in medium composition on the rate of glycolysis (1). In that study, the conditions under which fructose and glucose levels could limit glycolysis were defined. Evidence was also presented that indicated that the transport of sugars into the cell did not ordinarily limit glycolysis and that the sites of glycolytic control were present beyond the hexokinase step. The main sites of control of glycolysis are related to the regulation of the activity of glycolytic enzymes by an essential ion cofactor. Phosphofructokinase is involved in this control, as judged from its low concentration in sperm cells and its sensitivity to adenine nucleotides, which are substances known to be involved in the regulation in somatic cells. Inorganic phosphate, which stimulates phosphofructokinase in cell-free extracts, also stimulates glycolysis in intact sperm (2,3). This stimulation, however, only amounts to a 30% increase in rate, even at phosphate concentrations as high as 40 mM. This suggests that phosphate control of glycolysis may be less important than control by other cofactors.

The enzyme profile of human sperm is not typical of cells that exhibit a high rate of aerobic glycolysis, which suggests that metabolic changes may occur in human sperm cells after ejaculation. This hypothesis was prompted by analogies in the metabolism of bull sperm, where such changes are known to occur. Early work by Lardy et al. indicated that glycolysis in epididymal bull sperm is sharply decreased when the cells are exposed to oxygen, but are increased again when sperm are ejaculated, which suggests that a metabolic regulator may be released at the time of ejaculation that uncouples oxidative phosphorylation, which in turn decreases the respiratory inhibition of glycolysis (3). Like ram and bull spermatozoa, human sperm contain substantial levels of glucose-6-phosphate dehydrogenase and 6-phosphogluconate dehydrogenase, the first two enzymes in the hexose monophosphate shunt. The shunt pathway ordinarily has four major functions: (1) to provide reducing power in the form of NADPH, needed to drive biosynthetic reactions; (2) to provide the pentose needed for nuclei acid synthesis; (3) to provide an additional mechanism for the oxidative generation of ATP; and (4) to provide the NADPH needed to maintain functional the glutathione reductase/glutathione peroxidase protective system for reduction of lipid hydroperoxides (Storey et al. 1998, in press). In view of the absence of significant biosynthesis in sperm,

sperm. In addition, sperm is unable to metabolize compounds such as ribose-5-phosphate, adenosine, and uridine, the pentose moieties that are ordinarily converted to lactic acid at rapid rates in cells where the shunt pathway actively supports biosynthesis. The existence of the third function in human sperm is supported by the work of Sarkar et al., who found that sperm incubated in the presence of NADP and glucose-6-phosphate or 6-phosphogluconate produces high levels of NADPH (4). The significance of the low levels of a-glycerophosphate dehydrogenase in human sperm requires some consideration. This enzyme has an important role in oxidative metabolism because it catalyzes the conversion of dihydroxyacetone phosphate to a-glycerolphosphate that can be directly oxidized by mitochondria in most tissues. Furthermore, the enzyme competes with lactate dehydrogenase for NADH, the reduced form of NAD, and therefore can provide additional NAD for the oxidation of the glycolytic end product, pyruvic acid. It is clear, therefore, that differences in the activity of this enzyme could explain some of the observed differences in oxidative metabolism between human sperm and the sperm of other species, such as ram and bull. Higher levels of this enzyme in ram sperm, for example, could account for the higher rates of glucose oxidation observed in this species and also for the higher rates of sorbitol and glycerol oxidation.

The catalytic activity of glycolytic enzymes in human spermatozoa exceeds the rate of glycolysis, which indicates that glycolysis is not limited by the concentration of any one enzyme. Phosphofructokinase is present in the least concentration, which suggests a regulatory role for this enzyme in human sperm. Furthermore, the activity of phosphofructokinase in sperm homogenates is markedly affected by cofactors known to be involved in other cell types. High concentrations of ATP inhibit phosphofructokinase activity while AMP and inorganic phosphate stimulate enzyme activity. These observations also implicate phosphofructokinase as a site of glycolytic control.

The general character of the enzyme profile in epididymal human sperm is typical of cells that exhibit a pronounced Pasteur effect (oxygen inhibition of glycolysis). An important feature of ejaculated human sperm, however, is the absence of an appreciable Pasteur effect. Addition of dinitrophenol to sperm preparations, which is an agent known to release the inhibitory effect of oxidative metabolism on glycolysis, only slightly stimulates the aerobic rate of glycolysis. The absence of a significant Pasteur effect in human sperm also provides an explanation for the relatively small effect of inorganic phosphate on the rate of glycolysis.

The rate of formation of lactic acid from glucose by motile human spermatozoa suspended in plasma-free medium is constant over a 30-fold range in substrate concentration (1–30 mM), whereas lactic acid formation from fructose increases less than two-fold over the same concentration range. The additional observation that glucose-6-phosphate enters the sperm cells without prior dephosphorylation and is metabolized to lactic acid at the same maximum rate as fructose and glucose indicates that glycolysis in human sperm is ordinarily not substrate limited. This also indicates that the fructose levels commonly present in semen are sufficient to sustain a high rate of glycolysis even when considerably diluted, as is the case in the female reproductive tract.

Rabbit spermatozoa convert more than 70% of the glucose consumed to lactate under aerobic conditions through the Embden-Meyerhof pathway as shown by Murdoch and White (5), who used both measurements of glucose uptake and lactate production of $^{14}CO_2$ produced from glucose labeled at the 1- and 6-positions. One of the two enzymes in the Embden-Meyerhof pathway producing ATP from glycolysis is pyruvate kinase (6,7), which is readily assayed in hypotonically treated epididymal spermatozoa (8). Two major types of pyruvate kinase have been distinguished in various tissues by means of the effects on their kinetics by substrates, cofactors, and effectors (9,10). One is the type showing allosteric control by fructose-1-6-biphosphate. One isozyme of this type, designated L (11), is found in yeast (6) and in hepatocytes (12). Other isozymes of this type are M2 from liver nonparenchymal cells (12–14) and A from the kidney (15). The control characteristics of this type of enzyme, particularly the allosteric activation by fructose-1-6-biphosphate, are those expected for an enzyme operating in a pathway in which flux is closely controlled (7). The biosynthetic pathways operating in liver parenchymal cells, which include the pathway of gluconeogenesis, require maximal ATP with minimal utilization of glucose (16); the glucose used is effectively combusted to H_2O and CO_2 or converted to precursors for use in anabolic pathways. The same consideration applies to kidney cells that have the gluconeogenic pathway and the A isozyme of pyruvate kinase.

The second type of pyruvate kinase, represented by the muscle isozyme M (17), does not have this allosteric control characteristic. It is therefore suited for handling higher fluxes of glucose being catabolized to lactate through the Embden-Meyerhof pathway (7). The efficiency of ATP production, taken as moles of ATP produced per mole of glucose catabolized, is lowered, but a high rate of ATP production can be maintained. These control characteristics of the muscle enzyme are those needed for conversion of metabolic energy to mechanical work, in which efficiency of glucose utilization is subordinated to maximal rate of ATP production (16). The flux through the Embden-Meyerhof pathway is normally high to maintain speed and force of muscle contraction. The kinetic properties of the pyruvate kinase in a given cell type are therefore useful in inferring the regulatory properties of the glycolytic pathway characteristic of that cell type.

Oxidative Metabolism

Krebs Cycle

The presence of an oxidative metabolism in human sperm has been clearly established (2,18). It has also been shown that this metabolism can support sperm motility in the absence of glycolysis (19). Oxidative metabolism in human spermatozoa is less effective than glycolysis in maintaining cellular levels of ATP and in supporting sperm motility. In the absence of glucose, ATP levels decline steadily with a concomitant loss in motility, but they remain constant for several hours in the presence of glucose, and they decline if motility is small.

The inability of oxidative metabolism to generate high levels of ATP may explain the absence of a significant Pasteur effect in human sperm. This would assume that the Pasteur effect is mainly due to the feedback inhibition by ATP generated under aerobic conditions of key enzymes in the glycolytic pathway. The finding by Peterson and Freund that phosphofructokinase activity in human sperm homogenates is markedly inhibited by ATP and that this inhibition can be prevented or reversed by the addition of inorganic phosphate is pertinent to this (20). In the intact sperm cell, however, the addition of inorganic phosphate causes only a small increase in the aerobic glycolytic rate, which appears more to reflect a simple requirement for the ion as an enzymatic substrate than a phenomenon of glycolytic control (1). This suggests that the ATP generated aerobically in intact sperm is insufficient to cause significant inhibition of enzyme activity at the phosphofructokinase step.

With the exception of succinate, Krebs cycle intermediates, glucose, and pyruvate do not significantly increase respiration over the endogenous rate. The possible causes for these low oxidation rates could be as follows. The pathway to oxygen is common at coenzyme Q for the oxidation of succinate and pyridine nucleotide-linked substrates. The high rate of succinate oxidation, therefore, eliminates this portion of the electron-transfer chain as limiting the oxidation of other substrates. This assumes that succinate-stimulated respiration is not caused by exposure and activation of succinate dehydrogenase as a result of the washing procedure. Hamner and Williams reported that the level of glucose oxidation by human sperm could be increased to the level of succinate oxidation by the addition of bicarbonate (21). A possible interpretation of this could be that bicarbonate speeds the turnover rate of the cycle and, with it, acetyl CoA oxidation, by providing increased amounts of a limiting reactant (e.g., oxaloacetate via CO_2 fixation to pyruvate). Murdoch and White, however, reported that the addition of 6 mM bicarbonate only slightly stimulated human sperm respiration, and Peterson and Freund found comparable results using polarographic measurements. When tested in the presence of 1–10 mM sodium bicarbonate, the rate of oxidation of succinate was consistently two- to four-fold greater than was the rate of glucose oxidation (2,22). Furthermore, in whole semen, where the bicarbonate concentration is high, the respiration rates for sperm were low but could be stimulated by succinate. This indicates that factors other than bicarbonate are limiting the oxidation of pyridine nucleotide-linked substrates.

Several considerations also indicate that the concentration of phosphate acceptors (e.g., ADP and AMP) do not ordinarily limit the oxidation of pyridine nucleotide-linked substrates. The increased rate of oxidation in the presence of succinate alone suggests this because the succinate pathway crosses two of the three potentially limiting sites involved in ATP synthesis. Furthermore, the absence of any appreciable depression of endogenous respiration by glucose also argues against a phosphate acceptor limitation for oxidation since such depressed respiration has been explained in terms of competition by glycolysis by adenine nucleotides.

Citrate and other Krebs cycle intermediates are readily formed from pyruvate in human spermatozoa, provided that a source of oxaloacetate is present. In washed spermatozoa, entrance into the cycle appears to be limited merely by the availability of oxaloacetate. The conversion of acetate to citrate, however, is not increased in the presence of substrates that increase oxaloacetate levels and, apparently, the rate of formation of acetyl CoA from acetate limits entry into the cycle in this instance. This interpretation is in accordance with the report of Terner who found that acetate was oxidized by human spermatozoa at much lower rates than either glucose or pyruvate (18).

Although the increased rate of citrate formation may increase the rate of oxidation of a particular substrate, the total rate of respiration is not increased by stimulation in citrate synthesis, and other factors obviously dominate the control of oxidation of pyridine nucleotide-linked substrates. The high rate of succinate oxidation indicates that the major portion of the respiratory chain is capable of supporting a high rate of electron transfer. Moreover, the generation of high levels of tricarboxylic cycle intermediates from exogenous precursors suggests that most Krebs-cycle enzymes are present in more than adequate concentrations to handle the substrate loads sperm may ordinarily encounter. Oxidation, therefore, may be limited by the catalytic capacity of mitochondrial pyridine nucleotide dehydrogenase or by some form of stringent cofactor control. Several metabolic peculiarities in human sperm are known to contribute to the near absence of a Pasteur effect in human spermatozoa. First, a-glycerolphosphate dehydrogenase activity is very low (23). This tends to increase the NADH available to lactic dehydrogenase for pyruvate reduction and lower the acetyl CoA available for mitochondrial oxidation. Second, high ATP/ADP ratios are not generated in these cells, perhaps due to a loose coupling of respiration to phosphorylation. This would tend to lessen feedback inhibition of glycolysis at several points in the glycolytic sequence.

Fatty Acid Oxidation

In order for the mitochondrial oxidation of long-chain fatty acids to take place, acids must be converted to acyl esters of CoA in the cytosol and this, in turn, must be converted to the carnitine esters by the appropriate transferase located on the outside of the inner mitochondrial membrane (24–27). The carnitine esters are acyl ester substrates whose oxidation by isolated mitochondria can be monitored using oxygen uptake measurements. The required transferase activity has been reported in bull sperm mitochondria. The other part of the lipid molecule, which can also be utilized to produce ATP, is the glycerol moiety which is known to be oxidized as L-3-glycerophosphate (L-3-GP) by mammalian spermatozoa (28,29).

The set of mitochondrial oxidative activities of human spermatozoa fall between the full set typical of somatic cell mitochondria (shown by bull sperm mitochondria) and the limited set shown by rabbit sperm mitochondria (30). A qualitative comparison of the activities in spermatozoa from these species is summarized in Table 2.1. One particular difference between bull sperm mitochondria and human sperm mitochondria is that the former have an active L-3-glycerophosphate activity, but the latter have low activity. Bull sperm, which are available in sufficient quantity to test for the activity of this enzyme, have been shown to be without it (28). Mouse sperm lack the necessary enzymes needed to utilize the malate/aspartate shuttle (31) for transfer of these equivalents, as shown by their inability to oxidize glutamate in the presence of malate (32). It is probable that the lactate/pyruvate shuttle, apparently common to all mammalian spermatozoa, plays a major role in transferring NADH equivalents from cytosol to mitochondria in the mouse sperm cell. Mouse spermatozoa can directly oxidize fatty acids through the CoA esters, which is missing from rabbit and bull sperm. These esters provide a supply of endogenous substrate which would enable mouse sperm to remain viable for long periods in the absence of exogenous energy-yielding substrates. Indeed, mouse sperm from random-bred Swiss mice do remain motile for more than 4 hours in a simple solution containing only NaCl, tris-HCl, and $CaCl_2$ (33,34). Sperm from BL/6 mice, which have high initial motility (35), maintain their motility for more than six hours in defined saline medium buffered with phosphate and bicarbonate but lacking oxidizable substrates.

The comparison of the mitochondrial activities of human, bovine, mouse, and rabbit spermatozoa suggests that the bovine gametes are much more self-sufficient with regard to substrates that they can utilize, particularly endogenous stores of lipids. If the hypothesis postulated by Storey is correct (e.g., that sperm mitochondrial activities can be used to predict the content of

TABLE 2.1. Comparison of mitochondrial oxidative activities in mammalian spermatozoa.

Substrate	Mouse	Bull	Rabbit	Human
Glutamate/malate	–	++	–	++
Pyruvate/malate	+++	+++	++	++
Lactate/malate	+++	++	+++	+
L-3-glycerol phosphate	+++	+++	–	++
Acetyl carnitine/malate	++	++	+	+
Palmitoyl carnitine/malate	–	+	–	+
Acetyl CoA/malate	+	–	–	+

Activities are as follows: +++, high activity; ++, moderate activity; +, low activity; –, no activity.

oviduct lumen energy sources), then the bovine oviduct lumen should have a low content of these sources. Data regarding the substrate content of oviduct lumen support this indication (36–38).

Impact of Sperm Metabolic Strategy on Sperm Motility

The energy metabolism of a cell type is, of necessity, related to its function; this relation has been termed *the metabolic strategy of the cell*. In the case of the sperm cell, the question may be asked: Is the cell's metabolic strategy geared to the series of reactions preceding and involved in fertilization, including motility, or does the maintenance of motility dominate the metabolic strategy? These questions can be clarified by looking at the kinetic properties of pyruvate kinase in sperm as compared with the liver and muscle enzymes, as well as its metabolic coupling with flagellar ATPase. In permeabilized epididymal sperm, pyruvate kinase has access to its substrates, but it remains bound to the cell structure and suffers minimal perturbation from the preparation procedure (8). Epididymal sperm are usually immotile, but motility is restored in KCl medium containing Mg2+ upon addition of 3 mM ATP, following the method of Gibbons and Gibbons (39) with 50 mM phosphoenolpyruvate (PEP) to maintain ATP levels (40). Under these conditions, phosphoenolpyruvate is consumed. This consumption is readily measured so that the activity of flagellar ATPase in permeabilized epididymal sperm can be quantitated and putative regulators can be assessed.

The flagellar ATPase in mammalian sperm has an activity comparable to that of somatic pyruvate kinase. The flagellar ATPase requires Mg^{2+} for activity (40). If Mg^{2+} is omitted from the medium, then sperm remain immotile in the presence of 3 mM ATP and 50 mM PEP, but motility is restored by addition of 3 mM Mg^{2+}. The calculated KM values for ATP and Mg^{2+} at 37°C were 0.22 mM and 0.25 mM, respectively, which indicates that the substrate is MgATP, as previously shown by Tibbs (41) for sperm tails from perch and by Gibbons and Gibbons (39) and Hayasi for sea urchin axonemes (42).

Pyruvate kinase in mammalian sperm is kinetically very similar to muscle pyruvate kinase, and it is affected by the same inhibitors and activators as is the muscle enzyme. The question of whether or not the similarity extends to the protein structure of the enzyme remains unanswered at present. The difficulty of extracting and purifying this and other enzymes and organelles from the sperm cell without damage to their structure (43,44) makes its characterization by immunological methods uncertain. Immunological cross-reactions can occur among some of the pyruvate kinase isozymes (45), so such a characterization is rendered even less useful. For the purposes of metabolic analysis, however, the similarity of the kinetic properties and control characteristics of the sperm and muscle pyruvate kinases implies that control of the glycolytic pathway in the sperm cell operates as it does in the skeletal muscle cell. Both cells require ATP for mechanical work done by contractile proteins. Both cells have access to glucose reserves:

the muscle cell through glycogenolysis and the sperm cell through an effectively inexhaustible supply of glucose in the oviduct (46). In mature sperm cells, the energy-producing and energy-utilizing enzyme pathways seem fairly well balanced; the activities of pyruvate kinase and flagellar ATPase and of lactate dehydrogenase are all of the same order of magnitude. In any given sperm sample, these activities are an order of magnitude higher than the activity of mitochondrial lactate or pyruvate oxidase system (8). The metabolic strategy of mature spermatozoa depends on a high rate of glycolysis to provide ATP for motility as do skeletal muscle cells for contractibility (7,16).

Envoy

The enzymatic activities in sperm cells, which produce and utilize ATP, have kinetic properties and respond to regulators in a manner that closely parallels the same activities in muscle cells. Although the ATP-utilizing enzymes in these two types of cells are very different at the molecular level, they both produce contractile force, an activity to which the cellular metabolism is geared. This suggests that the major use of the sperm cell's metabolic machinery is maintenance of energy for the contractile work of motility; only minor amounts of metabolic energy appear to be consumed in other reactions, including those involved in fertilization.

The preferential conversion of glucose to lactate, under aerobic conditions, through the Embden-Meyerhof pathway may be an important evolutionary feature of mammalian sperm, perhaps intended to minimize the accumulation of reducing equivalents in the mitochondria and therefore the increased production in oxygen radicals. It is well known that sperm produce oxygen radicals, that the bulk of these radicals are produced by the mitochondria, and that oxygen radical-induced damage could result in loss of sperm motility, loss of acrosomal contents, and oxidative DNA damage (47–52). Conversion of glucose to lactate under aerobic conditions would (1) decrease production of mitochondrial NADH- and FADH-reducing equivalents by the Krebs cycle and (2) decrease electron flow in the inner mitochondrial membrane, thereby downregulating oxygen radical formation. This metabolic feature is especially important outside the protective environment of the epididymis where oxygen radical-induced damage is minimized by a lower temperature and $pO2$.

In summary, it appears that the metabolic strategy of the spermatozoon is similar to that of a muscle cell in that (1) it depends on a high rate of glycolysis (and low utilization of the Krebs cycle) to provide ATP for motility and (2) the hexose monophosphate shunt is almost exclusively devoted to produce NADPH to maintain functional the glutathione reductase/glutathione peroxidase protective system for reduction of lipid hydroperoxides. Spem's metabolic strategy, therefore, is both geared to maintain high rates of glycolysis to produce ATP for motility and to ensure that DNA integrity and motility are preserved during the sperm cell's long journey to the oviduct.

References

1. Peterson RN, Freund M. Glycolysis by washed suspensions of human spermatozoa. Effect of substrate, substrate concentration and changes in medium composition on the rate of glycolysis. Biol Reprod 1969;1:238–46.
2. Murdoch RN, White IG. Studies on the metabolism of human spermatozoa. J Reprod Fertil 1968;16:351–61.
3. Lardy HA, Parks RE. In: Gaehler O, editor. Enzymes: units of biological structure and function. New York: Academic Press, 1956:584–92.
4. Sarkar S, Nelson AJ, Jones OW. Glucose-6-phosphate dehydrogenase activity in human sperm. J Med Genet 1977;14:250–55.
5. Murdoch RN, White IG. The metabolism of labeled glucose by rabbit spermatozoa after incubation in vitro. J Reprod Fertil 1967;14:213–23.
6. Hess B, Brand K. Enzyme and metabolite profiles. In: Chance B, Estabrook RW, Williamson JR, editors. Control of energy metabolism. New York: Academic Press, 1965:111–21.
7. Newsholme EA, Start C. Regulation of metabolism. New York: John Wiley and Sons, 1973:88–145.
8. Storey BT, Kayne FJ. Energy metabolism of spermatozoa. V. The Embden-Meyerhof pathway of glycolysis: activities of pathway enzymes in hypotonically-treated rabbit epididymal spermatozoa. Fertil Steril 1975;26:1257–65.
9. Susor WA, Ratter WJ. Some distinctive properties of pyruvate kinase purified from rat liver. Biochem Biophys Comm 1968;18:527–36.
10. Carminatti HL, Jiménez de Asúa L, Leiderman B, Rozengurt E. Allosteric properties of skeletal muscle pyruvate kinase. J Biol Chem 1971;246:7284–88.
11. Seubert W, Schoner W. The regulation of pyruvate kinase. Curr Top Cell Regul 1971;3:237–67.
12. Crisp DM, Pogson CI. Glycolytic and gluconeogenic enzyme activities in parenchymal and nonparenchymal cells from mouse liver. Biochem J 1972;126: 1009–23.
13. Jiménez de Asúa L, Rozengurt E, Devalle JJ, Carminatti H. Some kinetic differences between the M isozymes of pyruvate kinase from liver and muscle. Biochim Biophys Acta 1971;135:326–34.
14. Imamura K, Taniuchi K, Tanaka T. Multimolecular forms of pyruvate kinase. II. Purification of M2 type pyruvate kinase from Yoshida ascitis hepatoma 130 cells and comparative studies on the enzymological properties of the three types of pyruvate kinase, L, M1, and M2. J Biochem (Tokyo) 1972;72:1001–15.
15. Berglund L, Humble E. Kinetic properties of pig pyruvate kinases type A from kidney and type M from muscle. Arch Biochem Biophys 1979;195:347–61.
16. Scrutton MC, Utter MF. The regulation of glycolysis and gluconeogenesis in animal tissues. Annu Rev Biochem 1968;37:249–302.
17. Kayne FJ. Pyruvate kinase. In: Boyer PD, editor. The enzymes, Vol. 8. New York: Academic Press, 1973:353–82.
18. Terner C. Oxidation of exogenous substrate by isolated human spermatozoa. Am J Physiol 1960;198:48–50.
19. Nevo A. Relation between motility and respiration in human spermatozoa. J Reprod Fertil 1966;11:19–26.
20. Peterson RN, Freund M. Profile of glycolytic enzyme activities in human spermatozoa. Fertil Steril 1970;21:151–58.

21. Hamner CE, Williams WL. Identification of sperm stimulating factor of rabbit oviduct fluid. Proc Soc Exp Biol Med 1964;117:240–43.
22. Peterson RN, Freund M. ATP synthesis and oxidative metabolism in human spermatozoa. Biol Reprod 1970;3:47–54.
23. Peterson RN, Freund M. Glycolysis by human spermatozoa: levels of glycolytic intermediates. Biol Reprod 1971;5:221–27.
24. Fritz IB, Yue KTN. Long-chain carnitine acyl-transferase and the role of acylcarnitine derivatives in the catalytic increase of fatty acid oxidation induced by carnitine. J Lipid Res 1963;4:279–88.
25. Bode C, Klingenberg M. Die veratmung von fettsauren in isolierten mitochondrien. Biochem Z 1965;341:271–89.
26. Haddock BA, Yates DW, Garland PB. The localization of some coenzyme A dependent enzymes in rat liver mitochondria. Biochem J 1970;119:565–73.
27. Yates DW, Garland PB. Carnitine palmitoyl-transferase activities of rat liver mitochondria. Biochem J 1970;119:547–52.
28. Mohri H, Mohri T, Ernster L. Isolation and enzymic properties of the midpiece of bull spermatozoa. Exp Cell Res 1965;38:217–46.
29. Mohri H, Masaki J. Glycerokinase and its possible role in glycerol metabolism of bull spermatozoa. J Reprod Fertil 1967;14:179–94.
30. Carey JE, Olds Clark P, Storey BT. Oxidative metabolism of spermatozoa from inbred and random bred mice. J Exp Zool 1981;216:285–92.
31. Borst P. Hydrogen transport and transport of metabolites. In: Karlson P, editor. Funktionelle und Morphologishe Organization der Zelle. Berlin: Spreinger Verlag, 1963:135–58.
32. LaNoue KF, Wadajtys EI, Williamson JR. Regulation of glutamate metabolism and interactions with the citric acid cycle in rat heart mitochondria. J Biol Chem 1973;248:7171–83.
33. Saling PM, Storey BT, Wolf DP. Calcium-dependent binding of mouse epididymal spermatozoa to the zona pellucida. Dev Biol 1978;65:515–25.
34. Heffner LJ, Saling PM, Storey BT. Separation of calcium effects on motility and zona binding ability in mouse spermatozoa. J Exp Zool 1980;212:53–59.
35. Carey J, Olds-Clark P. Differences in sperm function in vitro but not in vivo between inbred and random-bred mice. Gamete Res 1980;3:9–15.
36. Hamner C. Oviductal fluid-composition and physiology. In: Greep RO, editor. Handbook of physiology, Section 7 (endocrinology), Vol. 2, Part 2. Washington, DC: American Physiological Society, 1973:141–52.
37. Brackett BG, Mastroianni L. Composition of oviductal fluid. In: Johnson AD, Foley CW, editors. The oviduct and its functions. New York: Academic Press, 1974:133–59.
38. Blandau RJ, Brackett B, Brenner RM, et al. The oviduct. In: Greep RO, Koblinsky MA, editors. Frontiers in reproduction and fertility control, Part 2. Cambridge MA: MIT Press, 1977:132–45.
39. Gibbons BH, Gibbons IR. Flagellar movement and adenosine triphosphatase activity in sea urchin sperm extracted with Triton X-100. J Cell Biol 1972;54:75–97.
40. Keyhani E, Storey BT. Energy conservation capacity and morphological integrity of mitochondria in hypotonically-treated rabbit epididymal spermatozoa. Biochem Biophys Acta 1973a;305:557–69.
41. Tibbs J. Adenosine triphosphate and acetylcholinesterase in relation to sperm motility. In: Bishop DW, editor. Spermatozoan motility. Washington, D.C.: Am Assoc Adv Sci 1962:233–50.

42. Hayasi M. Kinetic analysis of axoneme and dynein ATPase from sea urchin sperm. Arch Biochem Biophys 1974;165:288–96.
43. Calvin HI. Isolation and subfractionation of mammalian sperm heads and tails. In: Prescott DM, editor. Methods in cell biology, Vol. 13. New York: Academic Press, 1976:85–104.
44. Hrudka F. A morphological and cytochemical study of isolated sperm mitochondria. J Ultrastruct Res 1978;63:1–19.
45. Osterman J, Fritz PF. Pyruvate kinase isozymes from rat intestinal mucose. Characterization and the effect of fasting and refeeding. Biochemistry 1974;13:1731–36.
46. Holmdahl TH, Mastroianni L. Continuous collection of rabbit oviduct secretions at low temperature. Fertil Steril 1965;16:587–95.
47. Alvarez JG, Storey BT. Spontaneous lipid peroxidation in rabbit epididymal spermatozoa. Biol Reprod 1982;27:1102–8.
48. Holland MK, Alvarez JG, Storey BT. Production of superoxide and activity of superoxide dismutase in rabbit epididymal spermatozoa. Biol Reprod 1982;27:1109–18.
49. Alvarez JG, Holland MK, Storey BT. Spontaneous lipid peroxidation in rabbit spermatozoa: a useful model for the reaction of O2 metabolites with cells. In: Lubbers DW, Acker H, Leninger-Follert E, Goldstick TK, editors. Oxygen transport to tissue – V. New York: Plenum, 1984:433–43.
50. Alvarez JG, Storey BT. Assessment of cell damage caused by spontaneous lipid peroxidation in rabbit spermatozoa. Biol Reprod 1984;30:323–32.
51. Alvarez JG, Touchstone JC, Blasco L, Storey BT. Spontaneous lipid peroxidation and production of hydrogen peroxide and superoxide in human spermatozoa. Superoxide dismutase as major enzyme protectant against oxygen toxicity. J Androl 1987;8:338–48.
52. Fraga CG, Motchnik PA, Shigenaga MK, Helbock HJ, Jacob RA, Ames BN. Ascorbic acid protects against endogenous oxidative DNA damage in human sperm. Proc Natl Acad Sci 1991;88:11003–6.

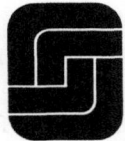

3

Extrinsic Factors Affecting Sperm Motility: Immunological and Infectious Factors and Reactive Oxygen Species

CLAUDE GAGNON AND EVE DE LAMIRANDE

Sperm motility requires the interaction of intracellular factors, including an adequate level of adenosine triphosphate (ATP), functional axonemal dynein ATPases, and an intact axoneme bathing in a proper ionic environment. These factors also represent the minimal conditions required to initiate and maintain the motility of modeled spermatozoa (i.e., spermatozoa demembranated by a detergent treatment in which motility is initiated by the addition of ATP and ions (1–4). Extracellular factors that affect these minimal requirements will cause an arrest in sperm motility. Factors such as sperm agglutinating antibodies that act at the surface of cells by forming a physical network of spermatozoa bound to each other obviously act via different mechanisms. This chapter will not cover the effects of sperm immobilizing or agglutinating antibodies on sperm motility, but it will focus on the actions of factors, such as infections, proteins of the immune system, polymorphonuclear leukocytes, and reactive oxygen species (ROS).

Infection, Bacteria, and Bacterial Products

Several criteria were suggested as indicators of an infection in the male sex glands, including: (1) history of urogenital infection and/or abnormal rectal palpation, (2) presence of leukocytes or bacteria in expressed prostate secretions and/or urinary sediments after prostatic massage, (3) growth of pathogenic (> 1000/ml) or nonpathogenic (> 10,000/ml) bacteria in twofold diluted seminal plasma, (4) presence of leukocytes (> 106/ml) in semen, and (5) disturbed secretory function of the accessory sex glands (5). Any combination of two of these criteria makes the diagnosis of an accessory gland infection likely, but far from definitive (5,6). Many men are asymptomatic while having elevated levels of bacteria and leukocytes in semen.

Infection, which is a major cause of infertility in women, may have a similar deleterious effect in men, but the evidence is often conflicting and controversial (6) unless pathogens completely block any segment of the male reproductive tract, therefore causing azoospermia. The negative effect of *Escherichia coli* on sperm motility in vitro that were first reported by Schirren and Zander (7) were confirmed by several authors (8–12). A sperm-to-bacteria ratio of 1 clearly decreases sperm motility parameters (percentage and progressiveness). Bacteria themselves rather than their secretory products cause these effects. Adherence of *E. coli* to sperm would be mediated via a mannose-binding site and would be involved in the triggering of membrane damage to spermatozoa (12,13)

Cytokines

The immune response is modulated by several factors, such as cytokines and cytokine inhibitors (14). Cytokines are a family of polypeptide hormones that are produced primarily by cells of the immune system involved in response to various stimuli, including foreign antigens. Both male and female genital tracts are immunologically dynamic tissues that contain products of local, as well as systemic, immune responses, both humoral and cell mediated. Thus, spermatozoa could be affected by these products before (in the male genital tract) and after ejaculation (in the female genital tract) (15).

Incubation of spermatozoa with transforming growth factor-b (TGF-b), interleukins 1 and 2 (IL-1, IL-2), granulocyte macrophage colony-stimulating factor (GM-CSF), and B-cell growth factor (BCGF) did not affect sperm motility, sperm function, and subsequent fertilization, except when used at very high concentrations (16). On the other hand, two cytokines—interferon (INF)-a and g, and tumor necrosis factors (TNF-a)—had negative effects on sperm motility and penetration rates in zona-free hamster oocytes (17,18). Relatively high concentrations of INF-a and TNF-a, however, were required in short-term culture in order to observe such effects. Huleihel et al. (14) reported that sperm cells from fertile and oligoasthenoteratozoospermic infertile men constitutively produced IL-1. This report is surprising because motile spermatozoa, as selected from normal ejaculated semen by swim-up technique, should be devoid of cytoplasmic ribosomes, which makes it impossible for IL-1 to be constitutively synthesized by mature sperm cells. The presence of remnant leukocytes or immature germ cells in the sperm swim-up fraction may explain the result of Huleihel et al. (14).

IL-6 is probably the most specific marker for the detection of male accessory gland infection (95% sensitivity), and the correlation observed between the concentration of IL-6 and the level of reactive oxygen species (ROS) produced in semen (19) may be linked to the stimulating effect of cytokines on lipid membrane peroxidation in human spermatozoa (20), which is an ROS-mediated event. On the other hand, IL-6 also enhanced the fertilizing capacity of human spermatozoa by increasing capacitation and acrosome reaction (21). Other cytokines—IL-1, IL-6, and TNF-a—were also shown to decrease sperm motility and be involved in reduced male fertility (22).

Cells in Semen That Can Damage Normal Motile Spermatozoa

Two types of cells from semen produce ROS that potentially can damage normal motile spermatozoa: the white blood cells [i.e., the polymorphonuclear (PMN) leukocytes (23)] and abnormal spermatozoa (24,25).

Abnormal Spermatozoa

Up to 25% of semen samples from an unselected population of men consulting for infertility produced ROS. The levels of ROS generated in semen varied within three to four orders of magnitude and were inversely correlated to the percentage of motile spermatozoa and to the semen volume (24) as well as to the outcome of the hamster sperm-oocyte penetration assay and fertility in vivo (26). Higher levels of ROS were produced by morphologically abnormal than normal spermatozoa (24). This phenomenon was associated with higher glucose-6-phosphate dehydrogenase activity, probably due to the presence of residual cytoplasm in the sperm midpiece, which could supply the substrate for ROS formation (27). The presence of precursor germ cells or immature spermatozoa in semen could be a source of ROS and, therefore, be a threat to normal motile spermatozoa. Experiments performed in rats, hamsters, guinea pigs, and mice indicated that germ cells (pachytene spermatocytes, round and elongated spermatids) generated the same low levels of ROS, but that spermatozoa from the caput epididymis produced much higher levels of ROS than did mature spermatozoa (28). Normal spermatozoa also have the potential to generate ROS, but unless they are subjected to centrifugation–resuspension cycles (29), treated with various substances such as phorbol myristate acetate (30,31), formyl-Met-Leu-Phe, nerve growth factor, complement 5a (32), calcium ionophore (31), or incubated in capacitating conditions (33), their level of ROS production is extremely low.

ROS generated by damaged spermatozoa did not appear to be responsible for decreased function of normal spermatozoa because the combination of ROS-producing and non-ROS-producing spermatozoa did not consistently affect sperm motility, regardless of cell concentration, duration of incubation (up to 24 hours) or level of ROS produced (34). On the other hand, even if spermatozoa produce relatively low levels of ROS (as compared with PMN) and release only one third of these ROS in the extracellular milieu (34), it is possible that longer incubation periods might be detrimental to sperm function. The source of ROS generated by spermatozoa is presently not known. Possible candidates include an NADPH oxidase on the sperm plasma membrane (35) and a mitochondrial NADH-dependent oxidoreductase diaphorase (36).

White Blood Cells

The prevalence of leukocytospermia, which is defined as the presence of more than 1×106 white blood cells/milliliter by the World Health Organization and is considered as a possible indication of ongoing infection along the male reproductive tract, ranges from 10 to 20% of all infertile patients (37). The white blood cells found in semen appeared to originate from the epididymis and the prostate. The negative effects associated with leukocytospermia, such as decreased sperm number, impaired sperm motility, and failure of in vitro fertilization–embryo transfer procedures, could be mediated among other things by ROS, proteases, and cytokines.

PMN are present in semen samples of normal and infertile men and usually represent 60–70% of the white blood cell population. In the fulfilment of their role of defense against invading microorganisms they release superoxide anion (O_2o-), which by dismutation and/or reaction with other ROS and ions forms other toxic species such as hydrogen peroxide (H_2O_2), the hydroxyl radical (oOH), and hypochlorite (38). The NADPH oxidase of PMN can be stimulated 20- to 100-fold into secreting toxic ROS to the extracellular space in the presence of the complement C5a, chemotactic interleukins, or N-terminus bacterial protein fragments, which are expected to be present in semen if there is an infection along the male genital tract.

Stimulated PMN produce a concentration- and time-dependent decrease in the motility of Percoll-washed spermatozoa (23,34). Despite the fact that, under the conditions of the study, the oxidative burst of PMN lasted for about 60 min, the effects on sperm motility were better perceived at 3–5 hours later. A concentration of 0.6×106 PMN/ml was sufficient to decrease sperm motility by 35% after 5 hours of contact.

Effect of ROS Scavengers and Seminal Plasma on the Motility of Spermatozoa Incubated with Stimulated PMN

Addition of superoxide dismutase (SOD; scavenger of superoxide anion) had no effect on the decrease of motility observed in PMN-treated spermatozoa, whereas catalase (scavenger of hydrogen peroxide) and dimethyl sulfoxide (DMSO; scavenger of the hydroxyl radical) individually allowed a 50% prevention of this toxic effect (23). When combined, catalase and DMSO nearly completely prevented the drop in sperm motility, indicating that essentially all effects of stimulated PMN on sperm motility were caused by ROS and that hydrogen peroxide and the hydroxyl radical were responsible for the effects observed.

In addition to DMSO and catalase, human seminal plasma could also prevent some of the damage caused by ROS released by stimulated PMN, but the preservation of motility varied from 10 to 100%, depending on the individual seminal plasma sample used (23). These results suggested that some men may be more susceptible to a loss of sperm motility caused by infection or simply to high concentration of PMN in their seminal plasma. It also indicated that inflammations and infections of the epididymis and testis are likely to have the largest impact on spermatozoa. The protective agents present in seminal plasma originated both from pools of small (< 10 kDa) and large molecules (> 12 kDa) that have the capacity to scavenge both the superoxide anion and hydrogen peroxide (23,25). Albumin, taurine, hypotaurine (39), glulathione (38), pyruvate (4), vitamins E (40) and C (41), and the like which are present in semen, are potential scavengers for ROS produced by activated PMN.

Mode of Action of ROS on Sperm Motility

Although high levels of ROS in semen were for decades associated mainly with lipid peroxidation and damage to the cell membrane, leading to loss of cytosolic components and cell death, as reviewed by Storey (42), low levels of ROS appeared to act differently on spermatozoa. The mechanisms by which ROS exert their toxic effects on sperm motility were investigated by incubating spermatozoa with the combination of xanthine and xanthine oxidase, which produces the superoxide anion, which spontaneously dismutates to hydrogen peroxide. Even though conditions were chosen so that the ROS were produced for only the first 30 min of incubation (the substrate, xanthine, is completely consumed within that time), the percentage of motile cells did not change for 2–3 hours, after which it rapidly fell to zero within 30 min (4,43). The effects of ROS were concentration dependent: Low concentrations of xanthine and xanthine oxidase caused a complete arrest of sperm motility and allowed a recovery from this ROS injury within a few hours after the beginning of the treatment; higher concentrations of xanthine and xanthine oxidase, which overcome the cell defence against ROS, caused an irreversible immobilization and a decrease in sperm viability. The presence of catalase prevented any loss of sperm motility due to ROS generated by xanthine and xanthine oxidase, again indicating that hydrogen peroxide is responsible for the effects observed (4,43).

The first manifestation of ROS action in spermatozoa was the progressive decrease in flagellar beat frequency that was initiated during the first hour of incubation and was due to a drop in the intracellular ATP concentration. This ATP depletion triggered a cascade of events, leading to an insufficient axonemal protein phosphorylation related to the cAMP-protein kinase A-dependent pathways. The drop in ATP and sperm protein phosphorylation were among the first effects of ROS on spermatozoa.

Conclusions

In summary, factors and cells related to infection of the male reproductive tract can have deleterious effects on fertility. Through their adhesion to spermatozoa, bacteria such as *E. coli* can trigger membrane damage and a subsequent loss of motility. High concentrations of cytokines such as interferon-a and -g, tumor necrosis factors, IL-1 and IL-6, and TNF-a decreased sperm motility and/or penetration rates in zona-free hamster oocytes assays. Interleukin-6, the most specific marker of male accessory gland infection, was associated with lipid peroxidation of human sperm membrane. It also increased capacitation and acrosome reaction. ROS generated in semen originated mainly from PMN, and abnormal spermatozoa and the levels of these ROS were inversely correlated to the percentage of motile spermatozoa and fertility in vivo. ROS, of which hydrogen peroxide is responsible for the inhibition of sperm motility, acted by depletion of intracellular ATP and subsequently on the cAMP-dependent phosphorylation of axonemal proteins.

The impact of ROS on sperm motility depends of several factors, including the type of ROS involved, the site and the duration of exposure, and the types of ROS scavengers present. The time at which the effects produced by ROS are evaluated is also of paramount importance because ROS often initiate a cascade of events that will trigger a biological response. At high ROS concentrations, this response will be detrimental and may endanger sperm viability. On the other hand, very low concentrations of ROS may participate in biological processes such as sperm hyperactivation (44), capacitation (33,45), and acrosome reaction (46).

References

1. Gibbons BH, Gibbons IR. Flagellar movement and adenosine triphosphatase activity in sea urchin sperm extracted with Triton X-100. J Cell Biol 1972;54:75–97.
2. Gibbons IR. Cilia and flagella of eukaryotes. J Cell Biol 1981; 91:107s–24s.
3. Gagnon C. Regulation of sperm motility at the axonemal level. Reprod Fertil Dev 1995;7:811–24.
4. de Lamirande E, Gagnon C. Reactive oxygen species and human spermatozoa. II. Depletion of adenosine triphosphate plays an important role in the inhibition of sperm motility. J Androl 1992;13:379–86.
5. Comhaire FH, Verschaegen G, Vermeulen L. Diagnosis of accessory gland infection and its possible role in male infertility. Int J Androl 1980;3:32–45.
6. Purvis K, Christiansen E. Infection in the male reproductive tract. Impact diagnosis and treatment in relation to male infertility. Int J Androl 1993;16:1–13.
7. Schirren C, Zander HA. Genitalinfektionen des mannes und ihre auswirkungen auf die spermatozoenmotilität. Medizinische Welt 1966;45:45–47.
8. Teague NS, Boyarski S, Glenn JF. Interference of human spermatozoa motility by Escherichia coli. Fertil Steril 1971;22:281–85.
9. Del Porto GB, Derrick FC, Bannister ER. Bacterial effect on sperm motility. Urology 1975;5:638–39.

10. Paulson JD, Polakoski KL. Isolation of a spermatozoal immobilizing factor from Escherichia coli filtrates. Fertil Steril 1977;28:182–85.

11. Auroux MR, Jacques L, Mathieu D, Auer J. Is the sperm bacterial ratio a determining factor in impairment of sperm motility: an in-vitro study in men with Escherichia coli. Int J Androl 1991;14:264–70.

12. Diemer T, Weidner W, Michelmann HW, Schieffer H-G, Rovan E, Mayer F. Influence of Escherichia coli on motility parameters of human spermatozoa. Int J Androl 1996;19:271–77.

13. Wolff H, Panhans A, Stolz W, Meurer M. Adherence of Escherichia coli to sperm: a mannose mediated phenomenon leading to agglutination of sperm and E. coli. Fertil Steril 1993;60:154–58.

14. Huleihel M, Levy A, Lunenfeld E, Horowitz S, Potashnik G, Glezerman M. Distinct expression of cytokines and mitogenic inhibitory factors in semen of fertile and infertile men. Am J Reprod Immunol 1997;37:304–9.

15. Naz RK, Chaturvedi MM, Aggarval BB. Role of cytokines and proto-oncogenes in sperm cell function: relevance to immunologic infertility. Am J Reprod Immunol 1994;32:26–37.

16. Anderson DJ, Hill JA. Cell-mediated immunity in infertility. In: Naz RK, editor. Immunology of reproduction. Boca Raton: CRC Press, 1988:61–80.

17. Hill JA, Cohen J, Anderson DJ. The effect of lymphokines and monokines on human sperm fertilizing ability in the zona-free hamster penetration test. Am J Obstet Gynecol 1989;160:1154–59.

18. Naz RK, Kumar R. Transforming growth factor B1 enhances expression of 50 kDa protein related to 2'-5' oligoadenylate synthetase in human sperm cells. J Cell Physiol 1991;146:156–63.

19. Depuydt CE, Bosman E, Zalata A, Schoonjans F, Comhaire FH. The relation between reactive oxygen species and cytokines in andrological patients with or without male accessory gland infection. J Androl 1996;17:699–707.

20. Buch JP, Kolon TF, Maulik N. Cytokines stimulate lipid membrane peroxidation of human sperm. Fertil Steril 1994;62:186–88.

21. Naz RK, Kaplan P. Interleukin-6 enhances the fertilizing capacity of human spermatozoa by increasing capacitation and acrosome reaction. J Androl 1994;15:228–33.

22. Gruschwitz MS, Brezinschek R, Brezinschek H-P. Cytokine levels in the seminal plasma of infertile males. J Androl 1996;17:158–63.

23. Kovalski NN, de Lamirande E, Gagnon C. Reactive oxygen species by human neutrophils inhibit sperm motility: protective effect of seminal plasma and scavengers. Fertil Steril 1992;58:809–16.

24. Iwasaki A, Gagnon C. Formation of reactive oxygen species in spermatozoa of infertile patients. Fertil Steril 1992;57:409–16.

25. Zini A, de Lamirande E, Gagnon C. Reactive oxygen species in semen of infertile patients: levels of superoxide dismutase- and catalase-like activities in seminal plasma and spermatozoa. Int J Androl 1993;16:183–88.

26. Aitken JR, Irvine DS, Wu FC. Prospective analysis of sperm-oocyte fusion and reactive oxygen species generation as criteria for the diagnosis of infertility. Am J Obstet Gynecol 1991;164:542–51.

27. Aitken JR, Krauz C, Buckingham D. Relationship between biochemical markers for residual sperm cytoplasm, reactive oxygen species generation, and the presence of leukocytes and precursor germ cells in human sperm suspensions. Mol Reprod Dev 1994;39:268–79.

28. Fisher HM, Aitken JR. Comparative analysis of the ability of precursor germ cells and epididymal spermatozoa to generate reactive oxygen metabolites. Mol Reprod Dev 1997;277:390–400.
29. Aitken JR, Clarkson JS. Significance of reactive oxygen species and antioxidants in defining the efficacy of sperm preparation techniques. J Androl 1988;9:367–76.
30. Gavella M, Lipovac V, Marotti T. Use of pentoxifylline on superoxide anion production by human spermatozoa. Int J Androl 1991;14:320–25.
31. Aitken RJ, Buckingham DW, West KM. Reactive oxygen species and human spermatozoa: analysis of the cellular mechanisms involved in luminol- and lucigenin-dependent chemiluminescence. J Cell Physiol 1992;151:466–77.
32. Weese DL, Peaster ML, Hemandez RD, Leach GE, Laad PM, Zimmern PE. Chemoattractand agents and nerve growth factor stimulate human spermatozoal reactive oxygen species generation. Fertil Steril 1993;59:869–75.
33. de Lamirande E, Gagnon C. Capacitation-associated production of superoxide anion by human spermatozoa. Free Radic Biol Med 1995;18:487–95.
34. Plante M, da Lamirande E, Gagnon C. Reactive oxygen species released by activated neutrophils, but not by deficient spermatozoa, are sufficient to affect normal sperm motility. Fertil Steril 1994;62:387–93.
35. Aitken JR, Fisher HM, Fulton N, et al. Reactive oxygen species generation by human spermatozoa is induced by exogenous NADPH and inhibited by the flavoproteins inhibitors diphenylene iodonium and quinacrine. Mol Reprod Dev 1997;47:468–82.
36. Gavella M, Lipovac V. NADH-dependent oxido-reductase (diaphorase) activity and isozyme pattern of sperm in infertile men. Arch Androl 1992;28:135–41.
37. Wolff HW. The biological significance of white blood cells in semen. Fertil Steril 1995;63:1143–57.
38. Halliwell B, Gutteridge JMC, editors. Free radicals in biology and medicine, 2nd Edition. Oxford: Clarendon Press, 1989.
39. Alvarez JG, Storey BT. Taurine, hypotaurine, epinephrine and albumin inhibit lipid peroxidation in rabbit spermatozoa and protect against loss of motility. Biol Reprod 1983;29:548–55.
40. Chow CK. Vitamin E and oxidative stress. Free Radic Biol Med 1991;11:215–32.
41. Dawson EB, Harris WA, Teter MC, Powell LC. Effect of ascorbic acid supplementation on the sperm quality of smokers. Fertil Steril 1992;58:1034–39.
42. Storey BT. Biochemistry of the induction and prevention of lipoperoxidative damage in human spermatozoa. Mol Hum Reprod 1997;3:203–13.
43. de Lamirande E, Gagnon C. Reactive oxygen species and human spermatozoa. I. Effect on the motility of intact spermatozoa and on sperm axonemes. J Androl 1992;13:368–78.
44. de Lamirande E, Gagnon C. Human sperm hyperactivation and capacitation as parts of an oxidative process. Free Radic Biol Med 1993;14:157–66.
45. Leclerc P, de Lamirande E, Gagnon C. Regulation of protein tyrosine phosphorylation and human sperm capacitation by reactive oxygen species. Free Radic Biol Med 1997;22:643–65.
46. Griveau JF, Renard P, LeLannou D. Superoxide production by human spermatozoa as a part of the ionophore-induced acrosome reaction. Int J Androl 1995;18:67–74.

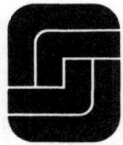

4

Intracellular Calcium and Sperm Motility

Haim Breitbart and Zvi Naor

Introduction

Several factors appear to be involved in the initiation and regulation of sperm motility (1), but it is unclear how these factors interact to coordinate flagellar motility.

Key second messengers in this process are calcium and cyclic AMP (cAMP) (2). Calcium is a major regulatory factor controlling sperm motility, although its effect may be inhibitory or stimulatory, depending on its concentration and on the species. Intracellular sperm calcium levels influence the flagellar shape and beating pattern (3). Relatively high free Ca^{2+} (>3 µM) imparts a hooklike bend to the midpiece region in the plane of the beat. Calcium and cAMP increase the amplitude of flagellar wave. Calcium and cAMP regulate motility by changes in sperm protein phosphorylation via activation of protein kinase A (PKA), which phosphorylate proteins on serine/threonine. Calcium could directly affect protein phosphorylation via calcium-activated protein kinases like protein kinase C (PKC) (4) or phosphatases (5), or directly through activation of sperm adenylate cyclase to produce cAMP from ATP (6). Calcium and PKA could also affect motility by regulation of tyrosine phosphorylation of motility-associated bovine sperm protein (7). In mouse sperm Ca^{2+} stimulates tyrosine phosphorylation (8,9); however, in human spermatozoa, extracellular calcium inhibited tyrosine kinases activity during capacitation (10).

Many studies have attempted to identify phosphoproteins involved in calcium and cAMP mediated changes in motility. Studies with demembranated sperm show the requirement for a cytosolic protein for cAMP-dependent motility activation (11,12). In trout sperm this 15 KDa soluble protein is phosphorylated on tyrosine (13). Two other phosphoproteins of 55 KDa and 220 KDa, which are associated with sperm motility, have been identified as well

(14,15). Studies have shown that sperm-specific serine/threonine phosphatase PP1γ2 is an important regulator of sperm motility (16,17). The activity of PP1 is known to be regulated by tyrosine phosphorylation (18). It was shown that the activity of sperm PKA is regulated by its interaction with A-kinase anchoring protein (AKAP) (19).

Calcium and Sperm Motility

Most of the data here represent collective motility of ram sperm, which is characterized in terms of periodic aggregation or cooperation among cells that are seen under the microscope as a continuous wave motion. Determination of collective motility is used for sperm quality analysis in artificial insemination centers, and it was found that it directly correlated with fertility (20).

We present data that concerns the effects of extracellular and intracellular Ca^{2+} concentration of collective sperm motion as well as individual sperm motility.

The collective motility of ram sperm was measured in sperm motility analyzer (RSG) that was developed in our department (21). Sperm cells at relatively high concentration (4×10^8 cells/ml) were excited at 450 nm, and the changes in the reflected light were recorded continuously on an eight-channel polygraph. Motility was measured in the presence or absence of added calcium, and under conditions by which sperm motility was made dependent on mitochondrial respiration only (glycolysis inhibited) or glycolytic activity only (mitochondrial respiration inhibited). Glycolytic-dependent motility was not affected by 1 mM extracellular calcium, but the mitochondrial-dependent motility was 75% inhibited under these conditions (Fig. 4.1; see also Ref. 22).

There is good correlation between the drop of cellular ATP and the decline of ram sperm motility (23). When we measured ATP levels under conditions by which mitochondrial-dependent motility is inhibited by extracellular Ca^{2+}, we found reduction of 25% only in ATP, which cannot explain the 75% inhibition in motility. The addition of 1 mM Ca^{2+} alone or 0.05 mM Ca^{2+} plus Ca^{2+}-ionophore to the cells, revealed an increase in intracellular Ca^{2+} concentration from 40 to 110 nM (Table 4.1). We also show that by inhibiting entry of Ca^{2+} into the mitochondria with ruthenium red, we could not eliminate the inhibitory effect of extracellular high Ca^{2+} on mitochondrial-dependent motility (Table 4.2). Thus, the increase in free Ca^{2+} in the cytosol and not reduction in ATP or influx of Ca^{2+} into the mitochondria is the cause for this inhibition in motility. Because there is no inhibition in glycolytic dependent motility at 110 nm $[Ca^{2+}]_i$ we suggest that the motility apparatus itself is not affected at this $[Ca^{2+}]_i$.

This difference in the sensitivity toward intracellular Ca^{2+} between mitochondrial- and glycolytic-dependent motility might be explained by considering the different localization of the two systems in the spermatozoon. Because the mitochondria are localized in the midpiece of the sperm, it is possible that ATP synthesized in the mitochondria drives motility by activat-

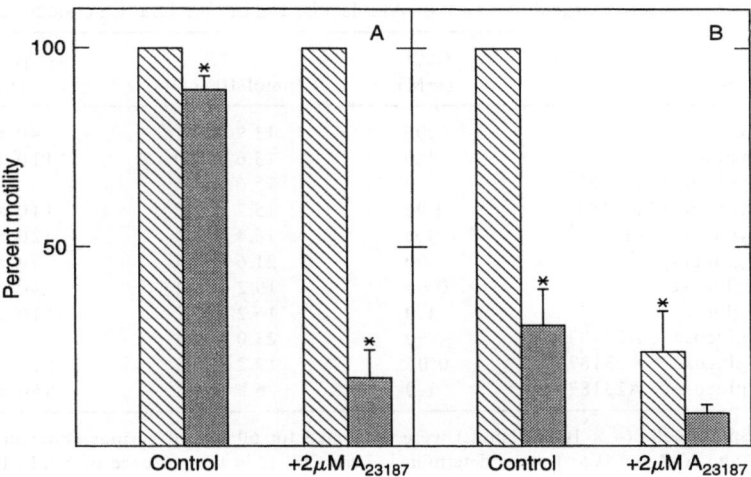

FIGURE 4.1. Effect of various intracellular Ca^{2+} concentration on sperm motility: Collective ram sperm motility was determined during 90 min, using the sperm motility analyzer. Wave frequencies were determined for each min and the percentage of motility was calculated by integration to the area under the lines. (A) Glycolytic dependent motility (cells treated with 1 μm antimycin A). (B) Mitochondrial dependent motility (cells treated with 20 mM deoxyglucose). The bars with the lines are without added Ca^{2+} (0.05 mM free Ca^{2+}) and those with circles are in the presence of 1 mM $CaCl_2$. Each point is the mean ± SEM from 4 determinations. Values with an asterisk represent significant differences compared to control with added Ca^{2+}, $p \leq 0.05$.

ing dynein ATPase localized close to the mitochondria, whereas ATP from the glycolysis activates dynein ATP along the tail. If this is the case, then the sensitivity of the dynein ATPase localized near the mitochondria toward changes $[Ca^{2+}]_i$ may be different from the dynein ATPase along the tail. Thus, the possible inhibition of dynein ATPase localized near the mitochondria by 110 mM $[Ca^{2+}]_i$ would inhibit mitochondrial-dependent motility. Glycolytic-dependent motility, however, which is driven by dynein ATPase along the tail is not affected unless the $[Ca^{2+}]_i$ is elevated to 420 nM, as described later.

When intracellular free Ca^{2+} concentration is elevated to 400 nM, there is an 80% inhibition of motility, independent of the source of ATP, mitochondrial or glycolytic. Under these conditions, the cellular level of ATP is not affected in antimycin-A treated cells (Table 4.1), which suggests that the motility machinery itself might be blocked at 400 nM $[Ca^{2+}]_i$. The inhibition of mitochondrial ATP synthesis shown at 550 nM $[Ca^{2+}]_i$ is caused by the entry of Ca^{2+} into the mitochondria, which resulted in reducing of the electrochemical proton gradient needed for ATP synthesis (24,25 and Table 4.1).

TABLE 4.1. Effect of extracellular Ca^{2+} on ATP levels, and intracellular Ca concentrations.

Treatment	$CaCl_2$ (mM)	ATP ($nmol/10^8$ cells)	$[Ca^{2+}]_i$ (nM)
Antimycin-A	0.05	13.9 ± 2.1	40 ± 20
Antimycin-A	1.0	13.6 ± 2.0	110 ± 30
Antimycin-A + A23187*	~0	15.6 ± 3.6	—
Antimycin-A + A23187*	0.05	15.2 ± 1.2	110 ± 15
Antimycin-A + A23187*	1.0	16.4 ± 2.4	420 ± 100
Deoxyglucose	~0	21.6 ± 2.4	40 ± 15
Deoxyglucose	0.05	19.2 ± 0.4	40 ± 10
Deoxyglucose	1.0	16.2 ± 0.2	110 ± 24
Deoxyglucose + A23187*	~0	23.0 ± 0.4	—
Deoxyglucose + A23187*	0.05	19.2 ± 0.8	115 ± 30
Deoxyglucose + A23187*	1.0	6.8 ± 1.6	550 ± 70

Note: Sperm cells (4×10^8 cells/mL) were incubated for 60 min at various concentrations of Ca^{2+} and ATP and $[Ca^{2+}]_i$ were determined. Zero Ca^{2+} is in the presence of 5 mM EGTA, and 0.05 mM without any addition. The concentrations for treatments are antimycin-A 1 μM, deoxyglucose 20 mM, and A23187 2 μM. The numbers represent the means ± SEM of duplicates from three experiments.
*In the $[Ca^{2+}]_i$ determinations the Ca^{2+} ionophore is iononycin (1 μM) instead of A23187.

The inhibitory effect of 1 mM extracellular Ca^{2+} is completely eliminated by chelating this Ca^{2+}. Under these conditions some Ca^{2+} binding sites on the cell surface and probably also inside the cells are no longer occupied by Ca^{2+} and the inhibition is relieved. The inhibition of motility by high extracellular Ca^{2+} can also be prevented by decreasing the medium pH from 7.6 to 6.5 (Table 4.2). This interesting result offers an explanation to the question of why high Ca^{2+} inhibits mitochondrial-dependent motility, but does not affect glycolytic-dependent motility. We previously reported that acidic products of the glycolysis pathway, mainly lactic acid, cause fast acidification of the medium in which the sperm cells are incubated (23,26). We also showed that

TABLE 4.2. The effect of ruthenium red and pH on mitochondria-dependent motility.

Treatment	pH 7.6				pH 6.5	
	Control frequencies	% I	1 μM Ruthenium red frequencies	% I	Control frequencies	% I
Control	1910 ± 85	—	1870 ± 37	—	1890 ± 54	—
1mMCaCl₂	611 ± 49	68	654 ± 66	65	1795 ± 90	5

Note: Sperm (4×10^8 cells/mL) were treated with 20 mM deoxyglucose, and the motility was determined. Each point represents the mean ± SEM of duplicates from three experiments. $p < 0.05$ (student's t-test) represents significant difference compared to the control at each pH. The values represent integration of frequencies from a complete experiment. %I = percentage of inhibition.

Ca^{2+} uptake by ram spermatozoa treated with antimycin-A is stimulated approximately twofold by quercetin, which inhibits glycolysis and prevents acidification of the medium (22). Thus, when the collective motility is made dependent on glycolytic activity only (antimycin-A-treated cells), the acidification of the medium prevents the binding of Ca^{2+} to some negative sites, which are now protonated. Under conditions in which the motility depends on mitochondrial activity (deoxyglucose-treated cells) the pH is kept at 7.6 and the Ca^{2+} binding sites are mostly not in the protonated form, which allows the binding of Ca^{2+} and motility is inhibited.

When glycolysis and mitochondrial respiration are both active, extracellular Ca^{2+} (1 mM) causes only very small (~10%) inhibition in ram sperm motility (22). It was shown elsewhere (27) that no net ATP synthesis in glycolysis occurs in bull sperm incubated under aerobic conditions at 37°C, but the glycolysis is still producing lactate. Assuming that it is also the case in ram sperm, we suggest that under aerobic conditions, the motility is mainly dependent on mitochondrial ATP synthesis. The fact that motility is not inhibited by high extracellular Ca^{2+} under these aerobic conditions and that glycolytic activity is blocked indicate again that acidification of the medium due to lactate secretion prevents this inhibition.

In our studies over the years with ram spermatozoa, we have found that from July to September the mitochondrial-dependent motility is reduced in comparison to the rest of the year. During these months, motility can be significantly improved by adding the Ca^{2+}-chelator EGTA to the incubation medium. Thus, our data have significant implications in terms of maintaining sperm motility over the year. Because sperm motility depends mostly on aerobic conditions (i.e., on mitochondrial activity) the extracellular Ca^{2+} concentration should be kept as low as possible.

PKC and Sperm Motility

Protein kinase C (PKC) plays an important role in cell signaling, in particular for calcium mobilization ligands (28,29). This multiisozyme family is involved in various cell functions including the regulation of ion channel activities. The PKC subspecies are classified into conventional PKCs (cPKC), novel PKSs (nPKC), and atypical PKCs (aPKC) (29). cPKC are activated by Ca^{2+}, diacylglycerol (DAG), and phosphatidylserine (PS). Two isoforms of this class, PKCα and βII, were identified in bovine sperm (30). nPKC are DAG- and PS-activated but Ca^{2+}-independent enzymes, and aPKC are DAG- and Ca^{2+}-independent enzymes and are activated by PS. The various PKC activators are produced by phospholipases. For example, phospholipase C (PLC) provides DAG and inositol triphosphate by the hydrolysis of phosphoinositides. Early publications on the absence of PKC in ram sperm (31) led us to investigate its presence and role in mammalian spermatozoa.

Human sperm PKC activity was found to be relatively low and was distributed in the soluble fraction (45%) and the particulate fraction (55%) (4,32). On the other hand, bull and ram sperm PKC was located mainly in the soluble fraction (80%) and only 20% in the particulate fraction (33). Concerning the localization of PKC, we found that in human sperm the enzyme was mainly in the equatorial segment (4,32), whereas in bull sperm PKC was located mainly in the postacrosomal region and in the upper region of the acrosome (33).

In many cells activation of PKC is associated with its translocation from the cytosol to the plasma membrane, which is a phenomena that was found in bovine sperm as well (30). Activation of human sperm PKC by phorbol ester 12-0-tetradecanoylphorbol-13-acetate (TPA) or by cell-permeable DAG analogue 1-oleoyl-2-acetylglycerol (OAG) resulted in enhancement of flagellar motility (4,32) (Fig. 4.2). Addition of the Ca^{2+}-ionophore ionomycin to incubated human sperm resulted in dose- and time-dependent increases in sperm motility (32). Removal of Ca^{2+} from the incubation medium abolished the effect of the Ca^{2+}-ionophore on sperm motility, but had no effect on TPA-stimulated motility. On the other hand, the use of PKC inhibitors revealed selective inhibition of the TPA, but not of the ionomycin elevated sperm motility (32). Thus, the separate signaling elicited by Ca^{2+} elevation or PKC activation can lead to stimulation of human sperm motility. Regression analysis revealed an excellent correlation between sperm motility and the percentage of PKC-stained cells from various semen donors (4), which supports the notion that PKC plays an important role in the regulation of human sperm flagellar motility.

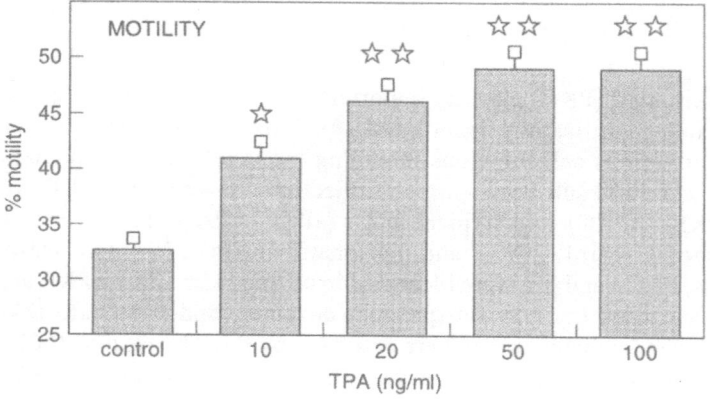

FIGURE 4.2. Effect of TPA on human sperm motility. Human sperm were incubated with increasing concentrations of TPA for 30 minutes, and motility was determined. Results are mean ± SEM. One asterisk $p < 0.05$; two asterisks $p < 0.02$.

Integration of Signaling (See Model)

Sperm display a ligand-independent increase in cAMP, which depends upon elevation of intracellular Ca^{2+} and activation of adenylate cyclase (AC) to produce cAMP from ATP. As a result PKA is activated and there is a PKA-dependent protein tyrosine phosphorylation (9). The activated PKA stimulates Ca^{2+}-channel of intracellular membrane to release Ca^{2+} into the cytosol.

The elevated $[Ca^{2+}]_i$, together with the increase in tyrosine-phosphorylation of PLC, activates the PLC to hydrolyze phosphoinositides to produce DAG and IP_3 (inositol triphosphate). IP_3 can further release Ca^{2+} from intracellular stores to further elevate $[Ca^{2+}]_i$. This elevated Ca^{2+}, together with DAG, activates PKC to phosphorylate Ca^{2+}-channel of the plasma membrane (34), resulted in further increase in $[Ca^{2+}]_i$. This elevated $[Ca^{2+}]_i$, together with other proteins phosphorylated by PKC, regulate sperm motility. The elevated Ca^{2+} is thereafter reduced by the activity of the plasma membrane Ca-ATPase and Ca^{2+}/Na^+ exchanger, the mitochondria, and Ca ATPase of intracellular membranes.

A Model: Regulation of Intracellular Calcium for Sperm Motility

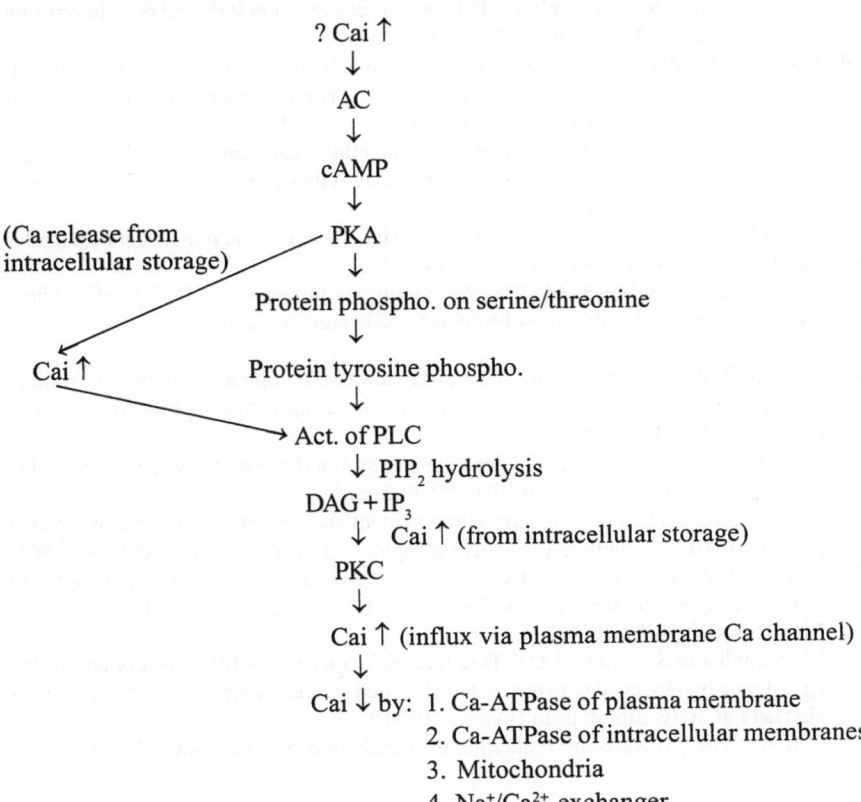

References

1. Yanagimachi R. Mammalian fertilization. In: Knobil E, Neil JD, editors. The physiology of reproduction. New York: Raven Press, 1994:189–317.
2. Garbers DL, Kopf GS. The regulation of spermatozoa by calcium and cyclic nucleotides. Adv Cyclic Nucl Res 1980;13:251–305.
3. Lindemann CB, Goltz JS. Calcium regulation of flagellar curvature and swimming pattern in Triton-X-100 extracted rat sperm. Cell Motil Cytoskeleton 1988;10:420–31.
4. Rotem R, Paz GF, Homonnai ZT, Kalina M, Naor Z. Protein kinase C is present in human sperm: possible role in flagellar motility. Proc Natl Acad Sci USA 1990;87: 7305–8.
5. Tash JS, Krinks M, Patel J, Means RL, Klee CB, Means AR. Identification, characterization and functional correlation of calmodulin-dependent protein phosphatase in sperm. J Cell Biol 1988;106:1625–33.
6. Gross MK, Toscano DG, Toscano WA, Jr. Calmodulin-mediated adenylate cyclase from mammalian sperm. J Biol Chem 1987;262:8672–76.
7. Vijayaragharan S, Traitman KD, Goueli SA, Carr DW. A tyrosine-phosphorylated 55-Kilodalton motility-associated bovine sperm protein is regulated by cyclic adenosine 3',5'-monophosphates and calcium. Biol Reprod 1997;56:1450–57.
8. Visconti PE, Bailey JL, Moore GD, Pan D, Old-Clarke P, Kopf GS. Capacitation in mouse spermatozoa. I. Correlation between the capacitation state and protein tyrosine phosphorylation. Development 1995;121:1129–37.
9. Visconti PE, Moore GD, Bailey JL, et al. Capacitation of mouse spermatozoa. II. Protein tyrosine phosphorylation and capacitation are regulated by a cAMP-dependent pathway. Development 1995;121:1139–50.
10. Luconi M, Krausz C, Forti G, Baldi E. Extracellular calcium negatively modulates tyrosine phosphorylation and tyrosine kinase activity during capacitation of human spermatozoa. Biol Reprod 1996;55:207–16.
11. Tash JS. Protein phosphorylation: the second messenger signal transducer of flagellar motility. Cell Motil Cytoskeleton 1989;14:332–39.
12. Tash JS, Kakar SS, Means AR. Flagellar motility requires the cAMP dependent phosphorylation of a heat-stable mp-40-soluble 56 KDa protein, axokinin. Cell 1984;38:551–59.
13. Hayashi H, Yamamoto K, Yonekowa H, Marisawa M. Involvement of tyrosine protein kinase in the initiation of flagellar movement in rainbow trout spermatozoa. J Biol Chem 1987;262:16692–98.
14. Brandt H, Hoskins DD. A cAMP-dependent phosphorylated motility protein in bovine epididymal sperm. J Biol Chem 1980;255:982–87.
15. Carr DW, Acott TS. The phosphorylation of a putative sperm microtubule-associated protein 2 (MAP2) is uniquely sensitive to regulation. Biol Reprod 1990;43:795–805.
16. Smith GD, Wolf DP, Trautman KC, da Cruze e Silva EF, Greengard P, Vijayaragharan S. Primate sperm contain protein phosphatase 1, a biochemical mediator of motility. Biol Reprod 1996;54:719–27.
17. Vijayaragharan S, Stephens DT, Trautman KC. Sperm motility development in the epididymis is associated with decreased glycogen synthase kinase-3 and protein phosphatase 1 activity. Biol Reprod 1996;54:709–18.
18. Cohen P. The structure and regulation of protein phosphatases. Annu Rev Biochem 1989;58:453.

19. Vijayaragharan S, Goueli SA, Davey MP, Carr DW. Protein kinase A-anchoring inhibitor peptides arrest mammalian sperm motility. J Biol Chem 1997;272:4747–52.
20. Bishop MWH, Campbell RC, Hancock JL, Walton H. Semen characterization and fertility in bull. J Agric Sci 1959;44:227–35.
21. Bar-Sagie D, Mayevsky A, Bartoov B. A new optical technique for evaluating collective motility of ram and bull ejaculated spermatozoa. Int J Androl 1980;3:198–209.
22. Breitbart H, Rubinstein S, Nass-Arden L. The role of calcium and Ca^{2+}-ATPase in maintaining motility in ram spermatozoa. J Biol Chem 1985;260:11548–53.
23. Nass-Arden L, Breitbart H. Modulation of mammalian sperm motility by quercetin. Mol Reprod Dev 1990;25:369–73.
24. Lehninger AL. Mitochondria and calcium ion transport. Biochem J 1970;118:129–38.
25. Mitchell P. Kelins respiratory chain concept and its chemiosmotic consequences. Science 1979;206:1148–59.
26. Breitbart H, Lardy HA. Effect of verapanil and sulfhydryl-reagents on calcium transport in bovine spermatozoa. Biol Reprod 1987;36:658–63.
27. Hammerstedt RH, Lardy HA. The effect of substrate cyclin on the ATP yield of sperm glycolysis. J Biol Chem 1983;258:8759–68.
28. Newton AC. Protein kinase C: structure, function and regulation. J Biol Chem 1995; 270:28495–98.
29. Nishizuka Y. Intracellular signaling by hydrolysis of phospholipids and activation of protein kinase C. Science 1992;258:607–14.
30. Lax Y, Rubinstein S, Breitbart H. Subcellular distribution of protein kinase C alpha and beta₁ in bovine spermatozoa, and their regulation by calcium and phorbol esters. Biol Reprod 1997;56:454–59.
31. Roldan ERS, Harrison RAP. Absence of active protein kinase C in ram spermatozoa. Biochem Biophys Res Commun 1988;155:901–6.
32. Rotem R, Paz GF, Homonnai ZT, Kalina M, Naor Z. Further studies on the involvement of protein kinase C in human sperm flagellar motility. Endocrinology 1990;127:2571–77.
33. Breitbart H, Lax Y, Rotem R, Naor Z. Role of protein kinase C in the acrosome reaction of mammalian spermatozoa. Biochem J 1992;281:473–76.
34. Spungin B, Breitbart H. Calcium mobilization and influx during sperm exocytosis. J Cell Sci 1996;109:1947–55.

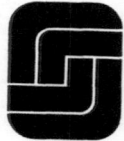

5

Genetic Aspects of Sperm Motility Disorders

JAMES M. CUMMINS

There is a clear link between impaired sperm motility and human male subfertility; however, in most cases the genetic causes (if there are any) are not known. In attempting to understand this, I argue that many aspects of sperm dysfunction in human reproduction may not necessarily be pathological in nature, rather, they may be inevitable outcomes of a mating system that has selected for reduced fecundity. We are thus faced with a paradox in that we need to seek medical and biotechnological solutions for a human dilemma that may be based in natural rather than pathological processes.

Introduction

In this chapter I will examine the nature and some of the genetic causes (where known) of human sperm motility, and how defects in motility can adversely affect fertility. As the medical genetics, biochemistry, and molecular biology of sperm motility have been exhaustively covered in other reviews (1–3), I will concentrate here on what we know about the underlying evolutionary processes that seem to lie behind motility disorders. Even though there are clear genetic influences on semen parameters and male infertility the precise causes of individual defects are obscure except for a minority of situations.

Evolution and Natural History of Sperm Motility

Sexual reproduction, specifically amphimixis (syngamy between gametes produced by different individuals), has been around for possibly 3000 mil-

lion years (4). There is still intense debate about the evolutionary significance and meaning of sex, but the essential significance lies in the production of genetically unique gametes by the recombination of DNA during
meiosis. This in turn allows for the generation of genetic diversity in the next
generation. Such diversity allows for evolution by natural selection, perhaps
to keep ahead of parasites or diseases in a genetic "arms race" (5). It is significant that much of this generation of diversity in mammals (and of course
humans) is driven by mutations that accumulate preferentially in the testicular germ cell line—possibly in concert with rapid changes to the Y chromosome (6). From this chapter's perspective the evolutionary processes that have
resulted in human reproductive patterns are clearly based in anisogamy. This
is the production of large sessile ova, with resources to fuel early embryo
development, and small motile spermatozoa with minimal cytoplasm, acting
as dispersal agents for the male's haploid contribution to the next generation
(7). The long evolutionary antecedents of this pattern of reproduction are
reflected in the near universal arrangement of microtubules in the sperm axoneme (see later), so that humans and flagellates such as *Chlamydomonas*
share a very similar pattern (1). This is convenient because we can learn from
basic biochemical studies on flagellar function in simple organisms and ex-
trapolate to the human from those findings. Much of what we know about
sperm movement in the human, therefore, is based on work in sea urchins and
other marine organisms (8).

  As gametes developing in a hormonally controlled testis, sperm can generally be considered to be a special subset of secondary sexual characteristics.
Many of their characteristics appear to be driven by sperm competition—that
form of intrasexual competition that occurs when two or more males' ejaculates compete to fertilize eggs within the same female (9,10). Although humans can be characterized as "moderately polygamous omnivores" (11), when
compared with our chimpanzee cousins we have relatively small and inefficient testes that produce low sperm numbers with high natural levels of
pleiomorphism (6,12,13). We share the latter "abnormal" feature with gorillas
and with some other species of animals who also have mating systems with
low levels of sperm competition (9,14). Even though the potential for sperm
competition certainly exists in humans (15,16), the slow generation time of
humans means that the overall intensity of selection for high fertility in men
has never been very high. Indeed, if anything, human evolution has favored
low fecundity with a preponderance of reproductive effort devoted to child
rearing and education rather than conception per se. Women exhibit a "natural" birth spacing of around 4 years, combined with a unique genetically
programmed period of infertility in mature life (the menopause) (17). Moreover, humans show an unusual mating pattern compared with other primates,
with no advertisement of the oestrus state, and copulation being usually a
private affair. This contrasts strikingly with the flamboyant oestrus vulvar
displays and public promiscuity of chimpanzees, even though we share 98%
of genes with them and probably only separated from their lineage around

5–7 million years ago (18). Humans have evolved a reproductive system with a monthly fecundity rate of only around 20% for young, fertile couples not practicing contraception (19). This is an order of magnitude below that seen in domestic animals that have been selected for fertility over many hundreds of generations.

It seems clear that low fertility has been tolerated (and perhaps even selected for) in the human male. The human testis is remarkably inefficient, producing only 25–35% of sperm per unit mass in comparison with nonhuman primates (20). Even "fertile" men (and *fertility* is very difficult to define for males) can show a two- to three-fold variation in daily sperm output. The "low output" periods coincide with loss of germ cells late in the meiotic process (21). Many sperm are released in an immature stage (22) and there is a close correlation between such immature sperm forms and infertility (23). Where the morphological appearance and maturity of spermatozoa can be improved with gonadotropin therapy in some infertile men (24), the etiology and genetics of this condition are generally largely unknown. We have suggested elsewhere that the human testis may be especially prone to accelerated aging, influenced by a combination of nuclear and mitochondrial genetics and accumulation of ischemic insult and free-radical mediated damage (25). This can only have come about, however, through a down-regulation in the intensity to which "quality control' mechanisms are effective in the testis (9).

One central problem facing any study of human male reproduction is that semen parameters (including motility) are only poorly correlated with fertility. Despite attempts to codify and standardize semen analysis (26), there are many examples of "normal" individuals who do not meet the official criteria (27). This makes the analysis of male fertility based on semen characteristics alone largely meaningless (28,29). Whereas Baker and Bellis (16) have argued that abnormal human spermatozoa may be adaptive in combating rival's sperm from fertilizing (the "Kamikaze sperm hypothesis"), Harcourt (30) has shown that the numbers of abnormal sperm in mammals do not correlate with their mating pattern. If the "kamikaze sperm" hypothesis were correct one would expect to see more abnormal forms in species with high intensity of sperm competition, whereas, if anything, the reverse is true. One suspects that Baker and Bellis have fallen into the Panglossian trap of assuming that every aspect of sperm biology is adaptive. Indeed, abnormal sperm cannot even be considered to be "exaptations" (features that may enhance fitness but that were not designed by natural selection for their current role) (31) because they do not normally participate in fertilization. Although abnormally shaped sperm (in mice) can generate normal embryos when microinjected into oocytes (32), amorphous human sperm heads injected into mouse oocytes showed significant increases in structural chromosomal anomalies (33). In normal circumstances barriers in the reproductive tract such as cervical mucus and the zona pellucida actively select against abnormal and poorly motile forms (34,35), and they are probably the major selective mechanisms for defining the heredity of sperm biology (36).

One can speculate that women may unconsciously have selected for subfertile men as a means of ensuring widely spaced births. Mate choice by women certainly seems driven much more by perceptions of capacity to attract and retain resources (e.g., status and ambitiousness) than by physical factors per se (17). By contrast, men primarily choose mates based on youth (hence potential fertility) and physical attractiveness using features that advertise successful child-rearing potential, such as breasts (37). The widespread evidence for false paternity rates—ranging up to 30% in some communities—suggests that extra-pair copulations (EPCs) are a normal if not socially sanctioned component of human sexuality (15,16). This is tacitly recognized by the near universal prevalence of male-written laws that paradoxically and asymmetrically restrict female access to competing males while allowing or even encouraging the reverse. In birds EPCs are now recognized as a standard part of the reproductive game even in nominally monogamous forms (38). It has even been suggested that both men and women act subconsciously to maximize fertility in EPCs: men by maximizing ejaculate output; women by orgasm and by soliciting illicit sex at the most fertile period of their cycle (16). These theories, however, are based largely on poorly controlled or self-reported survey data and are not unequivocally accepted by biologists. Women can always compensate for a subfertile partner—even if he is a good provider—by seeking EPCs. Likewise, men can greatly improve their chances of reproductive success by EPCs, so there is a continuous tension within and between the genders and pair-bond stability is always a compromise.

All this, of course, is highly speculative. There are obviously many pathological causes of male infertility—even though no clear diagnosis of cause can be arrived at in the majority of cases (39). The modern human lifestyle, with very high population densities, widespread infertility associated with sexually transmitted diseases (40), and increases in exposure to environmental pollutants and "xeno-endocrine" factors (41,42), may be totally unrepresentative of the gathering–hunting lifestyle of our ancestors. Nevertheless, the genetic factors at work that influence human fertility and infertility are largely those set in place by natural selection processes leading up to the onset of the Industrial Revolution and modern urban societies; therefore, they must still underlie the present reproductive status of the human male.

Genetics of Sperm Assembly

Sperm formation in the testis involves a cascade of complicated morphological and functional changes as the germ cells transform from pluripotent spermatogonial stem cells to committed haploid gametes. This involves the activation and expression of a unique set of genes, some of which are only expressed in the haploid state (43), and some of which may have somatic homologues. During this process the molecular endpoints are phenotypically well established, but the genes that control the process are still only poorly defined in humans. The most significant changes include the formation of the axoneme and acrosomal cap, and replacement of nuclear histones with protamines, which results in a largely inactivated genome held within a distinctively shaped nucleus with very precise DNA packaging (44). One exciting new discovery is that the nuclei of mature mammalian spermatozoa contain a spectrum of messenger RNAs (mRNAs) that represent remains of the mRNAs used in spermatogenesis (45,46). Although it is still not clear how representative these mRNAs may be of the genes acting during spermatogenic cascade, this is clearly a potential experimental window that promises the capacity to examine and categorize those genes in great detail and to identify those that may cause problems in flagellar assembly or function.

Biochemistry of Sperm Movement

Although we now understand the biochemistry of sperm maturation and motility in great detail (3,47) the genetic controls involved are largely unknown. As the haploid genome is inactivated by the end of meiosis the biochemical mechanisms presumably rely on proteins encoded early in spermatogenesis. These are reflected in mRNAs associated with the sperm nucleus that apparently become evenly distributed between sibling spermatids through cytoplasmic bridges (45,46).

Spermatozoa have to survive a period of up to 2 weeks between release from the testis up to the time they enter the female tract. During this time they experience dramatic changes in environments, ranging from the nearly anoxic state of the seminiferous tubule and epididymis to transient exposure to the aerobic environment of the vagina. Max (48) has pointed out that the life cycle of the sperm is the equivalent of descending from 200,000 feet altitude to near sea level and then returning. It is not surprising that sperm possess considerable metabolic flexibility and can switch between aerobic glycolysis, anaerobic glycolysis, and oxidative respiration according to needs (3). There are also marked differences between species. Human sperm are quite happy in an anaerobic environment as long as they have access to an exogenous glycolyzable substrate and do not rely heavily on respiration; which contrasts strikingly with sperm of, say, the boar, for which respiration is essential (3).

The basic fuel for sperm motility is ATP produced by the biochemical pathways outlined earlier. ATP produced in the midpiece mitochondria is thought to be transported to the site of action in the axoneme by means of a creatine shuttle using a specific isoform of creatine phosphokinase (49). Human infertility is frequently associated with poor motility and immaturity reflecting premature Sertoli cell release. Huszar has shown that this can be correlated with elevated ratios of the immature brain-type isoform compared with the mature brain-type isoform (23). Although seminal ATP levels have been proposed in the past as a measure of fertility this is no longer accepted

(50). This is not surprising given the rapid dynamics of ATP production and utilization in the spermatozoon and semen (51).

Basis of Flagellar Action

The Axoneme

The archetypical pattern of the axoneme is that of a central pair of microtubules surrounded by nine doublets, running the full length of the flagellum. In mammals these are reinforced by nine auxiliary coarse fibers that have a rather variable termination: All are surrounded by a fibrous sheath. Each doublet consists of subunits A and B. Inner and outer dynein arms project from subunit A toward the next doublet subunit B. Doublets are also linked by nexin bridges and by radial spokes to a sheath that surrounds the central pair. The molecules involved have been described in detail elsewhere (52).

Regulation of Axonemal Activity

The axoneme is driven by sliding between the microtubules, driven by an attachment–detachment cycle of the dynein arms that are in turn powered by binding and hydrolysis of ATP (3). The final wave form is three-dimensionally complex and mechanically modulated by the coarse fibers and fibrous sheath. Biochemical control is centered around Ca^{++} influx (a key trigger for the acrosome reaction), intracellular pH, and cAMP-dependent protein phosphorylation (51).

Maturation, Capacitation, and Hyperactivation

Human sperm gradually acquire the potential for motility as they mature in the epididymis (53). This motility is normally repressed until ejaculation, when they mix with the seminal plasma. When in the female tract, mammalian sperm show an obligatory delay in the ability to undergo the calcium-dependent acrosome reaction. Capacitation is clearly a device driven by natural selection processes to ensure that sperm and oocyte meet at a mutually optimal time for fertilization. It involves changes to the composition of the sperm membrane such as cholesterol efflux (3). The final phase of capacitation is normally accompanied by hyperactivation. This is a dramatic increase in power output by the sperm thought to be necessary to break covalent bonds formed during sperm–zona attachment (54). In vitro, hyperactivation manifests as erratic high amplitude beating. Additional possible functions for this mode of motility include increased efficiency of movement through the viscous environment of the Fallopian tube and the cumulus mass, and increasing the "search path" of the sperm in seeking the oocyte. The genetic control of capacitation and hyperactivation is unknown: The timing is presumably predetermined by the assembly of specific membrane components as the sperm itself is transcriptionally inert.

Flagellar Dyskinesia

There is a heterogenous group of genetic defects that affect ciliary structure and function throughout the body, and typically affect respiratory and reproductive ciliated epithelia along with spermatozoa (55). As the cilium consists of around 200 polypeptides with presumably at least as many genes involved (56), there is clearly potential for misassembly. They are generally grouped as "immotile cilia syndrome" and include Kartagener's syndrome characterized by bronchiectasis and in about half of the cases of situs inversus (57). Most of these involve partial or total absence of dynein arms in the axoneme, which is therefore incapable of using ATP for movement. The inheritance, originally thought to be an autosomal recessive disorder, is complex: Autosomal dominance or even X-linked inheritance may be possible (52). Minor variants on this syndrome include cases where the outer dynein arm is missing but other flagellar structures are normal, which results in a halving of flagellar beat frequency and infertility due to inability to penetrate cervical mucus (58). On a less acute level, the general syndrome of asthenozoospermia (26) is commonly associated with infertility, morphological defects, and disturbances to the organization of the periaxonemal coarse fibers (59). The genetics of this heterogenous group of disorders is obscure, and indeed there is evidence that the assembly of cilia and spermatozoa may be controlled by a mosaic of common and unique genes (52). These men used to be regarded as medical curiosities; however, the ability to treat infertility even in Kartagener's syndrome using intracytoplasmic sperm injection (ICSI) means that there is renewed interest and concern in the underlying mode of transmission (60). The genes controlling the dyneins responsible for axonemal movement are now being mapped (61), and it is hoped that the Human Genome Project will allow us to make rapid progress in understanding the genetic basis of motility disorders.

Sliding Spermatozoa, Globozoospermia, and Minor Genetic Anomalies

Rarely presenting as causes of infertility, there are a variety of minor genetic problems that manifest as impaired motility. These include the "sliding spermatozoa syndrome," where periaxonemal dense fiber anomalies reduce the beat amplitude, and infertility results from an inability of sperm to penetrate cervical mucus (62). Globozoospermia, or rounded-head syndrome, is a rare form of infertility where the sperm lack acrosomes due to lack of an essential protein of the perinuclear theca (63). Lack of an acrosome means that sperm cannot fertilize. Even when microinjected into oocytes the abnormal perinuclear theca means that they do not activate oocytes normally, presumably due to lack of "oscillin" (64). The sperm, however, are karyotypically normal and have been used successfully to generate pregnancies by ICSI (65).

Conclusions

The development of mouse genetic models of human infertility (66), together with an ability to categorize the genes involved in spermatogenesis through a study of persistent mRNA in the mature sperm nucleus (45,46), will undoubtedly provide essential information on the genetic control of sperm motility. I am forced to conclude, however, that many aspects of sperm motility disturbances are not necessarily pathological in nature; rather, they may simply be "noise" in the human reproductive pattern, possibly exacerbated by a deteriorating environment.

References

1. Gagnon C. Regulation of sperm motility at the axonemal level. Reprod Fertil Dev 1995;7: 847–55.
2. Tash JS, Bracho GE. Regulation of sperm motility—emerging evidence for a major role for protein phosphatases. J Androl 1994;15:505–9.
3. Bedford JM, Hoskins DD. The mammalian spermatozoon: morphology, biochemistry and physiology. In: Lamming GE, editor. Marshall's physiology of reproduction, 4th Edition. London: Churchill Livingston, 1990:379–568.
4. Margulis L, Sagan D. Origins of sex. Three billion years of genetic recombination. New Haven: Yale University Press, 1986.
5. Hamilton WD, Axelrod R, Tanese R. Sexual reproduction as an adaptation to resist parasites (a review). Proc Natl Acad Sci USA 1990;87:3566–73.
6. Short RV. The testis—the witness of the mating system, the site of mutation and the engine of desire. Acta Paediatr 1997;86:3–7.
7. Bell G. The masterpiece of nature. The evolution and genetics of sexuality. Canberra: Croom Helm, 1982.
8. Gibbons IR. The role of dynein in microtubule-based motility. Cell Struct Funct 1996;21:331–42.
9. Cummins JM. Evolution of sperm form: levels of control and competition. In: Bavister BD, Cummins JM, Roldan ERS, editors. Fertilization in mammals. Norwell, Massachusetts: Serono Symposia, 1990:51–64.
10. Parker GA. Sperm competition and the evolution of animal mating systems. In: Smith RL, editor. Sperm competition and the evolution of animal mating systems. London: Academic Press, 1984:1–60.
11. Short RV. Sexual selection and its component parts, somatic and genital selection, as illustrated by man and the great apes. Adv Study Behav 1979;9:131–58.
12. Harcourt AH, Harvey PH, Larson SG, Short RV. Testis weight, body weight and breeding system in primates. Nature 1981;293:55–57.

13. Møller AP. Ejaculate quality, testis size and sperm competition in primates. J Hum Evol 1988;17:489–502.

14. Seuanez HN, Carothers AO, Martin DE, Short RV. Morphological abnormalities in the shape of spermatozoa of man and the great apes. Nature 1977;270: 345–47.

15. Smith RL. Human sperm competition. In: Smith RL, editor. Sperm competition and the evolution of animal mating systems. London: Academic Press, 1984:601–59.

16. Baker RR, Bellis MA. Human sperm competition. Copulation, masturbation and infidelity. London: Chapman and Hall, 1995.

17. Daly M, Wilson M. Sex, evolution and behavior. Boston: PWS Publishers, 1983.

18. Diamond J. The rise and fall of the third chimpanzee. London: Radius, 1991.

19. te Velde E, Beets G. Are subfertility and infertility on the increase? J Fertil Res 1992;6:5–8.

20. Johnson L. Review article: spermatogenesis and aging in the human. J Androl 1986;7:331–54.

21. Johnson L, Chaturvedi PK, Williams JD. Missing generations of spermatocytes and spermatids in seminiferous epithelium contribute to low efficiency of spermatogenesis in humans. Biol Reprod 1992;47:1091–98.

22. Lalwani S, Sayme N, Vigue L, Corrales M, Huszar G. Biochemical markers of early and late spermatogenesis: relationship between the lactate dehydrogenase-X and creatine kinase-M isoform concentrations in human spermatozoa. Mol Reprod Dev 1996;43:495–502.

23. Huszar G, Vigue L, Morshedi M. Sperm creatine phosphokinase M-isoform ratios and fertilizing potential of men: a blinded study of 84 couples treated with in vitro fertilization. Fertil Steril 1992;57:882–88.

24. Baccetti B, Strehler E, Capitani S, et al. The effect of follicle stimulating hormone therapy on human sperm structure (notulae seminologicae 11). Hum Reprod 1997;12:1955–68.

25. Cummins JM, Jequier AM, Kan R. Molecular biology of human male infertility—links with aging, mitochondrial genetics, and oxidative stress? Mol Reprod Dev 1994;37:345–62.

26. World Health Organisation. WHO laboratory manual for the examination of human semen and sperm—cervical mucus interaction. Cambridge, UK: Cambridge University Press, 1992.

27. Lemcke B, Behre HM, Nieschlag E. Frequently subnormal semen profiles of normal volunteers recruited over 17 years. Int J Androl 1997;20:144–52.

28. Cummins JM, Jequier AM. Treating male infertility needs more clinical andrology, not less. Hum Reprod 1994;9:1214–19.

29. Jequier AM, Cummins JM. Attitudes to clinical andrology—a time for change. Hum Reprod 1997;12:875–76.

30. Harcourt AH. Sperm competition and the evolution of nonfertilizing sperm in mammals. Evolution 1991;45:314–28.

31. Gould SJ, Vrba ES. Exaptation—a missing term in the science of form. Paleobiology 1982;8:4–15.

32. Burruel VR, Yanagimachi R, Whitten WK. Normal mice develop from oocytes injected with spermatozoa with grossly misshapen heads. Biol Reprod 1996;55:709–14.

33. Lee JD, Kamiguchi Y, Yanagimachi R. Analysis of chromosome constitution of

human spermatozoa with normal and aberrant head morphologies after injection into mouse oocytes. Hum Reprod 1996;11:1942–46.

34. Katz DF, Morales P, Samuels SJ, Overstreet JW. Mechanisms of filtration of morphologically abnormal human sperm by cervical mucus. Fertil Steril 1990;54: 509–12.

35. Liu DY, Baker HWG. Acrosome status and morphology of human spermatozoa bound to the zona pellucida and oolemma determined using oocytes that failed to fertilize in vitro. Hum Reprod 1994;9:673–79.

36. Bedford JM. The coevolution of mammalian gametes. In: Dunbar BS, O'Rand MG, editors. A comparative overview of mammalian fertilization. New York: Plenum Press, 1991:3–35.

37. Short RV. What the breast does for the baby, and what the baby does for the breast. Aust N Z J Obstet Gynaecol 1994;34:262–64.

38. Birkhead TR. Mechanisms of sperm competition in birds. Am Sci 1996;84:254–62.

39. de Kretser DM. Clinical male infertility. I. Prevalence of and progress in understanding male infertility. Reprod Fertil Dev 1994;6:3–8.

40. Khatamee MA. Infertility: a preventable epidemic? Int J Fertil 1988;33:246–51.

41. Toppari J, Larsen JC, Christiansen P, et al. Male reproductive health and environmental xenoestrogens. Environ Health Perspect 1996;104:741–803.

42. Smith EM, Hammondsehlers M, Clark MK, Kirchner HL, Fuortes L. Occupational exposures and risk of female infertility. J Occup Environ Med 1997;39:138–47.

43. Hecht N. Genetic control of spermatogenesis: where can things go wrong? In: Barratt C, De Jonge C, Mortimer D, Parinaud J, editors. Genetics of human male fertility. Paris: Editions E.D.K., 1997:11–24.

44. Ward WS, Coffey DS. DNA packaging and organization in mammalian spermatozoa: comparison with somatic cells. Biol Reprod 1991;44:569–74.

45. Miller D. RNA in the ejaculate spermatozoon—a window into molecular events in spermatogenesis and a record of the unusual requirements of haploid gene expression and post-meiotic equilibration. Mol Hum Reprod 1997;3:669–76.

46. Kramer JA, Krawetz SA. RNA in spermatozoa—implications for the alternative haploid genome. Mol Hum Reprod 1997;3:473–78.

47. Hoskins D, Vijayaraghavan S. A new theory on the acquisition of sperm motility during epididymal transit. In: Gagnon C, editor. Controls of sperm motility: biological and clinical aspects. Boca Raton: CRC Press, 1990:53–62.

48. Max B. This and that: hair pigments, the hypoxic basis of life and the Virgilian journey of the spermatozoon. Trends Pharmacol Sci 1992;13:272–76.

49. Tombes RM, Shapiro BM. Metabolite channeling. A phosphorylcreatine shuttle to mediate high energy phosphate transport between sperm mitochondrion and tail. Cell 1985;41:325–34.

50. World Health Organization Task Force on the Prevention and Management of Infertility. Adenosine triphosphate in semen and other sperm characteristics: their relevance for fertility prediction in men with normal sperm concentration. Fertil Steril 1992;57:877–81.

51. Ford WCL, Rees JM. The bioenergetics of mammalian sperm motility. In: Gagnon C, editor. Controls of sperm motility: biological and clinical aspects. Boca Raton: CRC Press, 1990:175–202.

52. Gagnon C. Genetic aspects of flagellar dyskinesia, globozoospermia. In: Barratt C, De Jonge C, Mortimer D, Parinaud J, editors. Genetics of human male fertility. Paris: Editions E.D.K., 1997:76–97.

53. Bedford JM. The status and the state of the human epididymis. Hum Reprod 1994;9:2187–99.
54. Green DPL. Sperm thrusts and the problem of penetration. Biol Rev 1988;63:79–105.
55. Afzelius BA, Eliasson R. Male and female infertility problems in the immotile-cilia syndrome. Eur J Respir Dis 1983;127(Suppl):144–47.
56. Luck DJL, Huang B, Piperno G. Genetic and biochemical analysis of the eukaryotic flagellum. Soc Exp Biol Symp 1982;35:399–419.
57. Afzelius BA. Situs inversus and ciliary abnormalities—what is the connection? Int J Dev Biol 1995;39:839–44.
58. Jouannet P, Escalier S, Serres C, David G. Motility of human sperm without outer dynein arm. J Submicrosc Cytol 1983;15:67–71.
59. Jouannet P, Serres C. Normal and pathological movement of human sperm. Med Sci 1995;11:555–62.
60. Cummins JM. Controversies in science: ICSI may foster birth defects. J NIH Res 1997;9:38–42.
61. Neesen J, Koehler MR, Kirschner R, et al. Identification of dynein heavy chain genes expressed in human and mouse testis—chromosomal localization of an axonemal dynein gene. Gene 1997;200:193–202.
62. Feneux D, Serres C, Jouannet P. Sliding spermatozoa: a dyskinesia responsible for human infertility? Fertil Steril 1985;44:508–11.
63. Escalier D. Failure of differentiation of the nuclear-perinuclear skeletal component in the round-headed human spermatozoa. Int J Dev Biol 1990;34:287–97.
64. Swann K, Lai FA. A novel signalling mechanism for generating Ca^{2+} oscillations at fertilization in mammals. Bioessays 1997;19:371–78.
65. Liu J, Joris H, Tournaye H, Devroey P, Van Steirteghem A. Successful fertilization and establishment of pregnancies after intracytoplasmic sperm injection in patients with globozoospermia. Hum Reprod 1995;10:626–29.
66. Chubb C. Genes regulating testis size. Biol Reprod 1992;47:29–36.

6

Necrospermia: Etiology and Management

PIERRE J. LECOMTE, CLAIRE BARTHELEMY, LEONARD NDUWAYO, AND SAMIR HAMAMAH

Necrozoospermia is still a poorly understood cause of male infertility. It is defined as a condition in which spermatozoa in the ejaculated semen are dead. According to sperm norms of the World Health Organization (WHO) (1), sperm viability is higher than or equal to 75% in human semen samples. Fertility of the semen is impaired below this percentage. Necrozoospermia is a rare condition with a reported prevalence of 0.2–0.48% in infertile subjects (2,3).

In this chapter, we will first discuss the possible mechanisms that lead the testis to produce dead mature cells and compare cell necrosis and apoptosis. We will then report our data concerning necrozoospermia in a population of infertile men who consulted our Center for treatment of infertile couples, dealing with a variety of causes and the explorations. We will conclude by suggesting practical guidelines and therapies to overcome this rare but difficult problem.

Necrozoospermia and Apoptosis

Two different types of cell death occur: accidental (and pathological), which leads to necrosis, and physiological (and programmed), named apoptosis. It seemed useful in this context to review our current knowledge of apoptosis in male reproduction while staying fully aware of the differences between necrosis and apoptosis. This could help us to understand so-called idiopathic necrozoospermia better in the future. "Accidental" cell death, termed *necrosis,* occurs in response to a wide variety of harmful conditions and toxic substances: hyperthermia, hypoxia, ischemia, metabolic poisons, and direct cell trauma (e.g., infection) (4). It is a passive process that does not require energy expenditure by the cell (5). A cell undergoing necrosis typically exhibits distinctive morphological and biochemical characteristics. The earliest changes include swelling of the cytoplasm and organelles, especially the mitochondria, with only slight changes in the nucleus. The morphologic changes are due to loss of control of selective permeability of the plasma membrane with early disappearance of membrane ion-pumping activities. The increased permeability of the membrane leads to cellular swelling and an influx of cations (mainly Ca^{++}), which activate membrane-bound phospholipases and cause disruption of membranes (5). In the late stages of necrosis, the release of hydrolases from ruptured lysosomes causes a rapid acceleration of cellular disintegration. Rapid decreases in protein, RNA, and DNA levels occur. DNA exposed by proteolytic digestion of histones is cleaved by lysosomal desoxyribonuclease into fragments that display a continuous spectrum of sizes (6). Necrosis typically affects groups of contiguous cells, and an inflammatory reaction (leucocyte infiltration) develops in the adjacent viable tissue (4).

In contrast, as early as 1972, Kerr et al. (7) reported the first description of a spontaneous form of cell death called *apoptosis*, which occurs in scattered cells and progresses so rapidly that it was difficult to observe. The Greek noun *apoptosis* means the "falling off" of petals from flowers or leaves from trees. This is an active process and ATP generation is needed (5). Thus, mitochondrial integrity is generally preserved until the final moments. The stimuli that provoke physiological cell death include biological (absence or presence of a hormone) or pharmacological agents (irradiation, genotoxicants) (8). The process is probably timed according to the pattern of genes expressed in the cell (8).

The detachment of an individual cell from its neighbors is followed by cell death occurring in two distinct stages. First, the cells undergo nuclear (pyknosis) and cytoplasmic condensation and eventually break up into a number of membrane-bound fragments that contain structurally intact organelles, leading to cell shrinkage (anoikis). At the second stage these fragments, called *apoptotic bodies* (spherical membrane fragments containing nuclear fragments), are phagocytozed by neighboring cells and rapidly degraded (4,5,7). ADN fragmentation is induced by a Ca^{++}- and Mg^{++}- endonuclease, which leads to fragments of 185–200 bp, including a small number of nucleosomes (4). The differences are summarized in Table 6.1.

The proteins involved in the process of apoptosis are little known (9). The *bcl*-2 gene family includes repressors (BCL-2) and facilitators (BAX) of cell death (10). The expression of *bcl*-2 and related genes may be modulated by the actions of the p53 tumor suppressor protein. Nuclear translocation of p53 in vitro and in vivo can repress expression of the *bcl* -2 survival gene while concomitantly increasing transcription of the *bax* death gene (11). Genotoxic agents, therefore, might stimulate p53 activation, thus inducing a shift towards greater BAX availability and susceptibility to cell death.

Necrozoospermia could be related to postnatal cell death in endocrine-dependent tissues. In this case, apoptosis can be subdivided into two catego-

TABLE 6.1. Main differences between necrosis and apoptosis.

Necrosis	Apoptosis
Passive process (no energy expenditure)	Active process (with ATP generation)
Swelling of cytoplasm/mitochondria	Nuclear (pyknosis) and cytoplasmic condensation
Hydrolases from lysosomes → cell disintegration	Cell shrinkage with apoptotic bodies
DNA decrease; small fragments of DNA with a continuum in size	DNA fragmentation leading to fragments of 185–200 bp
Hyperthermia, hypoxia, ischemia, infection	Biological (absence or presence of a hormone) or pharmacological agents (irradiation, genotoxicants)

ries (8): tissues that undergo involution upon removal of survival factors under nonphysiological conditions (suppression of gonadotrophins for the testis) and those that undergo cyclical growth and involution in response to physiological fluctuations of survival factors (considerable germ cell loss during specific stages of spermatogenesis for the testis). Both mechanisms are observed in the testis. It has long been known that suppression of gonadotrophins [by hypophysectomy (12,13) or GnRH agonists (14)] induces massive germ cell death. Under physiological conditions apoptosis is generally absent in somatic cells (Sertoli and Leydig) of the adult testis. This has been confirmed in the aging testis (15): All types of germ cells are involved in apoptosis, but Sertoli cell apoptosis has not been encountered. There is evidence of considerable germ cell loss during specific stages of spermatogenesis in rodents (16,17). Estimates of the number of male germ cells that normally undergo apoptosis have indicated that physiological cell death may actually be the fate of more than one-half of the spermatogonia produced in the adult testis. Following the second hypothesis, there is thus also apoptosis under normal physiological conditions (8).

Little is known about the mechanisms involved in testis apoptosis. *bcl-2* is an inner mitochondrial membrane protein that represents a unique class of oncogene that is able to interfere with cell death without promoting cell division. Analysis of *bcl-2* protein levels in human tissues demonstrated that the protein is restricted to long-lived or proliferating cell zones, including hormone/growth factor-dependent glandular epithelium (18). *bcl-2* may counteract apoptosis and confer longevity to progenitor cells (e.g., spermatogonia). The cell survival-promoting activity of *bcl-2* is opposed by Bax, a homologous protein that forms heterodimers with *bcl-2* and accelerates cell death (19). An in vivo study in mice found Bax in reproductive tissues (20): Bax immunostaining was found in the epithelial cells of the prostate and weakly in the germinal cells of the testis located near the basal membrane, but not in spermatids or mature sperm cells. In contrast, intense bcl-2 immunoreactivity was observed in mature sperm, but no reactivity could be found in testicular germinal epithelium. Bax immunostaining was present in the epithelial cells lining the ductuli efferenti and epididymis. In contrast to Bax, no *bcl-2* immunostaining was detected in the epithelial cells of the epididymis. Tumor suppressor p53 is a direct transcriptional activator of the human *bax* gene (11). *bcl-2* functions as an antioxidant pathway to prevent apoptosis (21).

The generation of reactive oxygen species (ROS) and their deleterious effects on sperm function have been studied extensively (22–24). There are two sources of oxidative stress that affect human spermatozoa: ROS generated by defective spermatozoa due to some defect in spermiogenesis and infiltration of leucocytes in the semen of patients with accessory gland infections (25). Among ROS, generation of nitric oxide (NO) should be mentioned. There are antioxidant properties in seminal plasma necessary to prevent the deleterious action of superoxide anions, and the epididymis plays an important secretory role (26). Some major antioxidants of an enzymal nature are found in seminal plasma: superoxide dismutase (SOD) (27,28), catalase (29), and glutathione peroxidase (30). Catalase activity, however, has been questioned and glutathione peroxidase activity is negligible. Other low-molecular weight substances found in seminal plasma have protective effects: albumin (28), taurine, ascorbate, urate, and pyruvate (23). A protective role of superoxide dismutase in human sperm motility has been proposed (27). In their study of the superoxide anion scavenging capacity of human seminal plasma, Gavella et al. (31) found a SOD-like activity that correlated positively with levels of citric acid, zinc, and acid phosphatase activity, suggesting an important role of prostate secretions as superoxide anion scavengers. When infertile men had accessory gland infections, SOD-like activity was significantly lower in seminal plasma. In the same study, protective effects were shown for ascorbate urate and albumin, with a good correlation with fructose, which suggests that low-molecular weight components with antioxidant capacity derive partly from seminal vesicles. These findings stress the role of infection of accessory sex glands (e.g., prostate, seminal vesicles, epididymis) in overcoming the antioxidant capacity of seminal plasma. This might generate alterations in sperm motility or viability (Fig. 6.1).

Tumopr necrosis factor (TNF) alpha and interferon-gamma are cytokines found in the semen of infertile men (32). TNF alpha is secreted by macrophages in interstitial tissue and by germ cells in seminiferous tubules (33). The levels are higher in male genital tract infections, and is associated with leucocytospermia and immunological abnormalities (34). Estrada et al. (35) were able to determine a 50% decrease in sperm motility and viability when washed spermatozoa from normal volunteers were treated with TNF alpha plus interferon-gamma. These compounds appear to cause, either directly or indirectly, the production of ROS (36), which induces negative effects on sperm motion (37). The lipid peroxidation might account for the decrease in sperm membrane integrity and cell viability (38). The Fas death factor is a cell-surface receptor protein that mediates apoptosis-inducing signals (39).

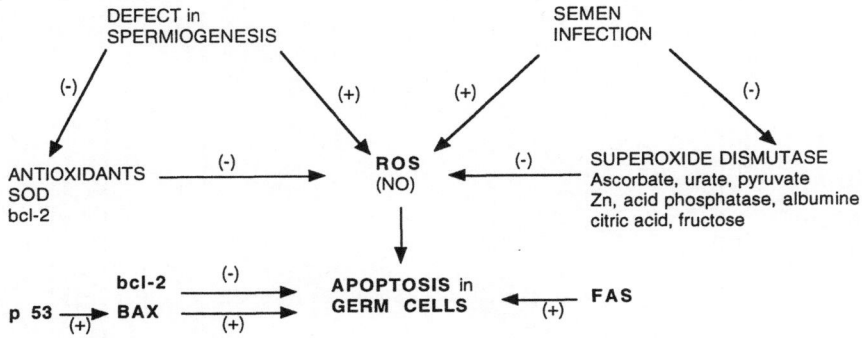

FIGURE 6.1. Relations between sperm alterations and apoptosis.

Retrospective Study

We approached the problem of necrospermia with a review of 5049 semen samples studied in our reproductive laboratory between January 1990 and December 1992. In this retrospective study, we looked for sperm viability lower than or equal to 50% in three semen samples to avoid transient necrospermia.

Eosin-nigrosin was used as live-dead staining technique, counting 100 spermatozoa with a light microscope. Medical histories, physical examination, endocrine profile, semen analysis after sexual abstinence of at least 3 days, seminal biochemical tests (e.g., seminal fructose, acid phosphatase, L-carnitine), sperm and urine culture, sperm antibodies evaluated by mixed antiglobulin reaction (MAR test), and, in some cases, electron microscopy and testicular biopsy allowed us to classify necrospermic subjects in different etiological groups. All semen analysis was performed using WHO criteria (1), with the exception of necrospermia defined as less than 50% live sperm instead of 75%. This threshold was chosen to be sure to be facing a pathology. It should be stressed that sperm viability is a parameter that is evaluated with a good precision and a low variation coefficient. Medical histories investigated smoking, stress, professional exposure to chemical radiation or heat, drugs, and recent episode of fever, history of urogenital disease, paraplegia, or infection (40).

Ultrasound rectal examination was performed in case of infection. Endocrine function was evaluated by measuring FSH, LH, and testosterone in serum. In 229 samples of 171 patients, necrospermia was observed at least once (4% of the total samples). The histogram of sperm viability in the different semen samples is shown in Figure 6.2. One hundred and thirty-one patients were followed in our reproductive unit (group P) and 28 of them had necrozoospermia in at least three semen samples (group P1). Fourteen had

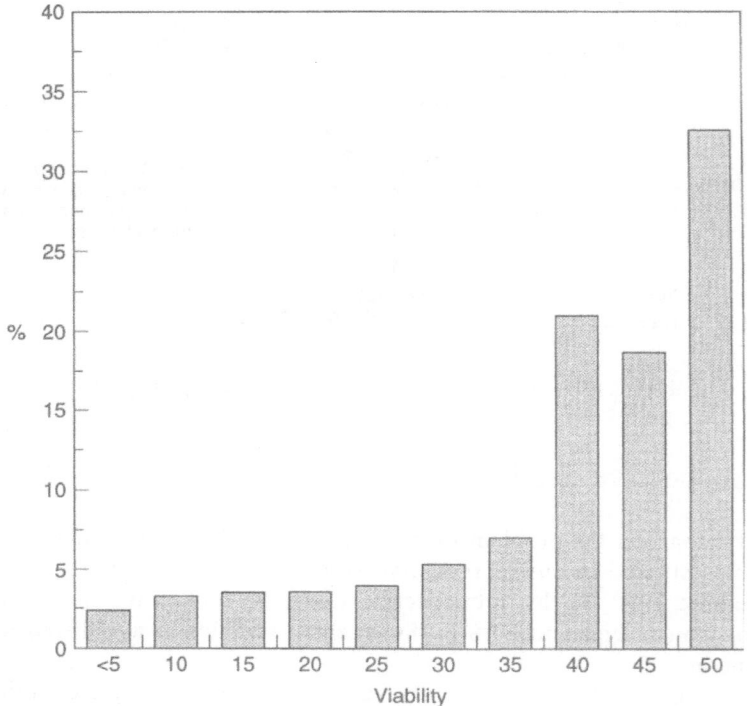

FIGURE 6.2. Histogram of sperm viability.

persistent necrospermia in all semen samples (group P3), and 14 had necrospermia in half the samples (group P2) (Table 6.2). Forty other patients
attended the reproductive laboratory for sperm analysis only and were followed by other physicians.

We observed two groups of patients with necrospermia, patients with transient abnormality, and patients with necrospermia observed in at least three
semen samples (P1). In this group, infection (acute or chronic) was the main
cause (40%), followed by testicular disease (21%), suspected epididymis abnormality (11%), and poor semen quality (11%). Urogenitary tract infection
was diagnosed by positive sperm or urinary culture. Infectious sequelae were
suspected according to medical history and decrease in routinely performed
biochemical markers: L-carnitine, fructose, or acid phosphatase (41,42). Testicular disease was clinically obvious with small testes or suspected due to
FSH increase or assessed by a bilateral testicular biopsy. We suspected epididymis dysfunction where there was no history of epididymis infection, but a
diminished level of L-carnitine. Poor seminal plasma quality was characterized by high viscosity, small volume of the ejaculate (< 1 ml) or high duration
of abstinence (> 8 days) (43), and electric semen collection in two paraplegic
men. Sperm antibodies and hyperthermia (i.e., professional exposure to heat,

TABLE 6.2. Frequency of etiologies in patients followed for necrozoospermia in our center.

Etiologies	P N	(%)	P1 N	(%)	P2 N	(%)	P3 N	(%)
Epididymal abnormality, 14.3%	11	8.4	3	10.7	1	7.1	2	
Seminal plasma quality, 21.4%	29	22.1	3	10.7	0	0	3	
Testicular pathology, 21.4%	33	25.2	6	21.4	3	21.4	3	
Hyperthermia	7	5.3	1	3.6	1	7.1	0	0
Infections, 35.7%	16	12.2	11	39.3	6	42.8	5	
Sperm antibodies	7	5.3	1	3.6	0	0	1	7.1
No etiology found	28	21.4	3	10.7	3	21.4	0	0
Total	131		28		14		14	

Note: n = 131. P = All patients followed for necrozoospermia (131/171) in our center. P1 = Group of 28 men with necrozoospermia in 2 or more semen samples. P2 = Group from P1 with an inconstant necrozoospermia in at least half of semen samples. P3 = Group from P1 with necrozoospermia in all semen samples.

fever) were rarely observed (3% each). No etiology could be found in 11% of our patients, leading to a tentative diagnosis of idiopathic necrozoospermia. In such cases, epididymis dysfunction responsible for sperm degeneration or death during transit or storage has been suggested (3).

In the group with persistent necrospermia (P3), the same causes were found: infection (36%), testicular pathology (21%), semen quality (21%), epididymis abnormality (14%), and sperm antibodies (7%), and a cause could be found for each case in this severe subgroup. Sperm antibodies are often associated with testicular trauma or infection (44). Viability of spermatozoa is seldomly impaired by fever and varicocele, but these rare causes were not observed in our study.

We also collected Assisted Reproductive Technology (ART) results for patients attending our infertility treatment unit: AID, AIH, IVF, and spontaneous success were recorded. Sixty-three of the 131 patients with necrozoospermia (P) were enrolled in our IVF program, and a pregnancy was achieved in 17 cases (27%). No success was observed in patients with autoantibodies or raised FSH, but intracytoplasmic sperm injection (ICSI) was not considered in this evaluation. In the group of 28 patients with necrozoospermia in at least three semen samples (P1), four wished to stop all kinds of treatment and two have been enrolled in our ICSI program. In the remaining 22, there have been three pregnancies in three couples who were selected for AID, four pregnancies in 17 couples treated with IVF, and two spontaneous pregnancies, leading to a 9 of 22, or 41%, pregnancy rate (Table 6.3). We could not find any correlation between the occurrence of pregnancy and the percentage of sperm viability nor any relation between success and etiology, but our groups of patients are small.

TABLE 6.3. Results of assisted reproductive technology.

	AID		AIH		IVF	
	P	P1	P	P1	P	P1
Patients	7	3	3	0	63	17
Pregnancy	4	3	0		17	4

Despite thorough research in the literature published on the subject, we have been unable to compare our results with other findings. From previously reported cases, we would like to stress some particular causes of necrospermia:

- Necrospermia was found in one in six drug addicts with severe degenerative changes of the sperm head seen by light and electron microscopy. Moreover, the entire sperm structure was modified by addiction (45). Addiction to drugs, therefore, has to be sought when looking for causes of necrospermia.
- Necrospermia was described in a patient infected with *Chlamydia trachomatis*. The sperm was studied by transmission electron microscopy, and intraepithelial vesicles containing *C. trachomatis* were present in remaining cytoplasmic droplets, contributing to decreased motility and necrospermia (46). In a cohort of patients with extensive and persistent disorder of motility, subclinical seminal infections were diagnosed in more than 20%. Using electron microscopy, a substantial number of acquired head abnormalities and necrospermia were observed (47). In a light and electron microscopy study of 25 patients with severe asthenospermia (no normal motility or complete immotility) nine cases of necrozoospermia were similarly observed. Mitochondrial defects were among the causes that might account for loss of sperm motility and necrospermia in this population (48). As we have seen in the first part and in our own findings, infection is very often involved in necrospermia.
- In workers exposed to 2,4-dichlorophenoxyacetic acid, an insecticide used by 32 male farm sprayers, significant levels of asthenospermia, necrospermia, and teratospermia were found in semen samples. The necrospermia diminished over time, but teratospermia continued (49). Toxic industrial drugs should be added to the list of causes of necrospermia. No definitive destruction of germinal cells can be observed with some toxins.
- Necrospermia was observed in one German patient with in situ carcinoma of the testis and azoospermia in two other patients (50). In the absence of a detectable cause, an ultrasound study of the testes could therefore be proposed, followed by a biopsy of a suspicious image. A tentative list of causes to be sought in cases of necrozoospermia is shown in Table 6.4.

What can be said about idiopathic necrospermia? It is clear from the first part of this chapter that infection is a leading cause, producing oxidative

TABLE 6.4. Causes of necrozoospermia.

1. Infection (oxidative stress, NO, TNF alpha)
2. Testicular abnormality (hypogonadal hypogonadism, aging, oxidative stress)
3. Abnormality of epididymis (partial obstruction, infectious sequelae)
4. Abnormality of seminal plasma (prolonged stay in the genital tract)
5. Sperm antibodies
6. Hyperthermia
7. Exposure to toxic products
8. Adiction
9. In situ carcinoma of testis
10. Abnormalities of mitochondrial function
11. Inactivating mutation of protecting factors against cell death (e.g., bcl-2)
12. Activating mutations of facilitating factors of cell death (e.g., BAX)
13. Other factors involved in sperm cell death (known, p53 protein, and unknown)
14. Idiopathic

stress (NO) able to alter sperm quality and viability. The protective role of bcl-2 and the opposite role of BAX has been emphasized. The role of protein p 53 in necrospermia needs to be clarified. TNF alpha and other cytokines will be further studied in the near future.

As seen in the histogram in Figure 6.2, 19% of our population had a sperm viability below 32%, and an etiology was found in all these cases. The threshold of 50% viability should be reduced to 30% if the goal is to find a cause of necrospermia.

We would like to emphasize the role of epididymis dysfunction in necrospermia. Sperm degeneration is frequently the expression of an inadequate epididymal environment with epithelial cells that are unable to maintain viable sperms in epididymal lumen (50). In our study, the epididymal group presented the lowest levels of living sperms. In vitro fertilization with spermatozoa obtained surgically from the epididymal caput was initially disappointing. This was explained by the low progressive motility of spermatozoa (around 6%) and marked necrozoospermia (around 20%) (51). The term *epididymal necrospermia* was proposed by Wilton et al. (3). Four patients with oligospermia and necrospermia were found to have severely degenerated sperm in the ejaculate. Testicular sperm of those examined, however, were ultrastructurally normal, which suggests that sperm degeneration and death occurred during epididymal passage or storage.

Another possibility might have been the occurrence of sperm degeneration and death upon mixing with the seminal plasma at ejaculation. The seminal plasma of these patients was found to be nontoxic to normal donor sperm. The presence of many lysosomes has been associated with necrospermia, which has been noted in other species such as marsupials, where the epididymis dysfunction is linked to anoxia in the distal part of epididymis (52). These drawbacks have been overcome by ICSI (53). The most recent paper on this subject is the work published by Van Steirteghem's team (54).

They made a retrospective study of five subjects presenting consistently with 100% dead spermatozoa in ejaculates. In such cases selection of immotile yet viable sperm by a hypoosmotic curl-tail medium may be a valuable solution. In these five patients, no viable sperm were found with this method. Assuming that spermatozoa from necrozoospermic patients lose their viability after release from the testicle, open testicular biopsy was then performed in four patients and three showed a normal testicular histology. Motile testicular sperm were recovered from the testicular biopsy in these three patients. The normal fertilization rate of metaphase II oocytes was 67%. One pregnancy was obtained on a total of five embryo transfers, and a healthy child was delivered.

As stated, this retrospective study ideally needs confirmation by a controlled study. It is questionable whether such a trial would be practically and ethically feasible. Testing viability of testicular sperm used for ICSI would theoretically be preferable, but it is not justified because the supravital staining methods used may compromise DNA integrity. The use of testicular sperm for ICSI may raise some concerns about the safety of this procedure (55). The testicular histology of these necrozoospermic patients, however, showed normal spermatogenesis. It is thus unlikely that their fertility problem had a genetic background. The use of viable yet immature testicular sperm in necrozoospermic patients even may be preferable over the use of apoptotic dysfunctional ejaculated spermatozoa that may have accumulated genomic damage (55).

Exploration of Necrospermia Proposed as a Practical Guide

We propose the following methods for the treatment of this sperm abnormality (see Fig. 6.3):

• Treat infection
• Treat hypogonadism
• Eliminate drug addiction and toxic products
• Activate spermatogenesis in shortening ejaculation delay
• Apply Van Steirteghem's current policy: In case of at least two fresh ejaculates collected at three months interval with a period of sexual abstinence of 5 days or less from a former oligozoospermic patient who do not show any viable sperm, it is recommended to perform a testicular sperm recovery procedure

Acknowledgments. The authors thank Serono Laboratories for their kind help in searching for references.

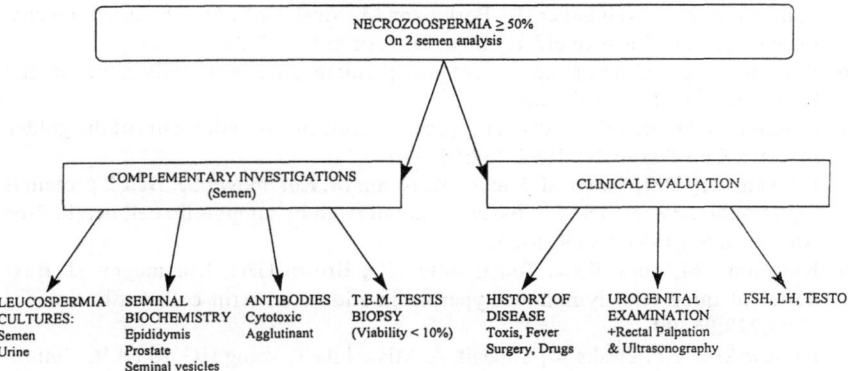

FIGURE 6.3. Proposed scheme for the management of an investigation of necrospermia.

References

1. World Health Organization. WHO laboratory manual for the examination of human semen and sperm cervical mucus interaction, 3rd Edition. London: Cambridge University Press, 1992.
2. Phadke AM, Samant NR, Dewal SD. Seminal fructose content in necrospermia. Fertil Steril 1975;26:1021–27.
3. Wilton LJ, Temple-Smith PD, Gordon Baker HW, de Kretser DM. Human male infertility caused by degeneration and death of sperm in the epididymis. Fertil Steril 1988;49:1052–58.
4. Schwartzman RA, Cidlowski JA. Apoptosis: the biochemistry and molecular biology of programmed cell death. Endocrinol Rev 1993;14:133–51.
5. Majno G, Joris I. Apoptosis, oncosis and necrosis. Am J Pathol 1995;146:3–15.
6. Duvall E, Wyllie AH. Death and the cell. Immunol Today 1986;7:115–19.
7. Kerr JFR, Wyllie AH, Currie AR. Apoptosis: a basic biological phenomenon with wide-ranging implications in tissue kinetics. Br J Cancer 1972;26:239–57.
8. Martimbeau S, Tilly JL. Physiological cell death in endocrine-dependent tissues: an ovarian perspective. Clin Endocrinol 1997;46:241–54.
9. Vaux DL. Toward an understanding of the molecular mechanisms of physiological cell death. Proc Natl Acad Sci 1993;90:786–89.
10. Reed JC. Bcl-2 and the regulation of programmed cell death. J Cell Biol 1994;124:1–6.
11. Miyashita T, Reed JC. Tumor suppressor p53 is a direct transcriptional activator of the human *bax* gene. Cell 1995;80:293–99.
12. Russell LD, Clermont Y. Degeneration of germ cells in normal, hypophysectomized and hormone-treated hypophysectomized rats. Anat Rec 1977; 87:347–66.
13. Tapanainen J, Tilly JL, Vikho KK, Hsueh AJW. Hormonal control of apoptotic cell death in the testis: gonadotropins and androgens as testicular cells survival factors. Mol Endocrinol 1993;7:643–50.
14. Sinha Hikim AP, Wang C, Leung A, Swerdloff R. Involvement of apoptosis in the induction of germ cell degeneration in adult rats after gonadotropin-releasing hormone agonist treatment. Endocrinology 1995;136:2770–75.

15. Brinkworth MH, Weinbauer GF, Bergmann M, Nieshlag E. Apoptosis as a mechanism of germ cell loss in elderly men. Int J Androl 1997;20:222–28.
16. Roosen-Runge EC. The generation of pre-spermatogonial germ cells in the rat after birth. Anat Rec 1964;148:328.
17. Miething A. Germ-cell death during prespermatogenesis in the testis of the golden hamster. Cell Tissue Res 1992;267:583–90.
18. Hockenberry DM, Zutter M, Hickey W, Nahm M, Korsmeyer SJ. BCL2 protein is topographically restricted in tissues characterized by apopototic cell death. Proc Natl Acad Sci 1991;88:6961–65.
19. Knudson CM, Tung KSK, Tourtellotte WG, Brown GAJ, Korsmeyer SJ. Bax-deficient mice with lymphoid hyperplasia and male germ cell death. Science 1995;270:96–99.
20. Krajewski S, Krajewska M, Shabaik A, Miyashita T, Wang HG, Reed JC. Immunohistochemical determination of in vivo distribution of Bax, a dominant inhibitor of Bcl-2. Am J Pathol 1994;145:1323–26.
21. Hockenberry DM, Oltvai ZN, Yin XM, Milliman CL, Korsmeyer SJ. Bcl-2 functions as an antioxidant pathway to prevent apoptosis. Cell 1993;75:241–51.
22. Aitken RJ. A free radical theory of male infertility. Reprod Fertil Dev 1994; 6:19–24.
23. de Lamirande E, Gagnon C. Reactive oxygen species and human spermatozoa. I. Effects on the motility and on sperm axonems. J Androl 1992;13:368–78.
24. Plante M, De Lamirande E, Gagnon C. Reactive oxygen species released by activated neutrophils, but not by deficient spermatozoa, are sufficient to affect normal sperm motility. Fertil Steril 1994;62:387–92.
25. Aitken RJ, Buckingham DW, Brindle J, Gomez E, Gordon Baker HW, Irvine DS. Analysis of sperm movement in relation to the oxidative stress created by leukocytes in washed sperm preparations and seminal plasma. Hum Reprod 1995;10:2061–71.
26. Perry ACF, Jones R, Hall L. Isolation and characterization of a rat cDNA clone encoding a secreted superoxide dismutase reveals the epididymis to be a major site of its expression. Biochem J 1993;293:21–25.
27. Kobayashi T, Miyazaki T, Natori M, Nozawa S. Protective role of superoxide dismutase in human sperm motility: superoxide dismutase activity and lipid peroxide in human seminal plasma and spermatozoa. Hum Reprod 1991;7:987–91.
28. Zini A, De Lamirande E, Gagnon C. Reactive oxygen species in semen of infertile patients: levels of superoxyde dismutase- and catalase-like activities in seminal plasma and spermatozoa. Int J Androl 1993;16:183–88.
29. Jeulin C, Soufir JC, Webert P, Laval-Martin D, Calvayrac R. Catalase activity in human spermatozoa and seminal plasma. Gamete Res 1989;24:185–96.
30. Alvarez JG, Storey BT. Role of glutathione peroxidase in protecting mammalian spermatozoa from loss of motility caused by spontaneous lipid peroxidation. Gamete Res 1989;23:77–90.
31. Gavella M, Lipovac V, Vucic M, Rocic B. Superoxide anion scavenging capacity of human seminal plasma. Int J Androl 1996;19:82–90.
32. Benhamed M. Tumor necrosis factor in the male gonad. Contracept Fertil Sex 1997;25:569–71.
33. Comhaire FE, Bosmans W, Ombelet U, Punjabi H, Schoonjans F. Cytokines in semen of normal men and of patients with andrological diseases. Am J Reprod Immunol 1994;31:99–103.

34. Naz RK, Chaturvedi MM, Aggarwal BB. Role of cytokines and protooncogenes in sperm cell function: relevance to immunologic infertility. Am J Reprod Immunol 1994;32:26–37.
35. Estrada LS, Champion HC, Wang R, et al. Effect of tumour necrosis factor-alpha (TNF-alpha) and interferon-gamma (INF-gamma) on human sperm motility, viability and motion parameters. Int J Androl 1997;20:237–42.
36. Whitman ED, Doherty GM, Peplinski GR, Norton JA. Role of cytokines in oxydative damage. In: Aggarwal B, Puri R, editors. Human cytokines: their role in disease and therapy, Chapter 22. Oxford: Blackwell Science, 1995:333.
37. Sikka S, Rajasekaran M, Hellstrom W. Role of oxidative stress and antioxidants in male infertility. J Androl 1995;16:464–68.
38. Buch JP, Kolon TF, Maulik N, Kreutzer DL, Das DK. Cytokines stimulate membrane lipid peroxidation of human sperm. Fertil Steril 1994;62:186–88.
39. Nagata S, Goldstein P. The Fas death factor. Science 1995;267:1449–56.
40. Gerhard I, Lenhard K, Eggert-Kruse W, Runnebaum B. Clinical data which influence semen parameters in infertile men. Hum Reprod 1992;7:830–37.
41. Clavert A, Cranz C, Tardieu J. Epididymis and genital infections. In: Hamamah S, Mieusset R, Dacheux J-L, editors. Frontiers in endocrinology. Epididymis role and importance in male infertility treatment, Vol. 11. Rome: Ares Serono Symposia, 1995:203–10.
42. Cooper TJ. Functions of human epididymis. In: Hamamah S, Mieusset R, Dacheux J-L, editors. Frontiers in endocrinology. Epididymis role and importance in male infertility treatment, Vol. 11. Rome: Ares Serono Symposia, 1995:1–12.
43. Mortimer D, Templeton AA, Lenton EA, Coleman RA. Influence of abstinence and ejaculation-to-analysis delay on semen analysis parameters of suspected infertile men. Arch Androl 1982;8:2516–20.
44. Sinisi AA, di Finizio B, Pasquali D, Corini A, Apuzzo D, Bellastella A. Prevalence of antisperm antibodies by sperm MAR test in subjects undergoing a routine sperm analysis for infertility. Int J Androl 1993;16:311–14.
45. El Gothamy Z, El Samahy H. Ultrastructure sperm defects in addicts. Fertil Steril 1992;47:699–702.
46. Villegas H, Pinon M, Shor V, Karchmer S. Electron microscopy of Chlamydia trachomatis infection of the male genital tract. Arch Androl 1991;27:117–26.
47. Hustin J, Koulischer L. Microscopie électronique des spermatozoïdes. Indications et résultats. Acta Urol Belg 1989;57:17–28.
48. Gopalkrishnan K, Padwal V, D'Souza S, Shah R. Severe asthenozoospermia: a structural and functional study. Int J Androl 1995;18(Suppl 1):67–74.
49. Lerda D, Rizzi R. Study of reproductive function in persons occupationally exposed to 2,4-dichlorophenoxyacetic acid (2,4-D). Mutat Res 1991;262:47–50.
50. Kleinschmidt K, Weissbach L, Holstein AF. Fruherkennung des kontralateralen zweitkarzinoms bei hodentumorpatienten durch das carcinoma in situ testis. Urologe A 1989;28:281–84.
51. Jardin A, Izard V, Benoit G, Testart J, Belaisch-Allart J, Volante M, et al. Fécondance in vivo et in vitro de spermatozoïdes épididymaires humains immatures. Reprod Nutr Dev 1988;28:1375–85.
52. Cummins JM, Temple-Smith PD, Rentree MB. Reproduction in male honeypossum (Tarsipes rostratus Marsupialia): the epididymis. Am J Anat 1986;177:385–93.
53. Palermo G, Joris H, Devroey P, Van Sterteighem AC. Pregnancies after intracytoplasmic injection of single spermatozoon into an oocyte. Lancet 1992;340:17–18.

54. Tournaye H, Liu J, Nagy Z, Verheyen G, Van Steirteghem A, Devroey P. The use of testicular sperm for intracytoplasmic sperm injection in patients with necrozoospermia. Fertil Steril 1996;66:331–34.
55. Cummins JM, Jequier AM. Concerns and recommendations for intracytoplasmic sperm injection (ICSI) treatment. Hum Reprod 1995;10(Suppl 1):138–43.
56. Nduwayo L, Barthélémy C, Lansac J, Tharanne MJ, Lecomte P. Necrospermia and human male infertility. Contracept Fertil Sex 1995;23:682–85.
57. Skakkebaek NE, Giwercman A, De Kretser D. Pathogenesis and management of male infertility. Lancet 1994;343:1473–74.
58. Zamboni L. Sperm pathology and infertility. Fertil Steril 1987;48:726–31.

Part II

Therapeutic Possibilities for Motility Disorders

Part II

Therapeutic Possibilities for Motility Disorders

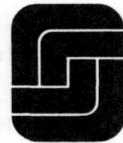

7

In Vivo Therapies for Asthenozoospermia

Roger Mieusset

Introduction

Motility is one of the major sperm characteristics needed to achieve a pregnancy in vivo. Several factors can affect sperm motility, some of which are relatively well known, such as ultrastructural tail defects (see previous chapters in this book). These are associated with various degrees of impaired motility from akinethozoospermia to sliding spermatozoa and lowered sperm motility. Impaired motility because of such ultrastructural defects should be considered as congenital because they arise during the development of the sperm, essentially throughout spermiogenesis; in such cases, no in vivo treatment will offer improvement in motility.

Abnormally low motility, however, may result from other factors, most of which are unknown, but with one of two main spermiologic patterns that can be distinguished. In the first, spermatogenesis seems normal, as indicated by a normal number of spermatozoa in the ejaculate, but with impaired motility. In the second, motility is just one of the sperm parameters impaired in an abnormal spermatogenesis inducing oligoasthenoteratozoospermia. Whatever the pattern, only live spermatozoa have the potential for motility, which indicates that sperm vitality should be assessed in any semen analysis. Indeed, viability assessment enables patients with necrozoospermia to be easily distinguished from other patients with low sperm motility. It also seems rather inadequate to deal with asthenozoospermia without indication of whether sperm viability is normal or abnormal.

In Vivo Treatment of Immotile Spermatozoa

There is no report in the literature of an in vivo treatment for immotile spermatozoa or for total necrozoospermia. In several publications dealing with in vivo treatment for low sperm motility or oligoasthenoteratozoospermia, however, individuals with immotile sperm have been included. Thus, the various controlled, uncontrolled, and empirical in vivo treatments for low sperm motility will be reviewed in this chapter, with the aim of showing how these treatments can be used before there is an indication for intracytoplasmic sperm injection (ICSI).

No In Vivo Drug Therapy for Asthenozoospermia

Because all pharmacological therapies designed to improve sperm production and fertility in idiopathic male infertility have been said to fail, variations in the times of abstinence and the frequency of ejaculations have been used as an alternative treatment method.

It is well documented that spermatozoa acquire motility as they pass through the epididymis, although the exact mechanisms by which this is achieved remain unknown. The transit time for spermatozoa through the human epididymis has been estimated to be 11–12 days (1), but with individual values ranging from 1 to 22 days. Such interindividual variation in the epididymal transit time of spermatozoa was suggested to be a consequence of the extremely low capacity of the human epididymis to store spermatozoa (2,3). In individuals with a high daily sperm production per testis, the epididymal transit time was very short, ranging from 1 to 5 days (3). Individuals with a low daily sperm production per testis (which could correspond to secretory oligozoospermia), however, exhibited a larger range of epididymal transit times from 1 to 15 days (3). The latter results seem to indicate that in certain (but not all) cases of low daily sperm production per testis, the transit time through the epididymis is three times greater than normal. In such cases, a longer time spent in the epididymis could be detrimental to sperm quality, with a reduction in the percentage of live and/or motile spermatozoa in the ejaculate.

Wilton et al. (4) reported that frequent ejaculations (2 ejaculates/day for 4 or 5 days) in four patients with necrozoospermia (< 45% live spermatozoa) and asthenozoospermia (0–30% motility), as well as moderate oligozoospermia or normozoospermia, resulted in a three- to sevenfold increase in the percentage of motile sperm associated with an increased sperm vitality when the baseline value was < 10% live spermatozoa. Supported by testicular biopsies from two of these men, this experiment suggests that normal, viable spermatozoa were produced in the testis, but most of them degenerated during passage through or storage in the epididymis, which appeared to act as a hostile environment for the spermatozoa. This hypothesis is supported in part by the results of Tur-Kaspa et al. (5), who reported an increased sperm motility in a second ejaculate collected 24 h after the first (with 3 days of sexual abstinence) in cases of asthenozoospermia ($n = 81$; sperm count $> 20 \times 10^6$/ml; motility 10–40%) and of oligoasthenozoospermia (sperm count $< 20 \times$

10^6/ml; motility 10–40%). Sperm motility was also reported to be increased in a second ejaculate collected 1 hour after the first one (with a 3-day abstinence period) in oligoasthenoteratozoospermic patients (6), an effect that could be explained by a decrease in potential suppressing sperm motility factor from vesicle secretion. Sperm count and total sperm count were not changed in these two studies (5,6), but they were reported to be increased in all cases of sperm counts of less than 10 million/ml (7). In another report, depletion of the extragonadal reserve was achieved by means of three successive ejaculations within a short period (1–4 hours), and three samples were collected (within 1–4 hours) after abstinence periods of 2, 7, or 10 days: Results seem to indicate that this experimental protocol could be of value in increasing the number of live and motile spermatozoa (8). Clinical studies of oligospermic men with necrozoospermia and asthenospermia, however, should be run for critical evaluation.

It should be noted that sperm vitality was not always assessed in these reports. In addition, these studies involved a mixture of true frequent ejaculation (4) and a second ejaculation collected 1, 2 (6,9), or 24 hours (5) after the first (i.e., a "repeated ejaculation"). Finally, when the effects of abstention times on spermatozoa have been examined, the unejaculated spermatozoa that remain in the ducts, and thus provide an older population of spermatozoa in the next ejaculate than would be anticipated from the abstention period, have usually been ignored.

These different conditions and results could correspond to various patterns of posttesticular sperm impairment, including the capacity of the epididymis to maintain the viability of the spermatozoa or to develop and maintain their motility, and the further secretions of the male genital glands to preserve both sperm viability and motility during the formation and expulsion of semen. In cases of immotile sperm with and without necrozoospermia, experiments using frequent and/or repeated ejaculations could be run before any ICSI attempt to exclude a potential functional disturbance of epididymal sperm transport or storage.

Antiinflammatory Treatment

Antiinflammatory (AI) drugs are usually used as an empirical therapy by many of the physicians dealing with male reproductive problems, however, there are no reports in the literature of controlled trials with such treatments. In a letter (10), the positive effects of AI therapy on sperm parameters (though only sperm numbers were reported) have been suggested in oligozoospermic and even in azoospermic infertile men, an effect supported by others (11). Such a positive effect was attributed to the treatment of either a partial obstruction of the epididymal tract (10) or to a functional disturbance of sperm transport caused by mediators of inflammation (11). Further clinical controlled trials are to be run to evaluate the efficiency of such a treatment. The diagnosis of chronic epididymal inflammation is difficult, however, and requires anamnesis, clinical examination as well as biological signs that were until now, without clear definition and/or support. In addition, the epididymal transit time of spermatozoa ranges from 1 to 15 days in cases of reduced sperm production, which is important for the duration of AI treatment. In addition, because the main problem is permanent necrozoospermia with asthenozoospermia, which is suggested to be indicative of a chronic inflammatory pattern, sequential AI treatments could be valuable.

Antibiotic Treatments

It has been recommended that the diagnosis of male accessory gland infection should be supported by at least two of several criteria (12). Seminal leukospermia or bacteriospermia, however, are usually considered to be indicative of infection and are therefore treated with antibiotics. Controversy exists over the possible effect of leukospermia on sperm motility and other semen parameters, with a detrimental effect found by some authors (13,14), but with no effect by others (15).

A patient with leukospermia ($> 10^6$ leukocytes/ml) clearly requires treatment for his infection. To minimize the potentially detrimental effects of the antibiotics (16), treatment should await the results of a semen culture. Antibiotics with demonstrated in vitro effectiveness and the minimum possible detrimental effects on fertility (16) may be used for treatment; however, this does not explain how to treat leukocytospermia without a positive sperm culture. A prospective, randomized, controlled study of two antibiotic regimens in both partners for leukocytospermia of unknown etiology indicated that no antibiotic regimen resulted in a significantly higher rate of resolution of the leukocytospermia than that seen in the untreated group (17). Because seminal leukocytes are not good Samaritans (18), however, previous results must be modulated as antibiotic treatment, coupled with frequent ejaculations, was the only effective treatment on the rate of leukocytospermia 3 months after the end of treatment in infertile patients with both prostatitis and leukocytospermia (19). Moreover, chronic abacterial prostatites are commonly associated with a greater impairment in sperm motility and morphology and a higher level of seminal white blood cells than normal males (20), and the existence of nonsymptomatic chronic prostatovesiculitis (21), as well as subclinical inflammation or infection in ejaculates (22), is said to be underdetected in the infertile population (21).

As antibiotic treatments have been reported to be ineffective in improving sperm motility in asthenospermic patients without sperm infection (23) or in infertile men with prostatitis (24) or with male accessory gland infection (25), antibiotic therapy should be used in asthenozoospermic patients only when sperm culture is positive. As the bacteriological quality of sperm culture can easily be improved by direct verbal counseling before semen collection (26), sperm microbial contamination, which is frequent in infertile men (27), should no longer be confused with sperm infection, particularly as an increased incidence of significant cultures of vaginal gram-negative bacilli was reported in patients with antibiotic-treated partners compared with untreated partners (28).

Pentoxifylline

Because methylxanthines were reported to have a potentially favorable effect on testicular microcirculation, as well as a stimulatory effect on sperm motility in vitro, the systemic application of pentoxifylline has been used for many years in the treatment of male infertility. In one report (29), the authors reviewed 10 trials that have studied the effect of oral therapy with pentoxifylline on sperm motility in idiopathic asthenozoospermia. Although eight of the studies demonstrated a significant increase in sperm motility, the efficacy of such a treatment is still considered as unproved because (1) the assessment and definition of asthenozoospermia are inadequate, (2) there is an absence of randomized, double-blind, placebo-controlled trials, and (3) the mechanism, if there is one, by which pentoxifylline could improve sperm motility is unknown (29). If the first two points are largely valid, then the third one should be reconsidered. Indeed, after determination of the levels of reactive oxygen species (ROS) and the identification of the source of such ROS formation (30), treatment with oral pentoxifylline had no effect on ROS production and sperm motility and motion parameters in the group of patients whose sperm preparation failed to generate detectable ROS levels ($n = 18$). Such a treatment, however, increased sperm motility and curvilinear velocity without altering ROS production in the group of patients ($n = 15$) whose sperm preparation generated detectable ROS levels that could be attributed to the spermatozoa themselves and not to coexisting leukocytes. This experiment indicates that orally administered pentoxifylline appeared to be effective for increasing sperm motility in the asthenozoospermic patients (about 21%) whose spermatozoa produced detectable levels of ROS (30).

Hormonal Treatments

Human Chorionic Gonadotropin/Human Menopausal Gonadotropin

The unique placebo-controlled double-blind trial of 2500 IU of human chorionic gonadotropin twice weekly in combination with 150 IU of human menopausal gonadotropin three times a week for 13 weeks in 19 oligozoospermic men (and 20 controls) with normal serum follicle-stimulating hormone (FSH) and testosterone values indicated no effect for such a treatment on sperm motility, either during therapy or within the following 4 months (31).

FSH Therapy

Long-term FSH treatment was reported to improve sperm-fertilizing ability in IVF couples with male factor infertility and a normal endocrine profile, but with no changes in the basic semen parameters (32,33). A daily FSH treatment administered for 30 days to assess, by means of transmission electron microscopy (TEM), only those morphological changes that occur during spermiogenesis and epididymal transport resulted in no changes in basic semen analysis parameters, and an ultrastructural improvement in the fine structure of sperm head subcellular organelles, but the axonema deteriorated with an 18% reduction of intact axonema after treatment (34). In a more recent work, a significant increase in the median value of morphologically normal spermatozoa was found, as analyzed with TEM, after 12 weeks of FSH treatment (35). These authors, however, failed to find any improvement of basic sperm parameters, including motility, although they did not confirm the axonemal deterioration previously reported (34). In another report of male FSH therapy in an intrauterine insemination program, 148 mainly asthenoteratozoospermic infertile men were randomly not treated or treated, with no change in the usual sperm characteristics (36). In a further study (37), 81 infertile patients were treated (15 subjected to placebo treatment and 66 to FSH therapy). Prior to therapy, five categories of major sperm defect were distinguished: immaturity, infection, apoptosis, autoantibodies, and azoospermia due to spermatogenic arrest. Each category responded differently to FSH therapy, which resulted in a decrease in the mean total number of spermatozoa devoid of ultrastructural defects (i.e., of healthy spermatozoa) in 19 (29%) patients (15 cases of infections, 1 of autoantibodies and 3 of immature spermatozoa), and in an improvement in the total number of healthy spermatozoa in 47 patients (23 cases of apoptosis, 4 of immature spermatozoa, and 20 of infections). With regard to the ultrastructural components involved in motility in the responders ($n = 47$), the proportions of spermatozoa with normal mitochondrial shape, regular mitochondrial assembly, normal axonemal pattern, normal arms in the axoneme, and of normal fibrous sheath shape were increased in the apototic group and in the immature group, even though less regularly, but never in the infections group. FSH therapy had no effect on the axonemic rolled up around the sperm body, or on the proportion of normal accessory fibers. Only the proportion of spermatozoa with regular mitochondrial assembly was improved in the infections group (37).

Evaluation of the effect of FSH therapy still gives conflicting information. The results of the six studies cited earlier (Table 7.1) clearly indicate that FSH therapy (whatever the frequency and dose of treatment) has no effect on sperm motility as assessed by manual analysis. The final study cited (37), however, indicates that inclusion in the selection criteria of parameters other than the usual sperm characteristics may be valuable in identifying those infertile men who could perhaps benefit from FSH therapy for potential in vivo fertilization.

TABLE 7.1. FSH therapy and sperm motility.

Authors	Sperm parameters	n	FSH therapy	Results
Acosta et al. (32)	Severe oligo- asthenozoospermia	36 [a]	150 IU×3/wk 3 months	No changes in sperm motility
Acosta et al. (33)	[b]	50	[b]	No changes in sperm motility
Bartoov et al, (34)	Teratospermia with astheno- or oligospermia	31 [c]	75 IU/day 30 days	No changes in sperm motility. Alteration. of the axoneme[d]
Strehler et al. (35)	Idiopathic oligo- asthenoteratospermia	46 [c]	150 IU/day 12 weeks	No changes in sperm motility. No alteration of the axoneme[d]
Matorras et al. (36)	Asthenoteratospermia and oligoasthenospermia	58 [e]	150 IU×3/wk 3 months	No changes in sperm motility
Baccetti et al. (37)	Not reported	66 [f]	150 IU/day 12 weeks	Improvement in most ultrastructural components of the tail in 41% of patients[d]

[a] Experimental clinical nonrandomized trial.
[b] Included are the data reported in the first quoted study.
[c] Prospective nonrandomized study without control group.
[d] Analysis assessed with transmission electron microscopy.
[e] Prospective randomized study with an untreated control group ($n = 78$).
[f] Prospective nonrandomized study with placebo-controlled group ($n = 15$).

Growth Hormone Therapy

Although the physiological significance of growth hormone (GH), insulinlike growth factor (IGF)-I and IGF-binding proteins in the male reproductive system still remains uncertain, the findings that subfertile men may suffer from relative GH insufficiency led to GH therapy in oligozoospermic men with partial or no results (38,39). GH secretion, however, was further evaluated in nine oligozoospermic men ($< 5 \times 10^6$/ml), nine asthenozoospermic infertile men (motility $< 30\%$; $> 15 \times 10^6$/ml), and nine age- and body mass index-matched fertile controls (40). Results showed similar basal levels of GH in all three groups, with an increase in GH in all groups after an arginine stimulation test, but with a significantly lower response in the two infertile groups compared with the controls (40), as already reported after a clonidine test (41). As these results were indicative of a relative GH insufficiency in the two infertile groups, the patients were treated daily with GH for 12 consecutive weeks (42). No increase in sperm count was observed in any of the groups. Sperm motility exhibited a nonsignificant increase in the oligospermic group and a significant increase in the asthenozoospermic patients, with a positive effect still observed 12 weeks after the end of treatment. Seminal plasma IGF-I was increased concomitantly with the increase in sperm motility during treatment (42). Further randomized trials are to be run to confirm these results.

Antioxidant Treatments

Cells that live in an anaerobic milieu and use oxygen generate some level of ROS. At the same time, however, they have developed defense mechanisms, the scavenger system, as the generation of ROS can result in peroxidative damage to cell membranes. The scavenger system acts as an antioxidant to detoxify the harmful ROS and prevent cell damage. Several studies have documented the possible role of spermatozoal ROS generation in defective sperm functions and infertility (43), with a negative correlation between the level of ROS formation and the percentage of motile spermatozoa, as well as linearity of sperm movement (44). The superoxide dismutase, glutathione peroxidase, and catalase have been reported to be protective enzyme scavengers in the sperm. As a result, the systemic application of antioxidative molecules has been used (Table 7.2).

Infertile men selected for unilateral varicocele or germ-free genital tract inflammation with various sperm anomalies including asthenozoospermia were treated with glutathione in a randomized placebo-controlled double-blind crossover trial (45), which resulted in improvement in sperm motility and morphology. In another, uncontrolled study of a similarly selected population, the same treatment resulted in improvements in both sperm count and motility (46).

In studies of vitamin E therapy, when patients were selected on high levels of ROS, there were no changes in sperm motility and no reduction in ROS level (47). When they were selected because of unexplained infertility, there were no ultrastructural changes in the tail components, but there was a reduction in lipid peroxidation (48). When they were selected because of asthenozoospermia (motility < 40%), there was no improvement in sperm motility and no change in lipid peroxidation in 40% of the treated patients, but there was an improvement in sperm motility with a reduction in lipid peroxidation in 60% (49). The discrepancy in the effects of vitamin E therapy in these trials could be the result of the basic sperm differences in the selected populations, the methods used for basic sperm ROS evaluation, or the differences in the dosage and duration of treatment because vitamin E concentration in seminal plasma was missing in two of the three studies.

Finally, in one study a potential antioxidant effect with pentoxifylline was reported to increase sperm motility without decreasing ROS levels in asthenozoospermic patients with high levels of ROS of spermatozoal origin (30). The selection of asthenozoospermic patients with high levels of ROS originating from spermatozoa seems to be an important selection criterion in antioxidant treatments.

TABLE 7.2. Effect of antioxidant treatments on sperm parameters.

Authors	Selection criteria	Nb of treated patients	Drugs	Dosage (mg) duration	ROS evaluation	Effects
Lenzi et al. (45)	Varicocele or germ-free genital tract inflammation	20 [a]	Glutathione (i.m.)	600 alternate day 2 months	No	No changes in sperm count. Improved sperm morphology, motility, and kinetics parameters
Lenzi et al. (46)	Varicocele or germ-free genital tract inflammation	10 [b]	Glutathione (i.m.)	600 alternate day 2 months	TBA method	Idem with a reduction in ROS levels
Kessopoulou et al. (47)	High levels of ROS	13 [a]	Vitamin E (α-tocopheryl acetate)	600/day 3 months	Chemo-luminescence	No changes in sperm parameters. No reduction in ROS levels
Geva et al. (48)	Unexplained infertility	15 [b]	Vitamin E (α-tocopherol acetate)	200/day 3 months	TBA method	Reduction in ROS levels. No changes in ultrastructural components of the tail (TEM)
Suleiman et al. (49)	Asthenozoospermia (motility[2] 40%)	52 [c]	Vitamin E	100/day 6 months	TBA method	Increased sperm motility with reduction in ROS levels in 60% of patients. No such changes in 40% of patients
Okada et al. (30)	Asthenozoospermia and high ROS levels from spermatozoa	15 [d]	Pentoxifylline	300/day for 3 months then 1200/day for 3 months	Chemo-luminescence	No decrease in ROS levels but improved sperm motility parameters at 1200 mg daily

[a] Randomized double-blind controlled-placebo crossover trial.
[b] No control groups.
[c] Randomized placebo-controlled double-blind trial.
[d] Control group made up of 23 asthenozoospermic patients without ROS.

Other Empirical Therapies

Folinic Acid

Sixty-five infertile men whose semen was characterized by an elevated concentration of round cells and oligoasthenozoospermia were treated daily with folinic acid over a period of 3 months in an uncontrolled trial (50). After treatment, the spermatozoa-round cells ratio was increased, as was sperm motility.

Magnesium

Magnesium concentration in the seminal plasma was found to decrease from normozoospermia to oligo- and asthenozoospermia, and eight oligoasthenozoospermic patients were treated daily for 3 months with per os magnesium citrate in an uncontrolled trial. Magnesium therapy resulted in an increased mean sperm count and motility, an effect that could result from an increase in activity of the enzymes that eliminate free oxygen radicals (51).

Mast Cell Blocker

Because mastocytosis was reported to occur in the testes of infertile men (52), mast cell blocker, which inhibits the release of histamine and other vasoactive substances from mast cells, was used in a placebo-controlled single-blind trial in 46 oligozoospermic patients. A daily treatment for 3 months resulted in a significant increase in sperm count and motility (53).

Acupuncture

In a prospective study (with an untreated control group) of 16 infertile men with mainly astheno- or asthenoteratozoospermia, 10 acupuncture treatments (one session twice weekly for 5 weeks) resulted in no differences in any of the biochemical semen parameters or in the existence of white blood cells and bacteriological contamination. Percentages of live and of motile sperm, however, were significantly increased after treatment, as was the percentage of intact axonema assessed by TEM (54).

Kallikrein

Since in vitro studies have shown a positive effect for kallikrein on sperm motility (55), as well as a stimulation of sperm metabolism (56), systemic application of kallikrein has been used for many years in the hope of improving sperm motility in infertile men. Clinical studies evaluating the effects of oral kallikrein therapy, however, have yielded contradictory results concerning sperm motility. Among these studies, only three double-blind, placebo-controlled trials resulted in a positive effect. One of these had just a small number of patients (57), and there was an absence of effect on sperm motility at 6 and 12 weeks after daily treatment in multicenter (58) and single-center (59) studies.

References

1. Rowley MJ, Teshima F, Heller CG. Duration of transit of spermatozoa through the human male ductular system. Fertil Steril 1970;21:390–96.
2. Aman RP, Howards SS. Daily spermatozoal production and epididymal sperm reserves of the human male. J Urol 1980;124:211–15
3. Johnson L, Vamer DD. Effect of daily spermatozoon production but not age on transit time of spermatozoa the human epididymis. Biol Reprod 1988;39:812–17.
4. Wilton LJ, Temple-Smith PD, Baker HWG, de Kretser DM. Human male fertility caused by degeneration and death of sperm in the epididymis. Fertil Steril 1988;49:1052–58.
5. Tur-Kaspa I, Maor Y, Levran D, Yanish M, Mashiah S, Dor J. How often should infertile men have intercourse to achieve conception? Fertil Steril 1994;62:370–75.
6. Gülmer A, Tatlisen M, Karacagil M, Kesekci S. Seminal parameters of ejaculates collected successively with sixty minutes interval in infertile men: effect of combination of prazosin and terbutaline on these parameters. Andrologia 1991;23:167–69.
7. Check HJ, Chase JS. Improved semen quality after short-interval second ejaculation. Fertil Steril 1985;44:416–18.
8. Cooper TG, Keck C, Oberdieck U, Nieschlag E. Effects of multiple ejaculations after extended periods of sexual abstinences on total, motile and normal sperm numbers, as well as accessory gland secretions, from healthy normal and oligozoospermic men. Hum Reprod 1993;8:1251–58.
9. Barash A, Lurie S, Weissman A, Insler V. Comparison of sperm parameters, in vitro fertilization results and subsequent pregnancy rates using sequential ejaculates, collected two hours apart, from oligoasthenozoospermic men. Fertil Steril 1995;64:1008–11.
10. Martin-Du Pan R, Bischof P, de Broccard G, Campana A. Is diclofenac helpful in the diagnosis of partial epididymal obstruction? Hum Reprod 1997;12:396–97.
11. Haidl G, Van der Ven H. Chronic genital inflammation in the male—an easily missed diagnosis. Hum Reprod 1997;12:2082.
12. Comhaire F, Verschraegen G, Vermeulen L. Diagnosis of accessory gland infection and its possible role in male infertility. Int J Androl 1980;3:32–35.
13. Auroux M. Non spermatozoal cells in human semen: a study of 1234 subfertile and 253 fertile men. Arch Androl 1984;14:335–42.
14. Wolff H, Politch JA, Martinez A, Haimovici F, Hill J, Anderson J. Leukocytospermia is associated with poor semen quality. Fertil Steril 1990;53:528–36.
15. Tomlinson MJ, Barratt CLR, Cooke ID. Prospective study of leukocytes and leukocyte subpopulations in semen suggests they are not a cause of male infertility. Fertil Steril 1993;60:996–1000.
16. Schlegel PN, Chang TSK, Marshall FF. Antibiotics: potential hazards to male fertility. Fertil Steril 1991;55:235–41.
17. Yanushpolsky EH, Politch JA, Hill JA, Andersen DJ. Antibiotic therapy and leukocytospermia: a prospective randomized, controlled study. Fertil Steril 1995;63:142–47.

18. Aitken RJ, Baker HWG. Seminal leukocytes: passengers, terrorists or good Samaritans? Hum Reprod 1995;10:1736–39.
19. Branigan EF, Muller ChH. Efficacy of treatment and recurrence rate of leukocytospermia in infertile men with prostatis. Fertil Steril 1994;62:580–84.
20. Leib Z, Bartoov B, Eltes F, Servadio C. Reduced semen quality caused by chronic abacterial prostatitis: an enigma or reality? Fertil Steril 1994;61:1109–16.
21. Purvis K, Christiansen E. Infection in the male reproductive tract. Impact, diagnosis and treatment in relation to male infertility. Int J Androl 1993;16:1–13.
22. Eggert-Kruse W, Probst S, Rohr G, Aufenanger J, Runnebaum B. Screening for subclinical inflammation in ejaculates. Fertil Steril 1995;64:1012–22.
23. Baker HGW, Straffon WGE, McGowan MD, Burger HG, de Kretser DM, Hudson B. A controlled trial of the use of erythromicin for men with asthenospermia. Int J Androl 1984;7:783–88.
24. Baker HGW, Straffon WGE, Murphy G, Davidson A, Burger HG, de Kretser DM. Prostatis and male infertility: a pilot study. Possible increase in sperm motility with anti-bacterial chemotherapy. Int J Androl 1979;2:193–97.
25. Comhaire F, Rowe PJ, Farley TMM. The effect of doxycycline in infertile couples with male accessory gland infection: a double blind prospective study. Int J Androl 1986;9:91–98.
26. Boucher Ph, Lejeune H, Pinatel MC, Gilly Y. Spermoculture: improvement of the bacteriological quality of samples by direct verbal counselling before semen collection. Fertil Steril 1995;64:657–60.
27. Eggert-Kruse W, Pohl S, Näher H, Tilgen W, Runnebaum G. Microbial colonization and sperm-mucus interaction: results in 1000 infertile couples. Hum Reprod 1992;7:612–20.
28. Liversedge NH, Jenkins JM, Keay SD, McLaughlin EA, Al-Sufyan H, Maile LA, et al. Antibiotic treatment based on seminal cultures from asymptomatic male partners in in-vitro fertilization is unnecessary and may be detrimental. Hum Reprod 1996;11:1227–31.
29. Tournaye H, Van Sterteighem AC, Devroey P. Pentoxifylline in idiopathic male-factor infertility: a review of its therapeutic efficacy after oral administration. Hum Reprod 1994;9:996–1000.
30. Okada H, Tatsumi M, Kanzaki M, Fujisawa M, Arakawa S, Kamidono S. Formation of reactive oxygen species by spermatozoa from asthenospermic patients: response to treatment with pentoxifylline. J Urol 1997;157:2140–46.
31. Knuth UA, Hölnigl W, Bals-Pratch M, Schleicher G, Nieschlag E. Treatment of severe oligospermia with human chorionic gonadotropin/menopausal gonadotropin: a placebo-controlled, double-blind trial. J Clin Endocrinol Metab 1987;65:1081–87.
32. Acosta AA, Œhninger S, Erfunc H, Philput C. Possible role of pure human FSH in the treatment of seven male-factors infertility by assisted reproduction: preliminary report. Fertil Steril 1991;55:1150–56.
33. Acosta AA, Khalifa E, Œhninger S. Pure human FSH has a role in the treatment of severe infertility by assisted reproduction: Norfolk's total experience. Hum Reprod 1992;7:1067–72.
34. Bartoov B, Eltes F, Lunenfeld E, Har-Even D, Lederman H, Lunenfeld B. Sperm quality of subfertile males before and after treatment with human FSH. Fertil Steril 1994;61:727–34.
35. Strehler E, Sterzick K, De Santo M, Abt M, Wiedermann R, Bellatti U, et al. The

effect of FSH therapy on sperm quality: an ultrastructural mathematical evaluation. J Androl 1997;18:437–39.

36. Matorras R, Pérez G, Corcostegui B, et al. Treatment of the male with FSH in intrauterine insemination with husband's spermatozoa: a randomized study. Hum Reprod 1997;12:24–28.

37. Baccetti B, Strehler E, Capitani S, Collodel G, De Santo M, Moretti E, et al. The effect of FSH therapy on human sperm structure (Notulae Seminologicae 11). Hum Reprod 1997;12:1955–68.

38. Radicioni A, Paris E, Dondero F, Bonifacio V, Isidori A. Recombinant-growth hormone (rec-hGH) therapy in infertile men with idiopathic oligozoospermia. Acta Eur Fertil 1994;25:311–17.

39. Lee KO, Ng SC, Lee PS. The effect of growth hormone therapy on men with severe idiopathic oligozoospermia. Eur J Endocrinol 1995;132:159–62.

40. Ovesen P, Jörgesen JOL, Kjaer T, Ho KKY, Orskov H, Christiansen JS. Impaired growth hormone secretion and increased growth hormone-binding protein levels in subfertile males. Fertil Steril 1996;65:165–69.

41. Shimonovitz S, Zacut D, Ben Chetrit A, Ron M. Growth hormone status in patients with maturation arrest of spermatogenesis. Hum Reprod 1993;8:919–21.

42. Ovesen P, Jörgesen JOL, Kjaer T, Ho KKY, Orskov H, Christiansen JS. Growth hormone treatment of subfertile males. Fertil Steril 1996;66:292–98.

43. Aitken RJ, Clarkson JS. Cellular basis of defective sperm function and its association with the genesis of reactive oxygen species by human spermatozoa. J Reprod Fertil 1987;81:291–98.

44. Iwasaki A, Gagnon C. Formation of reactive oxygen species in spermatozoa of infertile patients. Fertil Steril 1992;57:409–13.

45. Lenzi A, Culasso F, Gandini L, Lombardo F, Dondero F. Placebo-controlled, double-blind, cross-over trial of glutathione therapy in male infertility. Hum Reprod 1993;8:1657–62.

46. Lenzi A, Picardo M, Gandini L, et al. Glutathione treatment of dyspermia: effect on the lipoperoxidation process. Hum Reprod 1994;9:2044–50.

47. Kessopoulou E, Powers HS, Sharma KK, et al. A double-blind randomized placebo cross-over controlled trial using the antioxidant vitamin E to treat reactive oxygen species associated male infertility. Fertil Steril 1995;64:825–31.

48. Geva E, Bartoov B, Zabludovsky N, Lessing JB, Lerner-Geva L, Amit A. The effect of antioxidant treatment on human spermatozoa and fertilization rate in an in vitro fertilization program. Fertil Steril 1996;66:430–34.

49. Suleiman SA, Ali ME, Zaki ZMS, El-Malik EMA, Nasre MA. Lipid peroxidation and human sperm motility: protective role of vitamin E. J Androl 1996;17:530–37.

50. Bentiviglio G, Melica F, Cristoforoni P. Folinic acid in the treatment of human male infertility. Fertil Steril 1993;60:698–701.

51. Kiss AS, Viski S, Szöllösi J, Csikkel-Szonlnoki A. Effect of magnesium therapy on human semen and plasma Mg levels and on the volume of the ejaculate and the number and motility of spermia. Magnes Bull 1996;18:96–99.

52. Maseki Y, Miyake K, Mitsuya H, Kitamura H, Yamada K. Mastocytosis occurring in the testes from patients with idiopathic male infertility. Fertil Steril 1981;36:814–17.

53. Yamamoto M, Hibi H, Miyake K. New treatment of idiopathic severe oligozoospermia with mast cell blocker: results of a single-blind study. Fertil Steril 1995;64:1221–23.

54. Siterman S, Eltes F, Wolfson V, Zabludovsky N, Bartoov B. Effect of acupuncture on

sperm parameters of male suffering from subfertility related to low sperm quality. Arch Androl 1997;39:155–61.

55. Thompson W, Traub AJ, Earn Shaw JC. Effect of kallikrein on sperm motility. Arch Androl 1980;5(Suppl):A117.

56. Schill WB, Miska W. Possible effects of the kallikrein-kinin system on male reproductive functions. Andrologia 1992;24:69–75.

57. Izzo PL, Canale D, Bianchi B, et al. The treatment of subfertile men with kallikrein. Andrologia 1984;16:156–61.

58. Glezerman M, Lunenfeld E, Potashnik G, Huleihel M, Soffer Y, Segal S. Efficacy of kallikrein in the treatment of oligozoospermia and asthenozoospermia: a double-blind trial. Fertil Steril 1993;60:1052–56.

59. Keck C, Behre HM, Jockenhövel F, Nieschlag E. Ineffectiveness of kallikrein in treatment of idiopathic male infertility: a double-blind, randomized, placebo-controlled trial. Hum Reprod 1994;9:325–29.

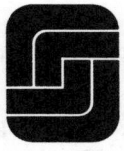

8

In Vitro Therapy for Sperm Motility: Specific and Nonspecific Treatments

SAMIR HAMAMAH, GENEVIÈVE GRIZARD, ALAIN FIGNON,
SHARON T. MORTIMER, AND DAVID MORTIMER

Introduction

Powerful assisted reproductive techniques (ART) have been developed to treat infertility. Intrauterine insemination (IUI) and in vitro fertilization (IVF) have been employed widely and allowed many couples the reward of children. With the improved ability to manipulate gametes precisely and routinely, intracytoplasmic sperm injection (ICSI) became possible and today represents one of the greatest technological advances in our capacity to treat various forms of infertility due to severe sperm defects. This highly technical treatment, however, is still not available in all ART centers and has been suggested to have a major drawback in that it bypasses the roocyte's natural barriers that might discriminate spermatozoa before fertilization.

All of these ART methods require a sperm population that is as clean as possible to increase the likelihood of successful fertilization. The human ejaculate is a mixture of dead and live spermatozoa mixed with cellular debris and nongametic cells such as lymphocytes suspended in the fluids coming from several regions of the male genital tract. Separation of motile spermatozoa from the other components of semen is essential because seminal plasma contains undesirable bioactive substances such as decapacitation factors (which prevent capacitation and hyperactivation) or proteolytic enzymes with deleterious effects on the sperm membrane that result in the loss of fertilizing ability (1,2). Before attempting IUI or IVF it is also necessary to increase the proportion of motile spermatozoa, as well as their mean velocity (although modern concepts of sperm movement analysis consider the kinematics of sperm subpopulations based upon functional criteria [e.g., hyperactivation (3,4)] because there is clear evidence for an association between the success of these treatments and these sperm motility parameters

95

(5–13). Improved motility is not the only factor involved because the physiological processes of sperm capacitation and hyperactivation must be achieved for successful IVF. *Hyperactivation* is the term used to describe changes in the movement of capacitating spermatozoa from a fairly rigid flagellar beat pattern into an asymmetric whiplash pattern reflected in an increased amplitude of lateral head displacement (14–20). This beating pattern is generally considered to be necessary in vivo for spermatozoa to migrate through the secretions of the female genital tract (21,22) as well as to penetrate the egg vestments (23–25).

This chapter is not intended to be an exhaustive review of all suggested in vitro treatments to improve sperm motility and the capacitation/hyperactivation steps; rather, it is meant to report and discuss some of the developments in (1) sperm preparation techniques for obtaining sperm suspensions from ejaculates with increased proportions of highly motile and morphologically normal cells without inducing any concomitant reduction in fertilizing capacity (e.g., swim-up, PureSperm), and (2) the use of specific or nonspecific biological and chemical factors that can stimulate sperm motility and/or fertilizing ability (e.g., human follicular fluid, oviduct fluid, prostasomes, human serum, 2'-deoxyadenosine, pentoxifylline, caffeine, cAMP, taurine).

Sperm Preparation Techniques

Various sperm preparation methods have been developed over the years, including simple centrifugation and washing, swim-up techniques, density gradient (continuous or discontinuous) centrifugation, and column filtration. Density gradient methods have become very popular because they both separate the spermatozoa from seminal plasma and simultaneously select a population of normal and highly motile spermatozoa. Simplified and microscale gradient methods have been introduced and developed for asthenozoospermic samples (26). Percoll gradients improve the fertilization rates in vitro (27–31), and higher clinical pregnancy rates have also been reported (26,32). Furthermore, excellent results have been obtained using Percoll gradients as the sperm preparation method for patients with male infertility. As a result, simple discontinuous density gradient methods are now the most commonly adopted by ART laboratories; however, because of the withdrawal of Percoll from all clinical applications by its sole manufacturer, Pharmacia Biotech, alternative methods must be used.

Simple Dilution and Washing Techniques

When spermatozoa are separated from seminal plasma by centrifugation the sperm pellet comprises both the good spermatozoa and the dead spermatozoa as well as the other cellular elements of the semen. In this case the functional potential of the motile cells, even after isolation, is impaired (33). Decreased sperm fertilizing capacity is due to both the physical effects of the *g* force applied and the production of reactive oxygen species (ROS) within the pellet, which cause irreversible damage to the spermatozoa (33). For this reason, any sperm preparation method that involves the centrifugal pelleting of unselected seminal sperm populations should be avoided (27).

Migration Techniques

Swim-Up from a Washed Pellet

In this technique the washed sperm pellet is overlayered with fresh medium and incubated so that the motile spermatozoa can swim out of the pellet into the upper layer. Although this approach had been used successfully in many ART programs, which demonstrated that the initial washing/centrifugation steps did not completely destroy the fertilizing capacity of spermatozoa, the IVF success rates obtained using this procedure were sometimes low, especially in male factor cases. This has been attributed to ROS-induced damage during the initial washing step (27).

Swim-Up from a Washed Sperm Preparation

In this swim-up method one or two washing steps are used to separate the unselected spermatozoa from seminal plasma and resuspend them in a culture medium from which they can then migrate into an overlayer of fresh medium (34). Although the method may produce a cleaner sperm preparation than swim-up from a washed pellet, it should be considered suspect for the same reasons of possible ROS-induced sperm dysfunction as swim-up from a washed pellet (27).

Direct Swim-Up from Semen

In this method liquefied semen is layered beneath culture medium, ideally in a round-bottom tube, and incubated for 15–60 min to allow the motile spermatozoa to migrate from the semen into the medium layer. After recovery of the upper medium layer, avoiding the interface, it is usually washed once (maximum 600 *g* for 10 min) and resuspended into fresh medium for use.

Sperm Select™

This alternative direct swim-up method uses a highly purified preparation of sodium hyaluronate at a final concentration of 1 mg/ml in culture medium. In an IVF program, swim-up from semen into Sperm Select™ gave a significantly higher percentage of motile spermatozoa compared with swim-up from a washed pellet as well as a higher pregnancy rate (35); however, it was not ascertained whether these improved results were due specifically to the use of the hyaluronate (perhaps by a capacitation effect) or to the use of a method that did not involve the intial pelleting of unselected spermatozoa.

Selective Washing Techniques

These methods are based on the use of centrifugation through continuous or discontinous density gradients to fractionate subpopulations of spermatozoa. Discontinous gradients are widely used in clinical IUI, IVF, and ICSI programs. Although the discontinous layers can lead to the problem of rafting of cells at the interface(s), passage through such interfaces may be advantageous for selecting only the best spermatozoa.

Percoll Gradients

Prior to mid-1996 density gradient centrifugation using Percoll (polyvinyl-pyrrollidone-coated silica particles) had gained widespread popularity, particularly for abnormal semen samples. The use of Percoll had been promoted for the rapid and efficient isolation of normal motile spermatozoa, which are freed of contamination by other seminal constituents. In the original paper by Berger et al. (30) isotonic Percoll (approximately 300 mOsm) was made by mixing 9 vol. of the commercial Percoll product with 1 vol. of modified (10 × strength) Ham's F-10, and, after adjusting the mixture to pH 7.4, diluting it with culture medium in order to obtain 30, 50, 60, 70, 80, and 90% (v/v) solutions were layered to form a discontinuous gradient. Only two layer Percoll gradients were used more recently: the upper layer was about 40–45% and the lower was between 80 and 90% (v/v). Liquefied semen, or semen diluted with medium, were placed onto the gradient and centrifuged at low speed (about 300 g) for 20 minutes. Spermatozoa separated on discontinuous Percoll gradients form distinct bands at the interfaces between the different Percoll concentrations with the fraction in the region between 80 and 90% containing optimal yields of motile, functional spermatozoa. With this procedure abnormal spermatozoa and seminal debris are largely eliminated, and there is a reduction in oxidative damage of sperm membranes by free radicals from contaminating cells or abnormal spermatozoa (27,33). After the first centrifugation the 80 to 90% layer or the soft pellet at the bottom of the tube were resuspended in fresh medium and centrifuged (maximum 600 g for 10 min). The final pellet was recovered, again resuspended into fresh medium, and used for insemination either in vivo or in vitro.

Although Percoll gradients produced a higher recovery than swim-up preparation for oligoasthenozoospermic patients, there were not always significant differences in the yield of spermatozoa with progressive motility between Percoll and direct swim-up (36). Swim-up, however, typically selected higher proportions of spermatozoa with improved characteristics, such as velocity, intact acrosome, and normal morphology (36).

Silane-Coated Colloidal Silica Gradients

Colloids made using silane-coated silica particles have become available from different vendors as replacements for Percoll (e.g., PureSperm from Nidacon International AB, Göteborg, Sweden, and ISolate from Irvine Scientific, Santa

Ana, CA, USA). These products are reported to have very low endotoxin levels, unlike Percoll, which has been reported as often showing very high levels of endotoxin contamination. When other colloids were compared with Percoll to determine its usefulness for separating cryopreserved human spermatozoa (37), it was found that although the sperm motility was almost the same, sperm recovery was higher using the other colloids. The colloid solutions also gave more variable results, and some had detrimental effects on the selected spermatozoa.

The commercial preparation PureSperm was evaluated for human spermatozoa as an alternative for Percoll. In this study no significant differences were found between the sperm populations obtained from either gradient material regarding the recovery yield, sperm kinematics, or hyperactivation rates (29). PureSperm apparently allows the preparation of selected, highly motile populations of human spermatozoa and now seems to be the most widely used Percoll replacement worldwide; however, published clinical results are needed before its use can be considered completely routine. Isolate is believed to be applicable in the same manner as PureSperm.

In routine use, PureSperm is used in very much the same way as Percoll, except that it is supplied as either ready-to-use 40 and 80% or 45 and 90% solutions, or as a 100% stock that is mixed with an appropriate culture medium to the required concentrations. It is recommended that the diluent for 100% PureSperm should be a HEPES-buffered medium to avoid pH shifts when used under an air atmosphere, and that it should contain a protein such as human serum albumin (HSA) at a concentration of at least 10 mg/ml. Prepared PureSperm solutions (like Percoll) can be filter-sterilized using 0.22 μm filters that do not release extractable wetting agents or other materials (e.g. Millipore Millex-GV). Two-step discontinuous gradients of 1.5- or 2.0-ml layers are prepared in conical-bottom centrifuge tubes (e.g., Falcon 2095) and semen, either diluted or not, is layered on top (up to about 1.5 ml of semen per gradient, but this is dependent upon the sperm concentration and debris, etc. content of the specimen that can cause excessive rafting at the interfaces). After a first centrifugation step at 300 g for 20 min in a swing-out rotor the seminal plasma, upper interface, 40/45% PureSperm and lower interface are removed carefully (do not remove the lower layer as this will cause substantial contamination of the pellet). Using a clean pipette the soft pellet at the bottom of the tube is then carefully aspirated, transferred to a clean tube, and mixed with about 10 ml of bicarbonate-buffered medium that contains at least 10 mg/ml HSA. This is then centrifuged at a maximum of 600 g for up to 10 min, the supernatant is aspirated, and the pellet is resuspended in fresh bicarbonate-buffered medium for use after determining the concentration of progressively motile spermatozoa and making any necessary adjustments.

Filtration Methods

Different types of filtration column have been used to separate motile from immotile spermatozoa (e.g., glass wool and Sephadex beads).

Glass Wool

Glass wool filtration has been used with several mammalian species spermatozoa to obtain a highly motile fraction. It has been reported that glass wool
filtration and a Percoll gradient gave equivalent results in that no difference
in fertilization was observed after ICSI using spermatozoa separated by either
method (38). It has also been suggested that this preparation method might be
used with oligozoospermic semen, although this was only demonstrated with
artificially created samples (39).

SpermPrep Column

This commercial column is based on sperm filtration through Sephadex beads
and should separate spermatozoa from the biological constituents of the surrounding medium. Several authors have tested its efficiency and compared the
results with the Percoll separation (e.g., 40–42). From these studies it appears that
the SpermPrep produces sperm populations with better morphology than swim-
up, and improved motility similar to two-layer Percoll gradients.

Stimulation of Sperm Motility

In vitro stimulation of sperm motility is aimed at enhancing sperm function,
primarily by increasing the level of intracellular cAMP that is believed to
play a key role in regulating sperm function. In addition, in vitro stimulation
may result in an appropriate change in cytosolic calcium levels that control
sperm flagellar bending and are involved in capacitation and hyperactivation.
Many substances have been suggested for the in vitro stimulation of human
sperm function, including poorly defined biological fluids such as serum
(43), peritoneal fluid (44), human follicular fluid (45–51), and prostasomes
(52,53), as well as well-defined agents such as hormones (e.g., prostagandins)
(54,55), and progesterone (56), enzymes (e.g., kallikrein and kinin) (57–59),
platelet activating factor (60,61), creatine phosphate (62), the calcium ionophore A23187 (63), calcium chelators (64), hyaluronic acid (65), glycosaminoglycans (66), cyclic nucleotide analogues (59), and adenosine analogues
(67–70). Most attention has probably been devoted to the methylxanthine
group, particularly caffeine, pentoxifylline (PTX), theophylline, and 3-isobu-
tyl-1-methylxanthine (IBMX).

Biological Stimulation of Human Spermatozoa

Human Follicular Fluid

Several studies have provided evidence for an effect of human follicular fluid
(HFF) on in vitro capacitation, mainly based on the changes of sperm motility
(45–51). Treatment of human spermatozoa with HFF can improve both pen-

etration rates in the hamster egg penetration test and fertilization rates in human in vitro fertilization (71,72). Hyperactivation has also been observed following HFF treatment and has been identified in human spermatozoa as well as in other species. Percoll-selected spermatozoa incubated with HFF for short periods (2 hours) showed significantly increased progressive motility, straight-line velocity (VSL), and hyperactivation than the untreated spermatozoa (51).

Various factors with a stimulatory effect on sperm motility and/or the acrosome reaction have been identified in HFF, including albumin, glycosaminoglycans, and progesterone (66,73,74, for review, see 75). Progesterone, and some of its derivatives, are able to induce capacitation and promote the acrosome reaction via an influx of calcium (73,76). It has been argued strongly that progesterone (or a protein-progesterone complex) acts via a specific membrane receptor that opens a chloride channel (77). Progesterone has also been incorporated into media used for sperm preparation in order to increase the quality of the selected sperm populations.

Prostasomes

Seminal plasma contains factors detrimental to sperm motility (78) as well as beneficial ones. A positive influence of prostate-derived organelles, designated prostasomes (see later), on various aspects of sperm motility have been described. For example, inclusion of prostasomes in swim-up media may increase the recovery of motile spermatozoa and have a beneficial effect on ALH and the proportion of hyperactivated spermatozoa for up to 6 hours (52). A positive effect of prostasomes on the motility of buffer-washed normal human spermatozoa exhibiting no forward motility was also demonstrated (53).

Prostasomes are multilamellar vesicles with a specific and characteristic lipid composition. They have a large proportion of cholesterol and a cholesterol-to-phospholipid ratio of about 2. Sphyngomyelin is the major phospholipid (about 50%) and the associated fatty acids are both saturated and unsaturated. In the ordered membrane of these organelles enzymes such as ATPases, both calcium- and magnesium-dependent, have been demonstrated. A protein kinase and phospholipase A_2 activities have also been demonstrated (79). Prostasome vesicles are rich in calcium and GDP. They can interact with spermatozoa either directly by a fusion process mediated by a slightly acidic mediator by an action on their surrounding environment (80,81). Heat treatment (100°C, 3 min) and ultrasonication do not diminish the beneficial effect of prostasomes on sperm motility, it is therefore unlikely that enzymatic systems are involved in their mechanism of action (52). This is also supported by the decreased sperm plasma membrane fluidity after fusion with prostasomes (82). A protective effect against peroxidation has also been suggested, with the lipids of the vesicle membranes acting as scavengers for the free oxygen radicals produced by leukocytes contaminating semen. Taken

together, these results suggest that prostasomes could be protective and mo-
tility-enhancing natural substances that may be clinically useful in ART, particularly for asthenozoospermic patients.

Prostasomes act in a dose- and time-related fashion and their effects can be
prolonged and improved by the addition of glucose, and by the addition of
adenine in the presence of magnesium ions (83,84). In one study, we also
observed a slight effect of prostasomes on the motility of washed human
spermatozoa (Table 8.1).

Glycosaminoglycans

Glycosaminoglycans (GAGs) have been isolated from bovine and human follicular fluid and have been suggested to play a role in the preservation of sperm
motility, as well as in the induction of the sperm acrosome reaction (85,86). GAGs
are composed of repeating disaccharide units that are generally covalently attached to a protein core to form a proteoglycan. Chondroitin-sulphates (CS) were
identified as the predominant GAGs among follicular proteoglycans. In addition,
HFF appears to contain a chondroitin-sulphate that improves the retention of
sperm motility (87). Hyaluronic acid (HA) was also identified as a component of
GAGs prepared from follicular fluid.

When spermatozoa were incubated in culture medium supplemented with
20% hFF treated by chondroitinase or hyaluronidase, a significant decrease
in sperm motility was observed (66). After short (2-hours) incubation in culture medium supplemented with chondroitin and hyaluronic acid the mean
values of the percentage of motility, VSL, ALH, and hyperactivation were
significantly increased as compared with the untreated group. After long incubation (24 hours), however, there were no significant differences. With human spermatozoa, hyaluronic acid has been shown to induce capacitation
(88) and to maintain sperm motility (89). More recently, a hyaluronan receptor has been described on the surface of human, rat, and bull spermatozoa
(90,91).

Pharmacological Stimulation of Sperm Motility

Sperm motility is believed to be controlled intracellularly by the level of
cAMP and the phosphorylation of several intracellular proteins (92). A subtle
equilibrium may exist between the cAMP production, phosphodiesterase activity, the different protein kinases, and phosphatases that act on the flagellar
proteins and cellular metabolism in order to maintain sperm movement (93).
These various factors are certainly also involved in regulating the different
physiological motility phases that occur during passage of the spermatozoon
from the male genital tract to the site of fertilization in the ampulla of the
oviduct. During sperm preparation in vitro, several pharmacological compounds have been tested for manipulating the second messenger pathways in
attempts to improve sperm motility and fertilizing ability.

TABLE 8.1. Effects of prostasomes on human sperm motility % (normozoospermic patients).

Parameters	Time (h)	PBS	PBS + Prostasomes	Supernatant (S)	S + Prostasomes
Total motility (%)	1	50 ± 3	54 ± 5	50 ± 3	51 ± 3
	4	40 ± 4	38 ± 5	41 ± 9	45 ± 4*
Forward motility (%)	1	28 ± 3	33 ± 4*	31 ± 3	35 ± 4
	4	16 ± 3	18 ± 3	23 ± 2	26 ± 3*
VCL (μm/s)	1	65 ± 4	68 ± 2	55 ± 3	62 ± 3*
	4	58 ± 3	66 ± 3*	54 ± 3	5 ± 3
VSL (μm/s)	1	32 ± 3	33 ± 2	34 ± 2	38 ± 2*
	4	29 ± 2	34 ± 4	31 ± 1	31 ± 1
ALH (μm)	1	3.2 ± 0.2	3.4 ± 0.1	2.7 ± 0.2	2.8 ± 0.2
	4	3.1 ± 0.1	3.4 ± 0.3	3.1 ± 0.1	3.2 ± 0.2

Values are mean ± SEM. * $p < 0.01$, * p 0.05

Methylxanthines

When added to human semen in vitro, caffeine, pentoxifylline (PTX), and several other phosphodiesterase inhibitors have been found to produce increases in intracellular cAMP, cellular glycosis, and ATP production. These substances can increase the proportion of motile spermatozoa and initiate motility in nonmotile vital spermatozoa. Caffeine and PTX were also reported to enhance the motility of frozen-thawed spermatozoa (94). In addition, PTX has been shown to improve sperm motion in samples obtained by electroejaculation (95), and to enhance sperm binding to the zona pellucida (96). PTX is also used in combination with 2'-deoxyadenosine, which potentiates its effect on phosphodiesterase.

Several reviews on the mode of action of these pharmacological compunds, and the results obtained in IVF, have been published (97–101), from which it can be concluded that the beneficial effect of these compounds on sperm fertilizing ability is highly dependent upon the individual, and that large discrepencies exist in the results of different studies. Tables 8.2 to 8.4 summarize the studies that deal with caffeine or pentoxifylline on either fresh or frozen-thawed spermatozoa obtained from normozoospermic or asthenozoospermic patients. The observed differences between studies may be due to: (1) the type of infertile male population studied; (2) the drug concentrations used; and (3) the duration of various incubation periods.

Conflicting data continue to be published, mainly on the use of pentoxifylline, because in vitro caffeine stimulation has been largely abandoned due to its detrimental effects on the acrosome reaction and on the quality of the sperm membrane counterbalancing its beneficial effect on mo-

TABLE 8.2. Effects of caffeine on human sperm motility (normozoospermic patients).

	Concentration (mM)	Incubation times	Significant improvement	Reference
Fresh sperm				
Semen	0.03–0.06–0.1–0.25–1.0	0–4 h	Motility%, VCL	122
Percoll	0.003–0.02–1.7–5.0–17	5 min, 4 h	Motility%, VCL, ALH	123
Washed	0.1–3.0	0, 1.5, 3, 4.5h	Motility%, VSL, ALHM	124
Frozen sperm				
Semen	7.5	15–30–45–60 mn	Motility%, linearity	59
Pellet	3.0	30mn, and 4h	ALH, HA%	70

TABLE 8.3. Effects of pentoxifylline on human sperm motility (normozoospermic patients).

Sperm	Concentration (mM)	Incubation times	Significant improvement	Reference
Fresh sperm				
Washed	0.1 to 3.0	0, 1.5, 3.0, 4.5 h	Motility %, VSL, VCL	124
Sperm-swim-up	3.6	10 min	VSL, VCL, ALH, HA %, LIN	105
Washed	5.0	30 min—4 h	Motility %, VCL, ALH	126
Swim-up	3.6	30 mn	VCL, ALH, LIN, HA %	125
Swim-up	3.6	1 h	ALH, HA %	127
Washed	3.6	1, 2, 4 h	HA %	106
Sperm-swim-up	3.6	0, 1.5, 3.0 h	Motility %	130
Frozen sperm				
Semen	3.6	15, 30, 45, 60 min	Velocity, motility %	59
Sperm-Percoll	3.6	15, 45, 75 min, 2, 4 h	HA %	125
Pellet	3.0	1 h	ALH, HA %	70
Washed	3.0	15 min	Motility %, ALH	25
Washed	3.0	30 min, 3 h, 24 h	Motility % VSL, VCL, ALH	128
Washed	1, 3, 10	30 min, 1 h	Motility%, progressive motility %	129

TABLE 8.4. Effects of pentoxifylline on human sperm motility (asthenozoospermic patients).

Sperm	Drug	Concentration (mM)	Incubation times	Significant improvement	Reference
Washed	Caffeine	0.1, 1.0, 3.0	0, 1.5, 3.0, 4.5 h	Motility %, VSL, VCL	95
Washed	PTX	0.1, 1.0, 3.0	0, 1.5, 3.0, 4.5 h	Motility %, VSL, VCL, LIN	95
Sperm-swim-up	PTX	3.6	10 min	VSL, VCL, LIN, VAP, HA %	105
Washed	PTX	3.6	1, 2, 4 h	HA %	106
Washed	PTX/2 DA	3.6/3.0	0, 3 h	HA %	99

tility. In addition, in a clinical trial, caffeine did not appear to improve the sperm fertility.

In vivo studies where infertile males were treated orally with PTX seemed to show improved sperm quality, and oral pentoxifylline treatment at high concentration has been reported to decrease the formation of ROS in asthenozoospermic samples (102,103). PTX as an oral medication had previously been reported to have no better effect than placebo (see Ref. 97).

In vitro, PTX acts as a phosphodiesterase inhibitor at the cellular level, but additional effects on sperm membrane fluidity via increased lipid peroxidation and inhibition of superoxide dismutase have been observed (104). An inhibitory effect of high concentration PTX on peroxide formation in asthenozoospermic samples has also been reported (101). Furthermore, the observation that PTX and PTX + 2'-deoxyadenosine can affect the development of mouse embryos adversely has raised questions as to the clinical usefulness of this drug (99). Because this effect is due to a direct action of PTX on the egg, an alternative could be to remove the drug from the medium that surrounds the spermatozoa before the fertilization step, especially because it was suggested that the effect on sperm motility after removal of the stimulant lasts for at least 3 hours (105) or 4 hours (106) in normozoospermic sperm samples, and for at least 2 hours in asthenozoospermic samples. One study indicated, however, that motility activation was lost rapidly after drug removal (96). Nonetheless, the detrimental effect of PTX on embryo development clearly indicates caution in its possible clinical use.

Reactive Oxygen Species

Reactive oxygen species (ROS) are generated by the human spermatozoa. Inadvertent generation of these harmful molecules during sperm preparation must be controlled because they have profound effects upon human spermatozoa, both detrimental and beneficial (107,108). Although ROS production in the environment surrounding the spermatozoa induces a decrease in sperm motility and viability, it also seems to play a role in promoting capacitation, hyperactivation, and the acrosome reaction. The beneficial effect of prostasomes, and the possible effects of pentoxifylline upon ROS formation, have been described earlier.

Alpha-tocopherol (vitamin E) is a known antioxidant agent. Administered orally, vitamin E was shown to improve sperm motility and decrease peroxide formation in a man with athenozoospermia (109). The in vivo pregnancy rate can also be improved by this treatment (109,110), although oral treatment with this vitamin did not increase its concentration in seminal plasma above the critical concenetration required for it to act as an ROS scavenger in vitro (111). In vivo, the vitamin E concentration in the seminal plasma was found to be related to both sperm motility and the presence of leukocytes (112), and is increased in cases of immunological infertility (113). Together, these data suggest that alpha-tocopherol plays a protective role in the semen in vivo in cases of immunopathology.

The role of alpha-tocopherol in vitro to preserve human semen quality requires further study. Only a small improvement in motility of frozen-thawed human spermatozoa has been reported (114), but a protective effect against the lipid peroxidation of boar spermatozoa in vitro has been reported (115).

Nitric Oxide

Nitric oxide (NO) is a cytotoxic free radical that is produced by nitric oxide synthase, an enzyme that has been immunolocalized in the head and midpiece of the human spermatozoon, and shown to be active (116). Nitric oxide may act to inactivate superoxide and increase intracellular cGMP. Low levels of NO seem necessary for sperm motility and capacitation/hyperactivation, and high levels are detrimental to spermatozoa (117,118). A high level of NO is also associated with poor motility in infertile men (119). Addition of sodium nitroprusside, a nitric oxide releaser, to the spermatozoa of asthenozoospermic infertile men improved their motility significantly (120).

It should be noted that polyamines, which are present in normal seminal plasma, become inhibitors of NO synthesis when converted into their aldehyde form by an oxidase (121). The complete elimination of seminal plasma could therefore be of importance in such cases of infertility.

The major factor that controls sperm motility is the availability of adenosine triphosphate (ATP), the energy substrate for the dynein-ATPase, produced by the mitochondria and transported to the axoneme through the mediation of phosphorylcreatinine (PCr). To produce ATP, human spermatozoa mainly metabolize exogenous energy substrates (e.g., fructose, lactate, pyruvate, or glucose) present in the seminal plasma, the female genital tract, or in the culture media used for in vitro sperm preparation for ART. Spermatozoa sustain their energy demands mainly from glycolysis, and to a lesser extent from mitochondrial oxidative phosphorylation (17). The availability of ATP, the key regulator of sperm motility, is controlled by calcium, cyclic nucleotides, and internal pH.

Conclusions

It is clear that motility is only one of many functional activities required for a spermatozoon to reach and fertilize the oocyte. The beneficial effect of in vitro sperm preparation (e.g., direct swim-up from semen, PureSperm density gradients) on sperm motility (percent motile) has been well documented. Choosing an appropriate sperm preparation technique should take into account the relative simplicity and rapidity of the method, for reasons of laboratory efficiency, as well as the quality of the semen samples and the selected sperm populations produced. One must also remember that there may well be substantial interindividual variability in which technique provides the optimum yield, even for samples of apparently comparable semen quality.

On the other hand there is some evidence to support the use of biological or chemical agents to improve sperm motility in samples obtained from asthenozoospermic patients. Whichever technique is used, however, any in vitro stimulation treatment of human spermatozoa in an attempt to increase motility must be aimed at improving sperm function, without creating any concomitant functional loss, either in sperm fertilizing capacity or in the developmental competence of resulting embryos.

References

1. Kanwar KC, Yanagimachi R, Lopata A. Effects of human seminal plasma on fertilizing capacity of human spermatozoa. Fertil Steril 1976;31:321–27.
2. Rogers BJ, Bastias C, Russell LD, Peterson RN. Cytochalasin-D inhibition of guinea pig sperm actin reduces fertilization. Ann N Y Acad Sci 1988;513:566–68.
3. Mortimer ST. A critical review of the physiological importance and analysis of sperm movement in mammals. Hum Reprod Update 1997;3:403–39.
4. ESHRE Andrology Special Interest Group. Guidelines on the application of CASA technology in the analysis of spermatozoa. Hum Reprod 1998;13:142–45.
5. Holt WW, Moore HDM, Hillier SG. Computer-assisted measurement of sperm swimming speed in human semen: correlation of results with in vitro fertilization assays. Fertil Steril 1985;44:112–19.
6. Hinting A, Comhaire F, Vermeulen L, Dhont M, Vermeulen A, Vandekerckhove D. Value of sperm characteristics and results of in vitro fertilization for predicting the outcome of assisted reproduction. J Androl 1989;13:59–66.
7. Grunert JH, De Geyter C, Bordt J, Schneider HPG, Neischlag E. Does computerized image of sperm movement enhance the predictive value of semen analysis for in vitro fertilization results? Int J Androl 1989;12:329–38.
8. Jeulin C, Feneux D, Serres C, et al. Sperm factors related to failure of human in vitro fertilization. J Reprod Fertil 1986;76:735–44.
9. Chan SYW, Wang C, Chan STH, et al. Predictive value of sperm morphology and movement characteristics in the outcome of in vitro fertilization of human oocytes. J In Vitro Fertil Embryo Trans 1989;6:142–48.
10. Bongso TA, Ng SC, Mok H, et al. Effect of sperm motility on human in vitro fertilization. Arch Androl 1989;22:185–90.

11. Oehninger S, Acosta R, Kruger T, et al. Relationship between morphology and motion characteristics of human spermatozoa in semen and the swim-up fractions. J Androl 1990;11:446–52.
12. Gerris J, Khan I. Correlation between in vitro fertilization and human sperm density and motility. J Androl 1987;8:48–53.
13. Talbert LM, Hammond MG, Halme J, O'Rand M, Fryer JG, Ekstrom RD. Semen parameters and fertilization of human oocytes in vitro: a multivariable analysis. Fertil Steril 1987;48:270–77.
14. Yanagimachi R. In vitro capacitation of hamster spermatozoa by follicular fluid. J Reprod Fertil 1969;18:275–86.
15. Barlow P, Devligne A, Van-Dromme J, Van-Hoeck J, Vandenbosch K, Leroy F. Predictive value of classical and automated sperm analysis for in vitro fertilization. Hum Reprod 1992;6:1119–24.
16. Hinney B, Wilke G, Michelmann HW. Prognostic value of an automated sperm analysis in IVF or insemination therapy. Andrologia 1993;25:195–202.
17. Ford WCL, Rees JM. The bioenergetics of mammalian sperm motility. In: Gagnon C, editor. Controls of sperm motility: biological and clinical aspects. Boca Raton, FL: CRC Press, 1990:175–202.
18. Gwatkin RBL, Anderson OF. Capacitation of hamster spermatozoa by bovine follicular fluid. Nature 1969;224:1111–12.
19. Burkman LJ. Characterization of hyperactivated motility by human spermatozoa during capacitation: comparison of fertile and oligozoospermic sperm populations. Arch Androl 1984;13:153–65.
20. Mortimer D, Courtot AM, Giovangrandi Y, Jeulin C, David G. Human sperm motility after migration into, and incubation in synthetic media. Gamete Res 1984;9:131–44.
21. Katz DF, Yanagimachi R. Movement characteristics of hamster spermatozoa within the oviduct. Biol Reprod 1980;22:759–64.
22. Demott RP, Suarez SS. Hyperactivated sperm progress in the mouse oviduct. Biol Reprod 1992;45:779–85.
23. Fraser L. Dibutyryl cyclic AMP decreases capacitation time in vitro in mouse spermatozoa. J Reprod Fertil 1981;62:63–72.
24. Katz DF, Cherr GN, Lambert H. The evolution of hamster sperm motility during capacitation and interaction with the ovum investments in vitro. Gamete Res 1986;14:333–46.
25. Wang C, Lee GS, Leung A, Surrey ES, Chan SYW. Human sperm hyperactivation and acrosome reaction and their relationships to human in vitro fertilization. Fertil Steril 1993;59:1221–27.
26. Ord T, Patrizio P, Marello E, Balmaceda JP, Asch RH. Mini-Percoll: a new method of semen preparation for in vitro fertilization in severe male factors infertility. Hum Reprod 1990;5:987–89.
27. Mortimer D. Sperm preparation techniques and iatrogenic failures of in vitro fertilization. Hum Reprod 1991;6:173–76.
28. Forster MS, Smith WD, Lee WI, Berger RE, Karp LE, Stenchever MA. Selection of human spermatozoa according to their relative motility and their interaction with zona-free hamster eggs. Fertil Steril 1983;40:655–65.
29. Kossakowski J, Morrison L, Mortimer D. Evaluation of PureSperm gradients instead of Percoll for human spermatozoa. Hum Reprod 1997;12:88 (Abs).

30. Berger T, Marrs RP, Moyer DL. Comparison of techniques for selection of motile spermatozoa. Fertil Steril 1985;43:268–73.
31. Hyne RV, Stojanoff A, Clarke GN, Lopata A, Johnston WIH. Pregnancy from in vitro fertilization of human eggs after separation of motile sperm by density gradient centrifugation. Fertil Steril 1986;45:93–96.
32. Guérin JF, Mathieu C, Lornage J, Pinatel MC, Boulieu D. Improvement of survival and fertilizing capacity of human spermatozoa in an IVF programme by selection on discontinuous Percoll gradients. Hum Reprod 1989;4:798–804.
33. Aitken RJ, Clarkson JS. Cellular basis of defective sperm function and its association with the genesis of reactive oxygen species by human spermatozoa. J Fertil Reprod 1987;81:459–69.
34. Russell LD, Rogers BJ. Improvement in the quality and fertilization potential of a human sperm population using the rise technique. J Androl 1987;8:25–30.
35. Wikland M, Wiko O, Quist K, Soderlund B, Janson PO. A self migration method for preparation of sperm for in vitro fertilization. Hum Reprod 1987;2:191–95.
36. Ng FLH, Liu DY, Gordon Baker HW. Comparison of Percoll, mini-Percoll and swim-up methods for sperm preparation from abnormal semen samples. Hum Reprod 1992;7:261–66.
37. Perez SM, Chan PJ, Patton WC, King A. Silane coated silica particle colloid processing of human sperm. J Assist Reprod Genet 1997;14:388–93.
38. Van-den-Bergh M, Revelard P, Bertrand E, Birmane J, Vanin AS, Englert Y. Glass wool column filtration an advantageous way of preparing semen samples for intracytoplasmic sperm injection: an auto-controlled randomized study. Hum Reprod 1997;12:509–13.
39. Johnson DE, Confino E, Jeyendran RS. Glass wool column filtration versus mini Percoll gradient for processing poor quality semen samples. Fertil Steril 1996;66:459–62.
40. Zavos PM, Correa JR, Sofikitis N, Kofinas GD, Zarmakoupis PN. A method of short term cryostorage and selection of viable sperm for use in the various assisted reproductive techniques. Tohoku J Exp Med 1995;176:75–81.
41. Smith S, Hosid S, Scott L. Use of postseparation sperm parameters to determine the method of choice for sperm preparation for assisted reproductive technology. Fertil Steril 1996;63:591–97.
42. Yamamoto Y, Maenosono S, Okada H, Miyagawa I, Sofikitis N. Comparisons of sperm quality, morphometry and function among human sperm populations recovered via SpermPrep II filtration, swim-up and Percoll density gradient methods. Andrologia 1997;29:303–10.
43. Makler A, Fisher M, Murillo O, Laufer N, DeCherney A, Naftolin F. Factors affecting sperm motility. IX. Survival of spermatozoa in various biological media and under different gaseous compositions. Fertil Steril 1984; 41:428–32.
44. Soldati G, Piffaretti-Yanez A, Campana A, Marchini M, Luerti M, Balerna M. Effect of peritoneal fluid on sperm motility and velocity distribution using objective measurements. Fertil Steril 1989;52:113–19.
45. Suarez SS, Wolf DP, Meizel S. Induction of the acrosome reaction in human spermatozoa by a fraction of human follicular fluid. Gamete Res 1986;14:107–21.
46. Mbizvo M, Burkman LJ, Alexender NJ. Human follicular fluid stimulates hyperactivated motility in human sperm. Fertil Steril 1990;54:708–12.
47. Mendoza C, Tesarik J. Effect of follicular fluid on sperm movement characteristics. Fertil Steril 1990;54:1134–39.

48. Siegel MS, Paulson RJ, Graczykowski JW. The influence of human follicular fluid on the acrosome reaction, fertilizing capacity and proteinase activity of human spermatozoa. Hum Reprod 1990;5:975–80.

49. Falcone L, Gianni S, Piffaretti-Yanez A, Marchini M, Eppenberger U, Balerna M. Follicular fluid enhances sperm motility and velocity in vitro. Fertil Steril 1991;55:619–26.

50. Hamamah S, Chevrier C, Royere D, Lansac J, Gatti JL, Dacheux JL. Follicular fluid: effects on survival/motility of human spermatozoa. Assist Reprod Technol Androl 1992;3:75–80.

51. Hamamah S, Lanson M, Barthelemy C, Garrigue MA, Lansac J, Royere D. Treatment of human spermatozoa with follicular fluid can influence the lipid content and the motility during in vitro capacitation. Reprod Nutr Dev 1993;33:429–35.

52. Fabiani R, Johanson L, Lundkvist Ö, Ronquist G. Enhanced recruitment of motile spermatozoa by prostasome inclusion in swim-up medium. Hum Reprod 1994;9:1485–89.

53. Fabiani R, Johanson L, Lundkvist Ö, Ulmsten U, Ronquist G. Promotive effect by prostasomes on normal human spermatozoa exhibiting no forward motility due to buffer washings. Eur J Obstet Gynecol Reprod Biol 1994;57:181–88.

54. Aitken RJ, Kelly RW. Analysis of the direct effects of prostaglandins on human sperm function. J Reprod Fertil 1985;73:139–46.

55. Colon JM, Ginsburg F, Lessing JB, et al. The effect of relaxin and prostaglandin E2 on the motility of human spermatozoa. Fertil Steril 1986;46:1133–39.

56. Uhler M, Leung A, Chan SYW, Wang C. Direct effects of progesterone and antiprogesterone on human sperm hyperactivated motility and acrosome reaction. Fertil Steril 1992;58:1191–98.

57. Schill WB, Haberland GL. Kinin induced enhancement of sperm motility. Hoppe-Seyler's Z Physiol Chem 1974;355:229–31.

58. Sato H, Hchill WB. Temperature dependent effects of the components of kallikrein-kinin system on sperm motility in vitro. Fertil Steril 1987;47:684–88.

59. Hammitt DG, Bedia E, Rogers PR, Syrop CH, Donovaan JF, Williamson RA. Comparison of motility stimulants for cryopreserved human semen. Fertil Steril 1989;52:495–502.

60. Ricker DD, Minhas BS, Kumar R, Robertson JL, Dodson MG. The effects of platelet activating factor on the motility of human spermatozoa. Fertil Steril 1989;52:655–58.

61. Wang R, Sikka SC, Veeraragavan K, Bell M, Hellstrom WJG. Platelet activating factor and pentoxifylline as human sperm cryoprotectants. Fertil Steril 1993;60:711–15.

62. Fakih H, MacLusky N, DeCherney A, Wallimann T, Huszar G. Enhancement of human sperm motility and velocity in vitro: effects of calcium and creatine phosphate. Fertil Steril 1986;46:938–44.

63. Pilikian S, Adeleine P, Czyba JC, Ecochard R, Guerin JF, Mimouni P. Hyperactivated motility of sperm from fertile donors and asthenozoospermic patients before and after treatment with ionophore. Int J Androl 1991;14:167–73.

64. Hong CY, Chiang BN, Ku J, Wei YH. Calcium chelators stimulate sperm motility in ejaculated human semen. Lancet 1984;i:460–61.

65. Huazar G, Willetts M, Corrales M. Hyaluronic acid (sperm Select) improves retention of sperm motility and velocity in normospermic and oligospermic specimens. Fertil Steril 1990;54:1127–34.

66. Hamamah S, Wittemer CH, Barthelemy C, et al. Identification of hyaluronic acid and chondroitin sulfates in human follicular fluid and their effects on human sperm motility and the outcome in vitro fertilization. Reprod Nutr Dev 1996;36:43–52.
67. Aitken RJ, Mattei A, Irvine S. Paradoxical stimulation of human sperm motility by 2-deoxyadenosine. J Reprod Fertil 1986;78:515–27.
68. Imoedemhe DAG, Sigue AB, Pacpaco ELA, Olazo AB. Successful use of the sperm motility enhancer 2-deoxyadenosine in previously failed human in vitro fertilization. J Assist Reprod Genet 1992;9:53–56.
69. Imoedemhe DAG, Sigue AB, Pacpaco ELA, Olazo AB. In vitro fertilization and embryonic development of oocytes fertilized by sperm treated with 2-deoxyadenosine. Int J Fertil 1993;38:235–40.
70. Mbizvo MT, Johnston RC, Baker GHW. The effect of the motility stimulants caffeine, pentoxifylline and 2-deoxyadenosine on hyperactivation of cryopreserved human sperm. Fertil Steril 1993;59:1112–17.
71. Yee B, Cummings LM. Modification of the sperm penetration assay using human follicular fluid to minimize false negative results. Fertil Steril 1988;50:123–28.
72. Ghetler Y, Ben-Nun I, Kaneti H, Jaffe R, Gruber A, Fejgin M. Effect of preincubation with follicular fluid on the fertilization rate in human in vitro fertilization. Fertil Steril 1990;54:944–46.
73. Blackmore PF, Beebe SJ, Danforth DR, Alexander N. Progesterone and 17 a-hydroxyprogesterone. Novel stimulators of calcium influx in human sperm. J Biol Chem 1990;25:1376–80.
74. Kulin S, Bastiaans BA, Hollanders HMG, Janssen HJG, Goverde HJM. Human serum and follicular fluid stimulate hyperactivation of human spermatozoa after preincubation. Fertil Steril 1994;62:1234–37.
75. Kopf GS, Kalab P, Leclerc P, Ning XP, Pan D, Visconti P. Signal transduction in mammalian spermatozoa. In: Verhoen G, Habenicht U-F, editors. Molecular and cellular endocrinology of the testis. Berlin: Springer, 1994:153–83.
76. Thomas P, Meizel S. An influx of extracellular calcium is required for initiation of the human sperm acrosome reaction induced by human follicular fluid. Gamete Res 1988;20:397–411.
77. Tesarik J, Mendoza C, Moos J, Fénichel P, Fehlmann M. Progesterone action through aggregation of a receptor on the sperm plasma membrane. FEBS Lett 1992;308:116–20.
78. Robert M, Gagnon C. Purification and characterization of the active precursor of a human sperm motility inhibitor secreted by the seminal vesicles: identity with semenogelin. Biol Reprod 1996;55:813–21.
79. Arvidson G, Ronquist G, Wikander G, Öjteg AC. Human prostasomes membranes exhibit very high cholesterol/phospholipid ratio yielding high molecular ordering. Biochim Biophys Acta 1989;984:167–73.
80. Ronquist G, Nilsson BO, Hjerten S. Interaction between prostasomes and spermatozoa from human semen. Arch Androl 1990;24:147–57.
81. Arienti G, Carlini E, Palmerini CA. Fusion of human sperm to prostasomes at acidic pH. J Membr Biol 1997;155:89–94.
82. Carlini E, Palmerini CA, Cosmi EV, Arienti G. Fusion of sperm with prostasomes: effects on membrane fluidity. Arch Biochem Biophys 1997;343:6–12.
83. Stegmayr B, Ronquist G. Stimulation of sperm progressive motility by organelles in human seminal plasma. Scand J Urol Nephrol 1982;16:85–90.

84. Fabiani R, Johanson L, Lundkvist Ö, Ronquist G. Prolongation and improvement of prostasome promotive effect on sperm forward motility. Eur J Obstet Gynecol Reprod Biol 1995;58:191–98.

85. Lenz RW, Ax RL, Grimek HJ, First NL. Proteoglycan from bovine follicular fluid stimulates an acrosome reaction in bovine spermatozoa. Biochem Biophys Res Commun 1982;106:1092–98.

86. Eriksen GV, Malmström A, Carlstedt I, Uldbjerg N. Human follicular fluid contains two large proteoglycans. In: Leppert PC, Woessner F, editors. The extracellular matrix of the uterus, cervix and fetal membranes: synthesis, degradation and hormonal regulation. Ithaca, New York: Perinatology Press, 1991:274–78.

87. Eriksen GV, Malmström A, Uldbjerg N, Huszar G. A follicular fluid chondroitin sulfate proteoglycan improves the retention of motility and velocity of human spermatozoa. Fertil Steril 1994;62:618–23.

88. Karlstrom PO, Bakos O, Bergh T, Lundkvist O. Intrauterine insemination and comparison of two methods of sperm preparation. Hum Reprod 1991;6:390–95.

89. Huazar G, Willetts M, Corrales M. Hyaluronic acid (sperm Select) improves retention of sperm motility and velocity in normospermic and oligospermic specimens. Fertil Steril 1990;54:1127–34.

90. Kornovski BS, McCoshen J, Kredentser J, Turley E. The regulation of sperm motility by a novel hyaluronan receptor. Fertil Steril 1994;61:935–40.

91. Ranganathan S, Ganauly AK, Datta K. Evidence for presence of hyaluronan binding protein on spermatozoa and its possible involvement in sperm function. Mol Reprod Dev 1994;38:69–76.

92. Yanagimachi R. Mammalian fertilization. In: Knobil E, Neill JD, Ewing L, Market CL, Greenwald GS, Pfaff DW, editors. The physiology of reproduction. New York: Raven Press, 1994:189–221.

93. Vijarayaghavan S, Trautman KD, Goueli SA, Carr DW. A tyrosine-phosphorylated 55-kDa motility associated bovine sperm protein is regulated by cAMP and calcium. Biol Reprod 1997;56:1450–57.

94. Barkay J, Zuckerman H, Sklan D, Gordon S. Effect of caffeine on increasing the motility of frozen human sperm. Fertil Steril 1977;28:175–77.

95. Sikka SC, Hellstrom WJG. The application of pentoxifylline in the stimulation of sperm motion in men undergoing electroejaculation. J Androl 1991;12:165–70.

96. Paul M, Sumpter JP, Lindsay KS. The paradoxical effects of pentoxifylline on the binding of spermatozoa to the human zona pellucida. Hum Reprod 1996;11:814–19.

97. Lanzafame F, Chapman MG, Guglielmino A, Gearon CM, Forman RG. Pharmacological stimulation of sperm motility. Hum Reprod 1994;9:192–99.

98. Matson PHL, Yovich JM, Edirisinghe WR, Junk SM, Yovich JL. An argument for the past and continued use of pentoxifylline in assisted reproductive technology. Hum Reprod 1995;10(Suppl 1):67–71.

99. Tournaye H, Devroey P, Camus M, Van-der-Linden M, Janssens R, Van-Steirteghem A. Use of pentoxifylline in assisted reproductive technology. Hum Reprod 1995;10(Suppl 1):72–79.

100. Schill WB. Survey of medical therapy in andrology. Int J Androl 1995;18 (Suppl 2):56–62.

101. Merino G, Martinez-Chequer JC, Barahona E, et al. Effects of pentoxifylline on sperm motility in normogonadotrophic asthenozoospermic men. Arch Androl 1997;39:65–69.

102. McKinney KA, Lewis SE, Thompson W. The effects of pentoxifylline on the generation of reactive oxygen species and lipid perioxidation in human spermatozoa. Andrologia 1996;28:15–20.
103. Okada H, Tatsumi N, Kanzaki M, Fujisawa M, Arakawa S, Kamidono S. Formation of reactive oxygen species by spermatozoa from asthenospermic patients: response to treatment with pentoxifylline. J Urol 1997;157:2140–46.
104. Nivsarkar M, Patel RY, Mokal R. Modulation of sperm membrane conformation by pentoxifylline in oligospermia: a biophysical investigation of sperm membrane in vitro. Bichem Biophys Res Commun 1996;225:791–95.
105. Tesarik J, Thébault A, Testart J. Effect of pentoxifylline on sperm movement characteristics in normozoospermic and asthenozoospermic specimens. Hum Reprod 1992;7:1257–63.
106. Pang SC, Chan PJ, Lu A. Effects of pentoxifylline on sperm motility and hyperactivation in normozoospermic and normokinetic semen. Fertil Steril 1993;60:336–43.
107. De Lamirande E, Gagnon C. A positive role for superoxide anion in triggering hyperactivation and capacitation of human spermatozoa. Int J Androl 1993;16:21–25.
108. Aitken J, Fisher H. Reactive oxygen species generation and human spermatozoa: the balance of benefit and risk. Bioessays 1994;16:259–67.
109. Suleiman SA, Ali ME, Zaki ZM, el Malik EM, Nasr MA. Lipid perioxidation and human sperm motility: protective role of vitamin E. J Androl 1996;17:530–37.
110. Geva E, Bartoov B, Zabludovsky N, Lessing JB, Lerner-Geva L, Amit A. The effect of antioxidant treatment on human spermatozoa and fertilization rate in an in vitro fertilization program. Fertil Steril 1996;66:430–34.
111. Moilanen J, Hovatta O. Excretion of alpha-tocopherol into human seminal plasma after oral administration. Andrologia 1995;27:133–36.
112. Therond P, Auger J, Legrand A, Jouannet P. Alpha-tocopherol in human spermatozoa and seminal plasma: relationships with motility, antioxidant enzymes and leukocytes. Mol Hum Reprod 1996;10:739–44.
113. Palan P, Naz R. Changes in various antioxidant levels in human seminal plasma related to immunoinfertility. Arch Androl 1996;36:139–43.
114. Askari HA, Check JH, Peymer N, Bollendorf A. Effect of natural antioxidants tocopherol and ascorbic acids in maintenance of sperm activity during freeze-thaw process. Arch Androl 1994;33:11–15.
115. Brezezinska-Slebodzinska E, Slebodzinski AB, Pietras B, Wieczorek G. Antioxidant effect of vitamin E and glutathione on lipid perioxidation in boar semen plasma. Biol Trace Elem Res 1995;47:69–74.
116. Lewis SE, Donnelly ET, Sterling ES, Kennedy MS, Thompson W, Chakravarthy U. Nitric oxide synthase and nitrite production in human spermatozoa: evidence that endogenous nitritic oxide is beneficial to sperm motility. Mol Hum Reprod 1996;2:873–78.
117. Zini A, De Lamirande E, Gagnon C. Low levels of nitric oxide promote human sperm capacitation in vitro. J Androl 1995;16:424–31.
118. Rosselli M, Dubey RK, Imthur B, Macas E, Keller PJ. Effects of nitric oxide on human spermatozoa: evidence that nitric oxide decreases sperm motility and induces sperm toxicity. Hum Reprod 1995;10:1786–90.
119. Nabunaga T, Tokugawa Y, Hashimoto K, et al. Elevated nitric oxide concentration in the seminal plasma of infertile males: nitric oxide inhibits sperm motility. Am J Reprod Immunol 1996;36:193–97.

120. Zhang H, Zheng RL. Possible role of nitric oxide on fertile and asthenozoospermic infertile human sperm functions. Free Radic Res 1996;25:347–57.
121. Szabo C, Southan GJ, Wood E, Thiemermann C, Vane JR. Inhibition by spermine of the induction of nitric oxide synthase in J774.2 macrophages: requirement of a serum factor. Br J Pharmacol 1994;112:355–56.
122. Ruzich JV, Gill H, Wein AJ, Van Arsdalen K, Hypolite J, Levin RM. Objective assessment of the effect of caffeine on sperm motility and velocity. Fertil Steril 1987;48:891–93.
123. Rogberg L, Fredricsson B, Poussette A. Effects of propanolol and caffeine on movement characteristics of human sperm. Int J Androl 1990;13:87–92.
124. Sikka SC, Hellstrom WJC. Functional evaluation and motility parameters of pentoxifylline-stimulated cryopreserved human sperm. Assist Reprod Technol Androl 1990;1:309–19.
125. Kay VJ, Coutts JRT, Robertson L. Pentoxifylline stimulates hyperactivation in human spermatozoa. Hum Reprod 1993;8:727–31.
126. Fuse H, Sakamoto M, Ohta S, Katayama T. Effect of pentoxifylline on sperm motion. Arch Androl 1993;31:9–15.
127. Lewis SEM, Moohan J, Thompson W. Effect of pentoxifylline on human sperm motility in normospermic individuals using computer assisted analysis. Fertil Steril 1993;59:418–23.
128. Aribarg A, Sukcharoen N, Jetsawangsri U, Chanprasit Y, Ngeamvijawat J. Effects of pentoxifylline on sperm motility characteristics and motility longevity of post-thaw cryopreserved semen using computer assisted semen analysis. J Med Assoc Thai 1994;77:71–75.
129. Brennan AP, Holden CA. Pentoxifylline supplemented cryoprotectant improves human sperm motility after cryoconservation. Hum Reprod 1995;10:2308–12.
130. Tarlatzis BC, Kolibianakis EM, Bontis J, Tousiou M, Lagos S, Mantalenakis S. Effect of pentoxifylline on human sperm motility and fertilizing capacity. Arch Androl 1995;34:33–42.

Part III

ICSI Option for Immotile Sperm

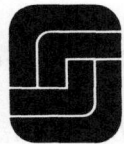

9

Injection Procedures of Immotile Sperm: Selection, Tail Breakage, and Viscous Solutions

SIMON FISHEL, STEVEN GREEN, ALISON HUNTER-CAMPBELL,
LOUISE GARRATT, HELEN McDERMOTT, SIMON THORNTON,
KENNETH DOWELL, AND JOHN WEBSTER

The early microinjection of mammalian eggs began around the 1950s and 1960s with the work of Lin (1–3), who studied the technical experimental nature of egg "micrurgy" (4). This preceded the early studies in the mid-1960s that investigated the early events of fertilization using sperm microinjection in different species (5–7). The clinical use of this procedure sprang from the work of Palermo et al. in 1992 (8); however, attempts by numerous groups to achieve consistent and efficient results with intracytoplasmic sperm injection (ICSI) proved difficult. Initial concerns were focused on the control required to aspirate motile sperm in culture medium and manipulate its injection into the cytoplasm. Two problems were apparent: gaining control of the injection process and the injection of a motile sperm per se. ICSI is now a highly reproducible, efficient, and effective method of procuring fertilization, even with retrieved gamete ratios at unity. This chapter will describe the conditions under which ICSI should be performed to guarantee a high efficiency of fertilization and a low incidence of oocyte damage.

Immobilization of Sperm

The idea of using viscous solutions to slow down and temporarily immobilize sperm motility stems from the early attempts to use sperm-immobilizing agents for human vaginal contraception (9–11). The immobilizing agents were generally metallic copper and iron, or salts of these heavy metals. Suitable vehicles for vaginal therapy were investigated, and these needed to present a physical barrier to sperm migration. The agents considered suitable for the purpose in studies performed during the 1970s were hydroxypropylmethylcelluloses (HMYC) and polyvinylpyrrolidone (PVP).

Immobilizing Sperm for ICSI

By 1995 ICSI was routine in most major units that utilized microinjection technology, but there was still considerable variation in the incidence of fertilization and outcome. There was a substantial "learning curve" to achieve successful ICSI. In 1995 we published the first and only study that systematically examined the treatment of sperm and its effect on sibling oocytes (12). This study evaluated different treatments of sperm from the same sample and compared the incidence of fertilization of each method using sibling oocytes. The data shown in Table 9.1 demonstrate a significant increase in the incidence of fertilization with sperm whose tails were permanently damaged (crimped) compared with temporarily immobilized or motile sperm. This work was confirmed by other studies (13,14), although Hoshi et al. (13) claimed that immobilizing sperm was unnecessary for achieving success with ICSI. In this study different patient groups were used to compare the different approaches, which included the use of A23187 or electroporation to activate the microinjected oocyte. Furthermore, the incidence of fertilization per oocyte injected ranged from 45 to 52%, which is considerably lower than what is generally achieved with immobilized sperm. Another study from Palermo et al. (14) compared two types of immobilization technique: "standard" and "aggressive," but different patients were evaluated rather than sibling oocytes. The "standard" approach was compression of the sperm flagellum, similar to that described by Fishel et al. (12) as "temporary immotile"; the "aggressive" approach was to damage the tail permanently, causing a kink posterior to the midpiece. The results from this study are shown in Table 9.2. Although fertilization rates in the region of 70% per oocyte were achieved, there was a significantly higher incidence of fertilization with the "aggressive" immobi-

TABLE 9.1. Pretreatment of injected sperm for ICSI[*] (53 patients 540 M^2 sibling oocytes).

Sperm treatment	%2 PN Fertilization
Group 1 (Sluggish)	25[†‡]
Group 2 (Temporary immotile)	36[†‡]
Group 3 (Inherent motility)	47[§]
Group 4 (Permanent damage)	62[‡§]

[*]C From Fishel et al. 1995 (12).
[†]NS   [‡]$p < 0.0001$ [§]$p < 0.02$

TABLE 9.2. Type of sperm immobilization* (N.B. Study per patient, not sibling oocytes).

| | Sperm treatment | | | |
| | "Aggressive" | | "Standard" | |
Sperm origin	No. Oocytes	% Fertilization	No. Oocytes	% Fertilization
Ejaculate	922	73[†]	5497	70[†]
Testicular	12	67[‡]	22	51[‡]

*From Palermo et al. 1996 (14).
[†]$P = 0.03$ [‡]NS

lization, which confirmed the study of Fishel et al. (12). The Palermo study (14) showed no statistical difference between the two methods using testicular sperm, the incidence of fertilization with the "aggressive" approach was 67%, but only 12 oocytes were injected, compared with 41% for the "standard" method ($n = 22$ oocytes). It would be wise to draw no conclusion from such small numbers of oocytes.

Evaluating the various studies in the literature (few established as randomized control studies), it appears necessary to permanently immobilize the sperm flagellum posterior to the midpiece to achieve the maximum incidence of fertilization. There is no data either way to establish whether there is an overall effect on the incidence of pregnancy once fertilization has been achieved. A study by Dozortzev et al. (15) to investigate the relevance of sperm immobilization demonstrated that the sperm plasma membrane is ruptured and becomes permeable for thiol-reducing agents, which may be involved in decondensation of the sperm nucleus in vivo (16). By permeabilizing the sperm membrane sperm-associated oocyte-activating factors may be released, as well as sensitizing the sperm nucleus to decondensing factors.

A potentially important aspect of the Dozortzev study (15) was the effect of the use of PVP during immobilization and sperm injection. PVP was shown to stabilize the sperm membrane and prevent thiol-reducing agents from gaining access to the nucleus. It is unclear whether this was a membrane stabilization effect or an effect on modification of other chemical substances. The suggestion, however, that the presence of PVP may prevent the beneficial effects obtained by damage to the plasma membrane led Dozortzev et al. (17) to conclude that care should be taken when transferring PVP to the oocyte. The presence of PVP during the transfer of sperm to oocyte may explain the delay between sperm injection and the beginning of calcium oscillations observed in some studies (18). No data have been provided on the approach of Dozortzev et al. (15) in washing off the PVP before injection into the oocyte. Whether this would be beneficial over and above minimal deposition of medium with the immobilized sperm needs to be evaluated.

In 1996, Hunter et al. (19) confirmed the observation of Dozortzev that the plasma membrane integrity was lost by permanently immobilizing the sperm tail. Further observations of Hunter et al., however, showed no significant difference in acrosomal status, indicating that sperm plasma membrane damage did not increase the incidence of acrosome-reacted sperm—a suggestion proffered by a number of workers.

Efficiency of ICSI

One method of defining the efficiency of the technique of ICSI is to compare the incidence of fertilization between different practitioners who adhere rigidly to protocol. Table 9.3 demonstrates the incidence of two pronucleate fertilizations and the percentage degeneration of oocytes between four different CARE practitioners who have utilized this technology in numerous units worldwide. The variation in the incidence of fertilization was between 61 and 69% (not significant), and there was an indistinguishable uniformity in the number of oocytes surviving the procedure. Hence, by adhering to a rigid protocol the intervariation between practitioners is extremely low, and to reduce the incidence of degeneration of oocytes (if possible) and to improve the incidence of fertilization (if possible) beyond these results would require a change to protocol rather than the skill of the practitioner. For example, if it were possible to reduce the incidence of degenerate oocytes after ICSI, attention ought to be given to the method of injection and its effects on the cytoskeleton of the oocyte. Attempts to increase the incidence of fertilization, if this can be achieved, should focus on the volume of medium injected, contamination with PVP, sperm quality, activation, and so on.

Table 9.4 demonstrates the results obtained by the four CARE practitioners, using the ICSI protocol of permanent immobilization, for different conditions of extreme male-factor infertility. In this particular cohort of patients, the incidence of fertilization using unselected nonmotile sperm was 23%, compared with 51% if the sperm was selected using hypoosmotic medium. It is clear from assessing individual patient data, however, that these results are extremely variable and it is likely that the outcome in such cases depends on flagella abnormalities and intrinsic centrosomal defects, rather than simply the vitality of the spermatozoon. There was a similarly significantly lower incidence of fertilization with globozoospermia and in patients with ciliary dyskinesia (Kartagener syndrome).

TABLE 9.3. Efficiency of ICSI with CARE practitioners.

Operator	No. Oocytes	% 2 PN	% Degenerate
A	2446	69	14
B	1965	65	14
C	1860	66	14
D	1748	61	14

TABLE 9.4. Incidence of fertilization in "extreme" cases of
male-factor infertility.

Condition	% Fertilization (per oocyte)
Azoospermic (testicular sperm)	64
Cryptozoospermia	58
Selected non-motile	51
Unselected non-motile	23
Globozoospermia	29
Kartagener syndrome	18

Sperm Control and Viscous Solutions for ICSI

Two systems of control were utilized: during the early developments of microinjection: pneumatic or hydraulic, of which the latter was based mainly on using paraffin oil. There are clear advantages and disadvantages to both systems, but the significant advantage of a hydraulic system is the immediate degree of control over the elements being manipulated. Extreme precision, however, can also be obtained by aspiration of the viscous solution into the tip of the microneedle.

By transferring sperm to a viscous solution, such as 10% PVP (w/v) or 3% MYC (w/v) motility will be severely impaired. This procedure simplifies the process of immobilization. Once immobilized, and according to the data of Dozortzev (15), the plasma membrane, although damaged, may be stabilized by the viscous solution and a number of immobilized sperm may be kept "on hold" before microinjection into the oocyte.

A study was performed to compare the use of MYC or PVP as a transport medium for sperm immobilization and microinjection for ICSI. We performed this study on 29 patients and inclusion criteria required each to have >9 M^2 oocytes for ICSI. The cohort for oocytes was split into two groups where either PVP or MYC was used for ICSI in each group. PVP was at a concentration of 100 mg/ml and MYC at 30 mg/ml. In order not to prejudice the patient's chance of pregnancy, our conventional criteria for deciding upon which embryo was to be transferred took precedence over selecting for a homogeneous group with either PVP or MYC. The results of the study are shown in Table 9.5 and indicate no significant difference in the incidence of fertilization using MYC or PVP. No significant difference between the morphological grade of the embryos existed when PVP and MYC were compared, although there was a trend to a higher percentage of grade 1/2 embryos in the former; however, the incidence of clinical pregnancy was 44% from nine embryo transfers in the PVP group compared to 28.6% from seven embryo transfers in the MYC group (Table 9.6). Although these numbers were far too small to draw any

TABLE 9.5. Comparison between MYC and PVP for ICSI: 1. Outcome of fertilization and cleavage (29 patients each with > 9 oocytes, PVP 100 mg/ml, MYC 30 mg/ml, sibling oocytes).

		Outcome			
Group	No. M^2 Ooyctes	% Fertilization	% Cleavage	% Grade 1/2	% Grade 3/4
MYC	151	61	95	74	26
PVP	150	59	86	68	32

conclusions, we now continue with PVP in preference to MYC, as the latter appears to confer no advantage over PVP.

PVP Toxicity

Although intracytoplasmic sperm injection had been used since 1990 (20–22), the first published clinical successes were by Palermo (8), who used PVP as a viscous transport medium for microinjection. In 1993 concerns were raised about the potential toxicity of PVP with ICSI (20). A study by Bras et al. in 1994 (23) used a mouse zygote bioassay for assessing the effects of small amounts of different media upon embryonic development. The study compared the injection of either medium alone or three solutions of 10% PVP obtained from different suppliers. Their results suggested that some commercially produced PVP solutions were toxic, inhibiting embryonic development. There has been some concern about a high incidence of sex chromosome aneuploidies after ICSI, and some commentators have implicated PVP as a potential culprit in destabilizing chromosome formation at syngamy. There is no evidence for this, however, and the mechanism by which this is likely to occur is difficult to imagine. Investigators have continued to study the poten-

TABLE 9.6. Comparison between MYC and PVP for ICSI: 2. Outcome of embryo transfer (ET).

No. patients	29
No. with ET	29 (100%)
No. with mixed MYC/PVP embryos	13
No. with MYC embryos only	7
No. clinical pregnancies	2 (28.6%)
No. with PVP embryos only	9
No. clinical pregnancies	4 (44.4%)

tial toxic effects of PVP. A study by Ray et al. (24) used human amniotic cells cultured in the presence of 100 mg/ml or 50 mg ml/ml MYC to evaluate the mutagenic effect upon the frequency of sister chromatid exchanges (SCE). As a positive control, the authors used Mitomycin at 0.33 µg/ml, and saline was used as a negative control. Thirty cells were examined and the median SCE for saline, PVP, and MYC was 6, 5, and 6, respectively; whereas Mitomycin induced a median SCE of 25 ($p<0.001$). The authors concluded from this data that neither PVP nor MYC caused DNA lesions resulting in SCE, and "provides reassuring evidence concerning their use in sperm injection procedures." The analogy with this study and ICSI, however, is the direct injection of PVP into the ooplasm during ICSI, whereas in the study of Ray et al. the human amniotic cells were cultured in the presence of PVP or MYC. The data would have been more convincing had they proven that these substances were actually incorporated into the cytoplasm.

In a more recent study by Motoishi et al. (25) these authors examined the embryonic development of bovine zygotes after the intracytoplasmic injection of 2–3 pl of PVP. Using conventional culture medium as a control, the authors demonstrated no significant difference in the numbers of bovine embryos that developed through to the blastocyst stage and subsequently hatched. The authors also examined the cell number at the blastocyst stage. The blastocysts resulting from the zygotes that had not been injected had a mean cell number of 155, compared with 101 and 110 for zygotes injected with culture medium or PVP, respectively. The data was not significant and the authors concluded that neither the ICSI procedure itself or the presence of 2–3 pl of PVP affected the number of cells per blastocyst, or the incidence of hatching.

Conclusions

Considerable experience from many units worldwide now demonstrate that permanent sperm membrane damage is a prerequisite for consistent optimal fertilization rates with ICSI. Using this approach and ensuring that the oolemma is penetrated, variation in interpractitioner results should be minimal. For ease of sperm manipulation and tail immobilization the viscous medium, such as PVP or MYC, is appropriate. There is currently no evidence that either PVP or MYC is detrimental to fertilization or subsequent development. Studies performed to date, however, have used animal models to reflect fertilization and embryonic development, or human cells cultured but not injected with PVP or MYC to examine sister chromatid exchange. The definitive experiments on human embryos have not been performed for obvious logistical reasons. It would be reassuring, however, to have such data. Finally, in consideration of any viscous solution, it is essential to evaluate the individual commercial product and each batch prior to use: It is clear that variations can exist and, as such, the risks of potential toxicity exist.

Acknowledgment. The authors are extremely grateful to Susan Corner for her expertise and support in the preparation of this manuscript.

References

1. Lin TP. D-L-Methionine (sulphur)-35 for labelling unfertilised mouse eggs in transplantation. Nature 1956;178:1175–76.
2. Lin TP. Microinjection in mouse eggs. Science 1966;151:33–37.
3. Lin TP. Micropipetting cytoplasm from the mouse eggs. Nature 1976;216:162–63.
4. Fishel SB, Symonds EM. Gamete and embryo micromanipulation in human reproduction. London: Edward Arnold, 1993.
5. Hiramato Y. Microinjection of the live spermatozoa into sea urchin eggs. Exp Cell Res 1962;27:416–26.
6. Graham CF. The regulation of DNA synthesis and mitosis in multi-nucleate frog eggs. J Cell Sci 1966;1:363–72.
7. Brun RB. Studies on fertilisation in Xenopus laevis. Biol Reprod 1974;11:513–18.
8. Palermo G, Joris H, Devroey P, Van Steirteghem AC. Pregnancies after intracytoplasmic injection of single spermatozoon into an oocyte. Lancet 1992;340:17–18.
9. White IG. The toxicity of heavy metals to mammalian spermatozoa. Aust J Exp Biol 1955;33:359–66.
10. Saito S, Bush IM, Whitmore WF, Jr. Effects of certain metals and agents on rat and dog epididymal spermatozoan motility. Fert Ster 1967;18:517–29.
11. Loewit K. In vitro immobilization of human spermatozoa with hydroxypropylmethylcellulose. Contraception 1977;15:233–37.
12. Fishel S, Lisi F, Rinaldi L, et al. Systematic examination of immobilizing spermatozoa before intracytoplasmic sperm injection in the human. Hum Reprod 1995;10:497–500.
13. Hoshi K, Yanagida K, Yazawa H, Katayose H, Satoa A. Intracytoplasmic sperm injection using immobilised or motile human spermatozoon. Fertil Steril 1995;63:1241–45.
14. Palermo GD, Schlegel PN, Colombero LT, Zaninovic N, Moy F, Rosenwaks Z. Aggressive sperm immobilisation prior to intracytoplasmic sperm injection with immature spermatozoa improves fertilisation and pregnancy rates. Hum Reprod 1996;11:1023–29.
15. Dozortzev D, Rybouchkin A, De Sutter P, Dhont M. Sperm plasma membrane damage prior to intracytoplasmic sperm injection: a necessary condition for sperm nucleus decondensation. Hum Reprod 1995;10:2960–64.
16. Perreault SD, Wolff RA, Zirkin BR. The role of disulphide bond reduction during mammalian sperm nuclear decondensation *in vitro*. Dev Biol 1984;101:160–67.
17. Dozortzev D, De Sutter P, Rybouchkin A, Dhont M. Oocyte activation and ICSI. Assist Reprod Rev 1995;5:32–39.
18. Tesarik J, Sousa M, Testart J. Human oocyte activation after intracytoplasmic sperm injection. Hum Reprod 1994;9:511–18.
19. Hunter AJ, Stoddart NR, Fishel SB, et al. Effects of immobilisation prior to ICSI on the viability and acrosomal status of human sperm. J British Fertility Society 1997;2 (1):35.
20. Fishel S, Dowell K, Timson J, Green S, Hall J, Klentzeris L. Micro-assisted fertilisation with human gametes. Hum Reprod 1993;8:1780–84.
21. Fishel S, Timson J, Lisi F, Jacobson M, Rinaldi L, Gobetz L. Micro-assisted fertilisation in patients who have failed subzonal insemination (SUZI). Hum Reprod 1994;9:501–5.

22. Fishel S, Timson J, Green S, Hall J, Dowell K, Klentzeris L. Micromanipulation. Rev Reprod Med 1993;2:199–222.
23. Bras M, Dumoulin JCM, Pieters MHEC, Michiels AHJC, Geraedtz JPM, Evers JLH. The use of a mouse zygote quality control system for training purposes and toxicity determination in an ICSI programme. Hum Reprod 1994;9:23–24, Abstract 042.
24. Ray BD, Howell RT, McDermott A, Hull MGR. Testing the mutagenic potential of polyvinylpyrrolidone and methyl cellulose by sister chromatid exchange analysis prior to use in intracytoplasmic sperm injection procedures. Hum Reprod 1995;10:436–38.
25. Motoishi M, Goto K, Tomita K, Ookutsu S, Nakanshi N. Examination of the safety of intracytoplasmic injection procedures by using bovine zygotes. Hum Reprod 1996;11:618–20.

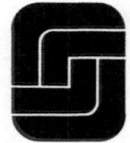

10

Fertilizing Capability of Frozen–Thawed Immotile Sperm

Raphael Ron-El, Deborah Strassburger, Yigal Soffer, Shevach Friedler, Daphna Komarovski, Orna Bern, Esti Kasterstein, Mory Schachter, and Arie Raziel

The introduction of intracytoplasmic sperm injection (ICSI) for severe male cases has made it possible to treat patients with azoospermia, in whom sperm is achieved from the epididymis and the testis (1–3). In some of the treated male patients, especially those with non-obstructive azoospermia, mainly immotile spermatozoa are available. Because it is assumed that the fertilizing potential of testicular sperm is lower (4) and motility is an important predictive factor for successful fertilization (5) it should be questioned whether ICSI perfomed with immotile sperm is justified.

Because the Microscopic Epididymal Sperm Aspiration (MESA), Percutaneous Epididymal Sperm Aspiration (PESA), Testicular Sperm Aspiration (TESA), and Testicular Sperm Extraction (TESE, namely, testicular biopsy) are all invasive methods, efforts are made to freeze supernumerary spermatozoa or testicular tissue. Several factors decrease the sperm quality derived from frozen testicular tissue: the very low concentration of the spermatozoa; the heterogeneous cell population that is frozen together with the sperm cells like red and white blood cells, cells from different stages of spermatogensis, and Sertoli cells. The preferable form of freezing testicular spermatozoa (whether as a whole tissue or by purification of testicular spermatozoa) is as yet unclear (6).

In view of all these limiting factors, the aim of the present study was to evaluate the fertilizing capability of thawed immotile sperm following ICSI.

Materials and Methods

Study Population

In all thawed sperm samples used in our IVF unit, a careful search for motile spermatozoa was performed on dozens of droplets of medium containing sperm

(Extended Sperm Preparation [ESP]) (7). Immotile spermatozoa were injected into the oocytes only when motile spermatozoa were not available.

All cases in which part or all the oocytes underwent ICSI with thawed immotile sperm were retrospectively analyzed. Because motile thawed sperm could be recovered in all ICSI cycles in which frozen thawed husband's ejaculated spermatozoa was used, the study group included only MESA–PESA–TESA and TESE cases.

Of the 31 cases with obstructive azoospermia, five underwent MESA in the beginning of our series. In the remaining 26 cases spermatozoa was retreived by PESA, and TESA was performed if no sperm was visible under the microscope. This means that in 31 treatment cycles fresh epididymal or testicular spermatozoa were used for ICSI. In addition, in 35 cycles frozen thawed sperm were used. Thawed immotile spermatozoa had to be injected in only 2 of these 35 cycles because not enough thawed motile spermatozoa were found.

Testicular sperm extraction was performed in 61 nonobstructive azoospermic patients. In 29 (48%) of them sperm could be retrieved from the testicular tissue. In 19 later occasions spermatozoa from the frozen thawed testicular tissue were used for ICSI. In 7 of these 19 treatment cycles thawed immotile spermatozoa also had to be injected into the oocytes because of lack of thawed motile sperm.

The ages of the two patients whose husband's spermatozoa was retrieved by PESA were 37 and 40. The mean age of the women whose husband underwent TESE was 34±4.4. Their controlled ovarian hyperstimulation was normally with the long protocol, starting the administration of the GnRH agonist either in the midluteal or early follicular cycle. Oocyte retrieval was performed about 36 hours after the administration of 10,000 units of human chorionic gonadotrophins.

The male patients underwent physical examination of their genitalia, testicular and transrectal sonography, assessment of hormonal profile, and cytogenetic counseling including karyotyping.

The methodology of PESA, TESA, and TESE is described in a previous study (8).

Freezing and Thawing of Sperm and Testicular Tissue

The remaining testicular tissue extract was cryopreserved, using a standard freezing protocol, with Test Yolk Buffer Freezing medium (Irvine Sceintific, Santa Anna, CA, USA.). The testicular extract was diluted dropwise 1:1 with the freezing medium, sealed in freezing straws (0.5 ml, Instruments de Medicine Veterinaire - IMV, l'Aigle, France). A simple two-step cryopreservation protocol was used. The straws were dropped in a nitrogen vapor chamber stabilized at -80°C for 20 minutes (cooling rate of -10°C/min) prior to immersion into liquid nitrogen for sperm storage at -196°C. Following removal of the straws from the liquid nitrogen, rapid thawing occurred at room temperature. The frozen-thawed sperm mixture containing cryoprotectant was then diluted with insemination medium, centrifuged at 300 g for 7 minutes, and the pellet processed for examination in multiple droplets.

Sperm collection and ICSI procedure was described in detail in our previous study (7).

Embryo Transfer, Luteal Support, and Pregnancy Evaluation

An assessment of fertilization, embryonic cleavage, and morphological quality ~24 hours later was performed. The morphological score was an average of our score system where the best morphological embryo is classified as 1 and the worst as 4. Embryo transfer was carried out into the uterine cavity. Luteal support included injections of either human chorionic gonadotrophin, every third day—2500 IU or progesterone in oil (50 mg/day, Gestone; Paines and Byrne, Surrey, UK). Serum βhCG measurement was 14 days following the embryo transfer, and only clinical pregnancies indicated by sonographic demonstration of a gestational sac were counted.

Results

Altogether 18 oocytes were injected with epididymal thawed sperm in two treatment cycles. Eight oocytes were injected with thawed immotile spermatozoa and the other 8 with thawed motile sperm. Only one egg among the former and 4 among the ones injected with thawed motile sperm fertilized. All of them cleaved. The morphology of the embryos and number of blastomeres is shown in Table 10.1.

In seven treatment cycles where thawed immotile and motile testicular sperm were used 51 oocytes were injected with thawed immotile spermatozoa and 63 with thawed motile ones. The outcome of the ICSI procedure in these

TABLE 10.1. The outcome of intracytoplasmic sperm injection in cases where thawed epididymal spermatozoon was used.

	Thawed immotile sperm	Thawed motile sperm
Injected oocytes	8	8
2 PN (fertilization)	1	4
1 PN	—	2
3 PN	1	—
Embryos	1	4
Morphology (mean)	2.5	2.2 ± 0.4
No. of blastomeres (mean)	3	2
Replaced embryos	1	4
Pregnancy	None	

TABLE 10.2. The outcome of intracytoplasmic sperm injection in cases where thawed spermatozoon was used.

	Thawed immotile sperm	Thawed motile sperm
Injected oocytes	51	63
Degenerated oocytes after ICSI	5 (10%)	7 (11%)
2 PN fertilization	16 (31%)	23 (37%)
1 PN	7 (14%)	4 (6%)
3 PN	0	4 (6%)
Embryos	12 (75%)	20 (87%)
Replaced embryos	10	20
Replaced embryos per transfer	2.3 ± 1.6	
Morphology (mean)	2.2 ± 0.6	1.8 ± 0.6
No. of blastomeres (mean)	3.6 ± 0.5	2.8 ± 0.6
Pregnancies	4	

*There were no statistically significant differences between the two groups.

cases is listed in Table 10.2. The fertilization rate of oocytes injected with thawed immotile spermatozoa was 31% and cleavage rate was 75% compared with 37% and 87%, respectively, in the oocytes that underwent ICSI with thawed motile sperm. These differences were statistically not significant. The occurrence of oocytes with single pronucleus was 14% in the oocytes injected with thawed immotile spermatozoa compared with 6% among those injected with thawed motile sperm. This difference was also not statistically different. Considering the embryo quality deriving from oocytes where thawed immotile spermatozoa were used, the morphology and mean number of blastomeres were not statistically different from the figures achieved with thawed motile spermatozoa (see Table 10.2).

In Table 10.3 the outcome of the ICSI procedure is compared between thawed immotile and motile spermatozoa in cycles leading to pregnancy.

TABLE 10.3. The comparison of ICSI outcome between oocytes injected with thawed immotile and motile spermatozoa in treatment cycles resulting in pregnancy.

	Thawed immotile sperm	Thawed motile sperm
Oocytes injected	42	17
2 PN (fertilization)	13 (31%)	6 (35%)
Embryos	10 (77%)	6 (100%)
Replaced embryos	10	6
No. of pregnancies	4	
No. of sacs	7	
No. of babies born	3	
Replaced embryos per injected oocyte	10/42 (24%)	6/17 (55%)

*There were no statistically significant differences.

Again, the fertilization and cleavage rates in the oocytes injected with thawed immotile sperm were lower than were those injected with thawed motile sperm, namely 31% and 77% compared with 35% and 100%, respectively. The differences are statistically not significant.

Embryos with acceptable morphology (I to III) were replaced into the uterine cavity. Embryo replacement was performed in all nine treated cases. Four cycles resulted with a clinical pregnancy, all of which belonged to the group where testicular thawed immotile sperm were injected. In three cases embryos deriving from thawed immotile and motile sperm were replaced together into the uterus. In the fourth case embryos developed only from oocytes injected with thawed immotile sperm and they were replaced. Three of the four pregnancies started as twin pregnancies, and the fourth had a single sac, meaning that altogether there were seven embryonal sacs. One of the twin pregnancies concluded with the birth of two healthy babies; in the second twin pregnancy only one fetus carried up to delivery whereas the other twin vanished. The third twin pregnancy and the fourth singleton pregnancy terminated as missed abortions. It can clearly be demonstrated that at least two embryonal sacs resulted from embryos where the oocytes were injected with thawed immotile spermatozoa, however, both of them terminated as missed abortions.

Discussion

The fertilizing capability of thawed sperm was already widely tested (9). The range of cryosurvival of the ejaculated sperm is huge (15–80%). Assuming that the survival of the testicular sperm is lower, questions have been raised about the usefulness of freezing testicular spermatozoa. Verheyen et al. (6) showed that testicular sperm can survive after freezing and thawing, although the motility is low—5% as mean value (range: 0–60%). Some of their thawed samples showed immediate motility after thawing but no motility after Percoll centrifugation, whereas other samples showed no motility in the beginning, but gained motility after Percoll centrifugation. The centrifugation of the sample through Percoll is to remove the cryoprotectant, which should select motile and vital sperm. The passage through the Percoll, however, induces an osmotic shock that damages the quality of the thawed testicular sperm (6). Thawed testicular sperm, unlike fresh testicular sperm, do not improve their motility after in vitro culture (10). Both motility and vitality of the sperm are affected by freezing and thawing. Both these parameters decreased to one third of their prefreeze levels (21:68 vs. 6:22) (6).

In our IVF program the sperm retrieved from patients with obstructive azoospermia had lower motility freezing–thawing. In all but two cases, however, there were always enough motile thawed spermatozoa to be injected into the oocytes. This situation was not true in the frozen–thawed spermatozoa originating from testes of patients with nonobstructive azoospermia.

Although numbers are small, the current study clearly demonstrates that the fertilizing capability of thawed immotile testicular sperm is somehow lower compared with thawed motile testicular sperm (31% vs 37%), although not statistically lower. In addition, the cleavage rate of the zygotes resulting from thawed immotile spermatozoa is lower than the rate achieved after the injection of thawed motile sperm (75% vs. 87%), with no statistically significant difference.

There are already some reports of pregnancies and deliveries resulting from the injection of fresh immotile testicular spermatozoa (11) and thawed motile testicular spermatozoa (12–14, Friedler S et al., unpublished observations); however, no one reported on pregnancies achieved from thawed immotile testicular sperm so far. In this study it was shown that the embryos achieved from the injection of thawed immotile testicular spermatozoa were not statistically different from the ones resulting from the injection of thawed motile testicular spermatozoon in terms of morphology and progress of cleavage. In two cases it was certain that the embryos resulting from thawed immotile testicular spermatozoa led to clinical pregnancy where a gestational sac was observed; however, both the twin pregnancy and the singleton terminated with a missed abortion.

Because the results are encouraging and the method to achieve testicular sperm is invasive and repeatable, this subject should be further investigated to see whether the fertilizing capacity of thawed immotile sperm can lead to viable pregnancies and deliveries.

References

1. Schoysman R, Vanderzwalmen P, Nijs M, et al. Pregnancy after fertilisation with human testicular spermatozoa. Lancet 1993;342:1237.
2. Devroey P, Liu J, Nagy Z, Tournaye H, Silber SJ, Van Steirteghem AC. Normal fertilization of human oocytes after testicular sperm extraction and intracytoplasmic sperm injection. Fertil Steril 1994;62:639–41.
3. Devroey P, Liu J, Nagy Z, et al. Pregnancies after testicular sperm extraction and intracytoplasmic sperm injection in non-obstructive azoospermia. Hum Reprod 1995; 10:101–4.
4. Nagy Z, Liu J, Janssenswillen C, Silber S, Devroey P, Van Steirteghem AC. Using ejaculated, fresh, and frozen-thawed epididymal and testicular spermatozoa gives rise to comparable results after intracytoplasmic sperm injection. Fertil Steril 1995;63:808–15.
5. Nagy Z, Liu J, Joris H, et al. The results of intracytoplasmic sperm injection is not related to any of the three basic sperm parameters. Hum Reprod 1995;20:1123–29.
6. Verheyen G, Nagy Z, Joris H, De Croo I, Tournaye H, Van Steirteghem AC. Quality of frozen-thawed testicular sperm and its preclinical use for intracytoplasmic sperm injection into in vitro-matured germinal-vesicle stage oocytes. Fertil Steril 1997;67:74–80.
7. Ron-El R, Strassburger D, Friedler S, et al. Extended sperm preparation: an alternative to testicular sperm extraction in non-obstructive azoospermia. Hum Reprod 1997;12:1222–26.

8. Friedler S, Raziel A, Strassburger D, Soffer Y, Komarovsky D, Ron-El R. Testicular sperm retrieval by percutaneous fine needle sperm aspiration compared with testicular sperm extraction by open biopsy in men with non-obstructive azoospermia. Hum Reprod 1997;12:1488–93.

9. Cohen J, Felten P, Zeilmaker GH. In vitro fertilizing capacity of fresh and cryopreserved human spermatozoa: a comparative study of freezing and thawing procedures. Fertil Steril 1981;36:356–62.

10. Edirisinghe RW, Junk SM, Matson LP, Yovitch JL. Changes in motility patterns during in-vitro culture of fresh and frozen/thawed testicular and epididymal spermatozoa: implications for planning treatment by intracytoplasmic sperm injection. Hum Reprod 1996;11:2474–76.

11. Kahraman S, Isik AZ, Vicdan K, Ozgur S, Ozgun OD. A healthy birth after intracytoplasmic sperm injection by using immotile testicular spermatozoa in a case with totally immotile ejaculated spermatozoa before and after Percoll gradients. Hum Reprod 1997;12:292–93.

12. Romero J, Remohi J, Minguez Y, Rubio C, Pellicer A, Gil-Salom M. Fertilization after intracytoplasmic sperm injection with cryopreserved testicular spermatozoa. Fertil Steril 1996;65:877–79.

13. Gil-Salom M, Romero J, Minguez Y, et al. Pregnancies after intracytoplasmic sperm injection with cryopreserved testicular spermatozoa. Hum Reprod 1996;11:1309–13.

14. Hovatta O, Foudila T, Siegberg R, Johansson K, von Smitten K, Reima I. Pregnancy resulting from intracytoplasmic injection of spermatozoa from frozen-thawed testicular biopsy specimen. Hum Reprod 1996;11:2472–73.

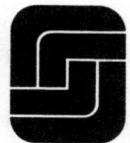

11

Clinical Aspects of ICSI
with Immotile Sperm

HERMAN TOURNAYE

The most dramatic improvement in assisted-reproductive technologies has been the introduction of intracytoplasmic sperm injection (1–3). Intracytoplasmic sperm injection (ICSI) uses only one single sperm cell in order to inseminate the oocyte. ICSI has proven to be an efficient treatment for quantitative and qualitative sperm disorders for which no specific cure exists; however, fertilization fails in about 3% of ICSI cycles (4). As can be seen from Table 11.1, fertilization fails in half of these cycles because of a given sperm factor (i.e., no motile spermatozoon available for injection) (38% of failed cycles). On the other hand, fertilization rates may also be reduced when immotile sperm are used for ICSI (Table 11.2).

Diagnosis of Absolute Sperm Immotility

An accurate clinical assessment may drastically reduce the incidence of cycles with only immotile spermatozoa available for ICSI.

Table 11.3 lists all the causes of sperm immotility and the key investigations for their diagnosis. Accurate and extensive examination of the ejaculate is needed to rule out the presence of any motile spermatozoon. The ejaculate should be produced after a standard duration of abstinence of 3 days (5). Longer abstinence intervals may lead to asthenozoospermia in oligozoospermic patients. Care should be taken to examine the semen samples at 37°C because lower temperatures may cause sperm immobilization.

The diagnosis of immotile sperm should be confirmed by at least a second semen analysis. At least two ejaculates should show absence of any motile spermatozoon, even after extended preparation and centrifugation (6,7).

If all these measures are implemented, the incidence of patients with only immotile sperm is extremely low. We analyzed 5380 ICSI cycles retrospectively and found absolute sperm immotility to be present in only 37 cycles (0.7%).

TABLE 11.1. Fertilization failure after 2732 ICSI cycles

	Cycles	Patients
Only 100% immotile spermatozoa present	29	28
Acrosomeless spermatozoa	8	6
Only one oocyte available for ICSI	14	14
Gross abnormalities in oocytes	5	5
All injected oocytes damaged	5	5
Unexplained fertilization failures	15	14

*Retrospective case series reprinted with permission from reference 2.

Investigating the absence of any sperm motility starts with history-taking and physical examination. Special inquiry should be made with regard to recurrent upper-respiratory-tract infections, history of sexually transmitted diseases and surgery of the genito-urinary tract. Familial history should also be taken because immotile-cilia syndrome may have a familial hereditary background (8). On physical examination, special attention should be paid to specific signs that may be associated with sperm immotility (e.g., dextrocardia or wheezing). Prostatic massage may be indicated whenever there is any suspicion of male accessory-gland infection (MAGI).

Additional laboratory tests may be performed. Vitality testing (5) may lead to the diagnosis of patients with absolute necrozoospermia, a condition in which all spermatozoa are dead. Patients with MAGI (e.g., chronic prostatitis) may also have absolute necrozoospermia. Patients with immotile dead sperm therefore need semen culture, urine culture after prostatic massage, and a transrectal ultrasonography (TRUS). Patients may occasionally present with 100% immotile but vital spermatozoa because of infection. *Escherichia coli*

TABLE 11.2. Results after ICSI in patients with extreme asthenozoospermia (from a retrospective case series including 901 ICSI cycles with ejaculated sperm).

	0% motility in the ejaculate and at ICSI	0% motility in the ejaculate
n of cycles (A)	12	54
n of oocytes injected oocytes	175	503
Normal fertilization (%)[†]	10.9 ± 12.1	60.2 ± 27.2
Transfer ratio[‡]	42	87
n of pregnancies (%)[§]	0 (0)	11 (20.3)

*Adapted from reference 2. Reproduced with permission.
[†]Average per cycle ± SD.
[‡]Percentage of A.
[§]Pregnancy rate per cycle between parentheses.

TABLE 11.3. Causes of complete asthenozoospermia and key investigations for diagnosis.

Immotile-cilia syndromes	Electron microscopy
ultrastructural axonemal defects	
periaxonemal ultrastructural defects	
Necrozoospermia (100% dead sperm)	Vitality testing
Enzymatic deficiencies	
Antisperm antibodies	MAR test*, IBT†
Infection (chronic prostatitis)	Culture, TRUS‡
Exposure of ejaculate to cold, spermicides	
Prolonged abstinence (?)	

*Mixed antiglobulin reaction test.
†Immunobead test.
‡Transrectal ultrasonography.

may cause complete immobilization of spermatozoa in the ejaculate. Whenever there is any evidence of MAGI, appropriate antibiotherapy should be given. Testing for antisperm antibodies should be performed in cases with viable spermatozoa. In cases with oligozoospermia, an indirect mixed antiglobulin-reaction test or immunobead test may be used (5).

If culture, antisperm antibody testing, vitality testing, and TRUS do not reveal the nature of the sperm immotility, then electron microscopy should be performed in order to diagnose axonemal defects or other functional sperm-tail defects. Electron microscopy may be performed directly whenever the patient has any signs of cilial dysfunction, such as chronic or recurrent sinopulmonary infections with or without situs inversus.

Most patients with occasionally 100% immotile spermatozoa have motile spermatozoa at subsequent ICSI cycles. Although the outcome is generally poor for ICSI in those cycles where they have only immotile sperm, they may have good fertilization in the subsequent cycles, and many of them will finally conceive. From 1991 to 1996, none but immotile ejaculated spermatozoa were used for injection in 20 ICSI cycles of 5380-TESE. The fertilization rate in these cycles was only 19.8%. No pregnancies were obtained after transferring 22 embryos in 10 transfer procedures. In nine of these cycles (eight couples) only immotile and presumably senescent spermatozoa were available. Six of these couples conceived during subsequent trials when motile spermatozoa were present in the ejaculate. In one couple (three cycles) the husband had necrozoospermia because of partial obstruction of the ejaculatory ducts. Spermatozoa were immotile in the eight remaining cycles (five couples) because of ultrastructural deficiencies, and pregnancies never ensued in subsequent cycles in these couples.

The Clinical Approach to Cases with Immotile Sperm

Whenever possible, patients with immotile sperm should be offered a specific treatment. Necrozoospermia caused by partial obstructions at the level of the ejaculatory ducts may be treated by appropriate antibiotherapy and antinflammatory drugs, which may occasionally lead to the presence of motile spermatozoa for ICSI in the ejaculate.

In other cases, transurethral resection of the prostatic verumontanum (deroofing) may improve sperm viability. If necrozoospermia is associated with vasectomy reversal, a repeat surgery may be indicated. If necrozoospermia is the result of a partial obstruction at the epididymal level a vasoepididymostomy may remedy the problem, but this surgery may also result in complete azoospermia (9).

Antisperm antibodies may be reduced by administration of corticosteroids. This treatment, however, may have serious side effects because it is estimated that it may cause aseptic necrosis of the femoral head in 1 out of 500 patients (10).

Few of these approaches may improve sperm quality to a level at which ICSI is no longer indicated but they may prevent a poor ICSI outcome.

When a patient is unexpectedly diagnosed as having 100% immotile sperm on the day of ICSI or no specific treatment is available by which to improve sperm quality, a second ejaculate should be delivered. In cycles where patients were asked to produce a second semen sample, this often contained enough motile spermatozoa to perform ICSI.

When both ejaculates contain only immotile spermatozoa, immotile but vital spermatozoa may be selected. Because most viable sperm cells have a chemically and physically intact membrane they will undergo tail swelling when exposed to a hypoosmotic medium. This hypoosmotic swelling (HOS) test may provide a simple method by which to select immotile yet vital spermatozoa. In our experience the best medium is composed of half milli-Q water and half Earle's medium containing 0.48% (v/v) HEPES and 1% human serum albumin (osmolality 285 mosmol/kg, final osmolality of the HOS medium 139 mosmol/kg) (11). The HOS-test is now increasingly used to select spermatozoa for ICSI even when the cells are motile. Casper et al. (12) reported a higher fertilization rate after ICSI with spermatozoa selected by the HOS-test than after ICSI with nonselected spermatozoa. In this small series, however, the fertilization rate after ICSI with selected spermatozoa was lower than generally reported. It is therefore far from clear whether this test may improve ICSI outcomes in general, and ICSI outcome with 100% immotile spermatozoa in particular.

Where no vital spermatozoa can be selected, we prefer to recover testicular spermatozoa. Because the majority of patients with necrozoospermia have normal spermatogenesis, testicular sperm can be recovered easily by simple percutaneous puncture or small open biopsy under local anesthesia. If spermatogenesis is normal, then these spermatozoa are often motile (13,14). Furthermore, the vitality of testicular spermatozoa is generally higher than their motility (15), and the use of testicular spermatozoa is therefore an attractive approach by which to overcome the poor fertilization rate when only senescent or dead spermatozoa are available for ICSI (16).

Table 11.4 shows the results of the 17 cycles in which the husbands were prepared to undergo a testicular sperm recovery procedure because only immotile senescent spermatozoa were available in their ejaculates. The overall fertilization rate was 63.6% and in 16 transfers a total of 45 embryos were replaced. Of the five pregnancies obtained, four resulted in the birth of a healthy child.

Testicular sperm recovery, however, will not be useful for those rare patients with axonemal defects or functional sperm-tail defects. Even if spermatozoa selected by the HOS-test are injected, results remain poor. In four couples with immotile-cilia syndrome, HOS-positive ejaculated spermatozoa were injected (seven cycles). The fertilization rate was only 29% and only seven embryos were transferred in three transfer procedures. No pregnancies ensued.

Many ultrastructural defects may have associated defects at the level of the sperm centrosome and deficiencies at this level may be involved in fertilization failure after ICSI and poor embryonic development (17,18).

Coda

Few patients will have no motile spermatozoon available for microinjection. This subgroup, however, requires special attention from a clinical andrologist to prevent poor ICSI outcomes. In the ART-laboratory, too, more attention should be paid to this subgroup. A rigorous search may be needed to reveal motile or vital spermatozoa. Patients whose ejaculate unexpectedly contains only immotile spermatozoa should produce at least a second ejaculate. Patients with absolute necrozoospermia may benefit from testicular sperm recovery whenever specific treatments to improve sperm vitality have failed. At present the overall outcome in patients with immotile-cilia syndrome is generally poor. A subpopulation selected by electron microscopy and microtubule-assays, however, may have a better ICSI outcome. In the future, centrosome transplantation may become a viable option by which to overcome the poor ICSI success rate.

TABLE 11.4. Results of ICSI cycles with testicular spermatozoa from patients with immotile ejaculated spermatozoa.

	n	% of A	% of B	% of C	% of D
Couples	12				
Cycles (A)	17				
M-II oocytes injected (B)	157				
2 PN embryos (C)	91		57.2%		
Cleaving embryos[*]	81			87.9%	
Transfers	16	94.1%			
Embryos transferred (D)	45				
Positive hCG	5	29.4%			
Positive heartbeat	4				8.8%

[*]Embryos with <50% anucleate fragments.

References

1. Palermo GP, Joris H, Devroey P, Van Steirteghem AC. Pregnancies after intracyto-plasmic injection of single spermatozoon into an oocyte. Lancet 1992;1:826–35.
2. Van Steirteghem AC, Nagy Z, Joris H, et al. High fertilization and implantation rates after intracytoplasmic sperm injection. Hum Reprod 1993;8:1061–66.
3. Van Steirteghem AC, Liu J, Joris H, et al. Higher success rate by intracytoplasmic sperm injection than subzonal insemination. Report of a second series of 300 consecutive treatment cycles. Hum Reprod 1993;8:1055–60.
4. Liu J, Nagy ZP, Joris H, et al. Analysis of 76 total-fertilization-failure cycles out of 2732 intracytoplasmic sperm injection cycles. Hum Reprod 1995;10:2630–36.
5. World Health Organization. WHO laboratory manual for the examination of human semen and sperm–cervical mucus interaction. Cambridge, UK: Cambridge University Press, 1992.
6. Nagy ZP, Liu J, Joris H, et al. The results of intracytoplasmic sperm injection is not related to any of the three basic sperm parameters. Hum Reprod 1995;10:1123–29.
7. Ron-El R, Strassburger D, Friedler S, et al. Extended sperm preparation: an alternative to testicular sperm extraction in non-obstructive azoospermia. Hum Reprod 1997;12:1222–26.
8. Afzelius BA. Genetical and ultrastructural aspects of the immotile-cilia syndrome. Am J Hum Genet 1981;33:852–64.
9. Schoysman R. L'oligozoospermie epididymaire: la recherche des difficultés du transit. In: Arvis G, editor. Andrologie, Tome II. Paris: Maloine, 1989.
10. Hendry WF. Bilateral aseptic necrosis of femoral heads following intermittent high dose steroid therapy (letter). Fertil Steril 1982;38:120.
11. Verheyen G, Joris H, Crits K, Nagy Z, Tournaye H, Van Steirteghem A. Comparison of different hypo-osmotic swelling solutions to select viable immotile spermatozoa for potential use in intracytoplasmic sperm injection. Hum Reprod Update 1997;3:195–203.
12. Casper RF, Meriano JS, Jarvi KA, Cowan L, Lucato ML. The hypo-osmotic swelling test for selection of viable sperm for intracytoplasmic sperm injection in men with complete asthenozoospermia. Fertil Steril 1996;65:972–76.
13. Jow WW, Steckel J, Schlegel P, Magid MS, Goldstein M. Motile sperm in human testis biopsy specimens. J Androl 1993;14:194–98.
14. Tournaye H, Liu J, Nagy Z, et al. Correlation between testicular histology and outcome after intracytoplasmic sperm injection using testicular sperm. Hum Reprod 1996;11:127–32.
15. Verheyen G, De Croo I, Tournaye H, Pletincx I, Devroey P, Van Steirteghem A. Comparison of four mechanical methods to retrieve spermatozoa from testicular tissue. Hum Reprod 1995;10:2956–59.
16. Tournaye H, Liu J, Nagy Z, Verheyen G, Van Steirteghem AC, Devroey P. The use of testicular sperm for intracytoplasmic sperm injection in patients with necrozoospermia. Fertil Steril 1996;66:331–34.
17. Sathananthan AH, Ratnam SS, Ng SC, Tarin JJ, Gianaroli L, Trounson A. The sperm centriole: its inheritance, replication and perpetuation in early human embryos. Hum Reprod 1996;11:345–56.
18. Hewitson LC, Simerly CR, Tengowski MW, et al. Microtubule and chromatin configurations during rhesus intracytoplasmic sperm injection: successes and failures. Biol Reprod 1996;55:271–80.

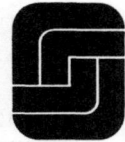

12

Intracytoplasmic Sperm Injection in Difficult Cases: The Egyptian Experience

MOHAMED A. ABOULGHAR, RAGAA T. MANSOUR, GAMAL I. SEROUR, YAHIA M. AMIN, AHMED KAMAL, AND NEVIN A. TAWAB

Introduction

The first successful pregnancies after intracytoplasmic sperm injection (ICSI) in human were reported by Palermo et al. (1). Since then, major developments occurred in this field and ICSI became a standard treatment for male factor infertility irrespective of the severity of the condition. The scope of ICSI widened to include a broad range of indications.

Despite the fact that the technique of ICSI is now more or less standardized and is being used as a routine treatment in most assisted reproductive technology centers, difficulties are still encountered by many patients for different reasons.

The objective of this chapter is to present some of the difficult aspects in the ICSI technique in our center and to discuss the difficult ICSI patients in general.

ICSI for Nonobstructive Azoospermia

Extraction of sperm in obstructive azoospermia is generally easy; however, with the introduction of testicular sperm extraction (TESE) for the treatment of nonobstructive azoospermia, great difficulties were encountered (2). In patients with Sertoli-cell-only syndrome or tubular sclerosis there may be a single seminiferous tubule producing spermatozoa, despite the rest of the testicular biopsy showing complete lack of spermatogenesis and no spermatozoa being found, even in the centrifuged specimen of the ejaculate (3). The knowledge that there could be a tiny point of normal spermatogenesis somewhere in the testicle led us to attempt TESE and ICSI, even with patients

TABLE 12.1. Histopathology of 106 patients with nonobstructive azoospermia.

Nonobstructive	106
Hypospermatogenesis	5
Partial spermatogenic arrest	28
Complete spermatogenic arrest (spermatid)	21
Complete spermatogenic arrest (primary spermatocyte)	9
Sertoli cell-only syndrome (mixed)	25
Sertoli cell-only syndrome (classical)	17
Hyalinization	1

whose testicle biopsy revealed no spermatogenesis. We were able to find sufficient number of spermatozoa, however rare, with which to perform ICSI successfully for the couple (4). If spermatozoa showed some motility, then they were preferentially used. If all spermatozoa were immotile, ICSI was performed successfully and 2PN fertilization and pregnancies were obtained (5). In some cases of nonobstructive azoospermia, even after extensive searches lasting up to 4 hours, no spermatozoa were found or their number was too few to inject all retrieved ova.

In our experience among 106 patients with the diagnosis of nonobstructive azoospermia, previous histopathology reports revealed the diagnoses listed in Table 12.1.

Our results in a series of 272 cycles are shown in Table 12.2. Spermatozoa could be found in testicular biopsy of non-obstructive azoospermia in 196 out of 272 cycles (72%).

Patients with nonobstructive azoospermia and severe oligozoospermia may be suffering from a genetic defect or a genetic barrier to reproduction (6). It is not surprising, therefore that despite succeeding in extracting live spermatozoa in nonobstructive azoospermia, the fertilization and pregnancy rates are significantly lower than those of obstructive azoospermia.

One of the most difficult points during counseling is assessment of the change of finding sperms in the testis. Different clinical criteria was used and study of the previous histopathology report of testis could not assess the prognosis.

TABLE 12.2. Outcome of intracytoplasmic sperm injection (ICSI) for patients with nonobstructive azoospermia.

No. of ICSI cycles	272
No. of injected oocytes (MII)	726
No. of fertilized oocytes (2PN)	275
Fertilization rate (%)	38
No. of ICSI cycles reaching embryo transfer stage (%)	180 (66)
No. of clinical pregnancies	35
Clinical pregnancy rate per cycle (%)	13
Clinical pregnancy rate per embryo transfer (%)	19.4

Table 12.3. Correlation between histopathology and injected germ cell type in nonobstructive azoospermia.

Histopathology of previous biopsy report	No. of cycles	Spermatogenic cell used on the day of oocyte retrieval			
		Spermatozoa	Spermatozoa + spermatids	Spermatids	None
Hyalinization	1	1	—	—	—
Sertoli cell-only (classical)	17	4	—	2	11
Sertoli cell-only (mixed)	25	19	2	1	3
Complete arrest at primary spermatocytes	9	2	—	2	5
Complete arrest at early spermatids	21	7	6	7	1
Partial spermatogenic arrest	28	22	3	3	—
Hypospermatogenesis	5	5	—	—	—
Total	106	60	11	15	20

Based on our experience in these 272 cycles of nonobstructive azoospermia we would counsel our patients that there is a 72% chance of finding spermatozoa and achieving a 19.4% pregnancy rate. On the other hand, we would stress the fact that there is a chance of 28% of not finding spermatozoa and the whole procedure will be canceled.

Analysis of 106 cycles and correlation between the histopathological testicular biopsy report and the type of injected germ cells in nonobstructive azoospermia are shown in Table 12.3. The timing of the biopsy in relation to the time of egg retrieval in nonobstructive azoospermia may affect the degree of difficulty. It was noticed that performing the biopsy 6–24 hours earlier may facilitate the search for sperms. It may be a problem, however, if we do the biopsy too early as only very few sperms may be found and it might be difficult to relocate them again before injection.

In conclusion, difficulties may arise during sperm extraction in nonobstructive azoospermia and complete failure to find sperm occurred in about 28% of our patients. Our embryologists continue their search for up to 4 hours before they stop and they consider injecting spermatids or they abandon injection completely.

Cryothawed Testicular Sperm

The minimal sperm requirements for obtaining high fertilization and pregnancy rates after ICSI open the possibility of cryopreservation of poor-quality sperm for performing ICSI after thawing. Cryopreservation becomes more and more important, especially in patients with nonobstructive azoospermia and small testis because multiple extracted testicular biopsies may represent a significant loss of testicular mass (7).

TABLE 12.4. ICSI using fresh and cryothawed testicular sperm in the same patient of nonobstructive azoospermia.

	Fresh	Cryothawed
No. of cycles	5	5
No. of MII oocytes	48	63
2 PN (%)	26 (54%)	43 (68%)
No. of embryo transfers	5	5
Cryo embryos	—	22
Clinical pregnancy	1	1

Our ICSI results document the successful use of surgically retrieved cryopreserved testicular and epididymal samples for ICSI (8). Cryopreservation of testicular tissue is an encouraging step for a group of men who would otherwise require repeated scrotal biopsies each time an ICSI cycle was attempted. It has been shown that testicular biopsies associated with multiple biopsy sites may devascularize the entire testis. In addition, local inflammation and recovery associated with TESE may adversely affect sperm production in men with nonobstructive azoospermia for up to 6 months after TESE procedure (9).

In nonobstructive azoospermia, cryopreservation of testicular tissue is more difficult as the testis in many patients contains very few sperms. In total, the use of cryothawed testicular spermatozoa in nonobstructive azoospermia was attempted in 10 cycles. In 6 out of 10 cycles, enough live spermatozoa could be found for the injection (60%). The fertilization and pregnancy rates were comparable to fresh cycles (Table 12.4).

Occult Azoospermia

Azoospermic patients occasionally show few sperm in their semen. This group of patients usually belong to the nonobstructive azoospermia group where foci of spermatogenesis are present and few sperms of their production can reach the ejaculated semen.

Routine centrifugation of the semen of azoospermic men is essential to exclude the presence of few sperms not detected by the routine semen analysis. Cryopreservation of the few sperms detected after centrifugation or the sperms that appear intermittently is important as there is no guarantee that sperm could be retrieved on day of egg retrieval. To overcome this difficulty, we routinely cryopreserve these samples and several pregnancies were achieved using this protocol. Semen collection and processing using Tea tube (based on migration and sedimentation phenomena) several hours (4–6 hours) before ICSI is recommended. This prolonged time allows separation of the few motile spermatozoa present in the sample.

ICSI in Difficult Cases: General Considerations

The present data show that in our laboratory, the most difficult problems with ICSI are encountered in patients with nonobstructive azoospermia. Cryopreservation of testicular tissue in these patients represents a major problem; however, ICSI in difficult cases can extend to other areas.

Spermatid Injection

In cases of nonobstructive azoospermia, no spermatozoa can be found in the testicular tissues, even after an extensive search. These cases represent about 30–33% of patients undergoing ICSI and TESE for nonobstructive azoospermia (4,5). The only hope for these patients is to look for spermatids to be used for intracytoplasmic injection. Spermatids are a unique source of haploid number of chromosomes (10). Fertilization as a result of the use of round spermatids (11) and elongated spermatids (12) was reported in humans. There has always been a debate about the certainty of identifying spermatids, in the live state without any stain, to be used for ICSI. Any experienced embryologist can easily identify round and elongated spermatids in a testicular sample from obstructive azoospermia. You can identify the round spermatids as a unique cell among any other round cells by its prominent condensed nucleus surrounded by a thin layer of cytoplasm. No other round cells contain such a dark condensed nucleus (13). You may also see a small dimple in the nucleus. Elongated spermatids have a darker condensed nucleus, which resembles the head of spermatozoa. You can also see the cytoplasm shed from around the nucleus surrounding only part of it which gives it a very characteristic shape, like an ice-cream cone (13).

The difficulty in identifying spermatids in nonobstructive azoospermia is due to the fact that they are very rare to be present in the first place (13). The two spermatid pregnancies in our program resulted from injection of elongated spermatids. They both resulted in the delivery of two healthy boys with normal karyotyping. There are still multiple areas to be explored in spermatid injection, as an immature cell still has not undergone histone protamin transition. Future research is needed before this technique can be widely adopted. Another cause of difficulty is the use of 100% immotile sperms. Absolute necrozoospermia, a condition in which all spermatozoa are dead, needs to be distinguished from patients with conditions such as immotile-cilia syndrome, enzymatic defects, or functional sperm-tail defects.

The use of viable, yet immature testicular sperm in necrozoospermic patients may be preferable to the use of apoptotic dysfunctional ejaculated spermatozoa that may have accumulated genomic damage (14). Testing the viability of the individual sperm injected during ICSI would not be justified because the supravital staining methods as used for accurate viability testing may compromise DNA integrity (15).

Immotile Spermatozoa

The high number of totally immotile spermatozoa in the ejaculate is mostly thought to be degenerative, whereas totally immotile testicular spermatozoa are probably immature and can become motile upon maturation. The totally immotile spermatozoa in the testis may therefore be immature and viable (16).

Finally, difficulties are met in counseling and assessing the long-term results.

Difficulties in Counseling the Couples Before ICSI

In patients with nonobstructive azoospermia, it is almost impossible to guarantee that sperms will be retrieved from the testicular biopsy. It was previously reported that FSH level, size of testicles, and even the pathological report of the previous biopsy cannot assess the chances of finding sperms in a future biopsy (5).

It is always very difficult to counsel these patients because the couple should be informed that sperm may not be retrieved after ovulation induction and oocyte retrieval. Although a testicular biopsy performed before the cycle is started might reveal the presence of few sperm that are extremely difficult to cryopreserve for future use, repeating the biopsy after a few weeks will not be welcomed by the male. This is particularly the case if there is no guarantee that sperm will be found during a repeat biopsy as occasionally we hit foci of spermatogenesis during the first biopsy simply by chance.

Difficulties in Counseling for Potential Risks of ICSI

The frequency of chromosomal anomalies is increased in infertile males (17). With the increasing use of testicular spermatozoa with ICSI in cases of nonobstructive spermatozoa, there might be a greater risk of sex chromosome aneuploidy because of the chromosomal nature of the underlying pathology. Another concern about ICSI is the use of epididymal or testicular spermatozoa from men with BCAVD. This has a major genetic implication because ICSI of BCAVD males is likely to result in an increased frequency of cystic fibrosis in the offspring (18). It has also been documented that a significant number of azoospermic men had translocation defects affecting the long arm of the Y chromosome (18).

In conclusion, there are many difficult cases of ICSI, and most of them could be predicted and counseled before the procedure is started. Improvement of the stimulation protocols, methods of retrieval, and cryopreservation of sperm and technique of ICSI could overcome many difficult cases (13).

References

1. Palermo G, Joris H, Devroey P, Van Steirteghem AC. Pregnancies after intracytoplasmic sperm injection of single spermatozoon into an oocyte. Lancet 1992;340:17–18.

2. Fahmy I, Mansour R, Aboulghar M, et al. Intracytoplasmic injection of surgically retrieved sperm and spermatids in obstructive and non-obstructive azoospermia: a comparative study. Middle East Fertil Soc J 1996;1:134–41.
3. Devroey P, Liu J, Nagy Z, et al. Pregnancies after testicular sperm extraction and intracytoplasmic sperm injection in nonobstructive azoospermia. Hum Reprod 1995;10:1457–60.
4. Mansour RT, Kamal A, Fahmy I, Tawab N, Serour G, Aboulghar MA. Intracytoplasmic sperm injection in obstructive and nonobstructive azoospermia. Hum Reprod 1997;12:1974–79.
5. Mansour RT, Aboulghar MA, Serour GI, Fahmi I, Ramzi AM, Amin Y. Intracytoplasmic sperm injection using microsurgically retrieved epididymal and testicular sperm. Fertil Steril 1996;65:566–72.
6. Vogt PH. Genetic aspects of human infertility. Int J Androl 1995;18:3–6.
7. Romero J, Remohi J, Minguez Y, Rubio C, Pellicer A, Gil-Salom M. Fertilisation after intracytoplasmic sperm injection with cryopreserved testicular spermatozoa. Fertil Steril 1996;65:877–79.
8. Kamal A, Mansour R, Aboulghar M, Fahmy I, Serour G, Tawab NA. Pregnancy after intracytoplasmic injection using cryothawed epididymal and testicular spermatozoa. Middle East Fertil Soc J 1997;2:30–34.
9. Schlegel PN. Physiological consequences of testicular sperm extraction. Abstract at the 12th Annual Meeting of the ESHRE, Maastricht. Hum Reprod 1996;11:74.
10. Edwards RG, Tarin JJ, Dean N, Hirsch A, Tan SL. Are spermatid injections into human oocytes now mandatory? Hum Reprod 1994;9:2217–19.
11. Tesarik J, Mendoza C, Testart J. Viable embryos from injection of round spermatids into oocytes. N Engl J Med 1995;333:525.
12. Mansour RT, Aboulghar MA, Serour GI, et al. Pregnancy and delivery after intracytoplasmic injection of spermatids into human oocytes. Middle East Fertil Soc J 1996;1:223–25.
13. Mansour RT. Intracytoplasmic sperm injection: a state of the art. Hum Reprod Update (in press).
14. Cummins JM, Jequier AM. Concerns and recommendations for intracytoplasmic sperm injection (ICSI) treatment. Hum Reprod 1995:10(Suppl 1):138–43.
15. Tournaye H, Verheyen G, Liu J, Van Steirteghem A, Nagy Z, Devroey P. The use of testicular sperm for intracytoplasmic sperm injection in patients with necrozoospermia. Fertil Steril 1996;66:331–34.
16. Kahraman S, Tasdemir M, Tasdemir I, et al. Pregnancies achieved with testicular and ejaculated spermatozoa in combination with intracytoplasmic sperm injection in men with totally or initially immotile spermatozoa in the ejaculate. Hum Reprod 1996;11:1343–46.
17. Chandley AC. The genetic basis of male infertility. Reprod Med Rev 1995;4:1–8.
18. Silber SJ, Nagy Z, Liu J, et al. The use of epididymal and testicular spermatozoa for intracytoplasmic sperm injection: the genetic implications for male infertility. Hum Reprod 1995;10:2031–43.

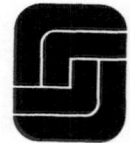

13

Difficult Cases in ICSI (Male Factors)

Martine Dumont-Hassan, P. Cohen-Bacrie, and A. Hazout

Intracytoplasmic sperm injection (ICSI) represents spectacular progress in the treatment of male infertility. This technique makes the conception of a child possible in cases where only a few living spermatozoa (mostly motile ones) can be obtained from the ejaculate or recovered from the male genital tract. The intra-oocyte injection of spermatozoa that originates from the ejaculate, the epididymis, or the testis can yield fertilization rates (2 PN zygotes/intact oocyte) of 62%, 65.6%, and 58%, respectively. The respective clinical pregnancy rates per transfer from the three sperm sources are 33.4%, 39.5%, and 35.8% (see Tables 13.1–13.4).

Despite these encouraging results, which corroborate those obtained by other international teams, it should not be forgotten that difficulties in producing a viable embryo by means of ICSI still persist with certain clinical indications. Examples of these conditions that are the most refractory to this treatment are: akinetozoospermia, some cases of severe teratozoospermia, and secretory azoospermia without testicular spermatozoa.

Akinetozoospermia

Sperm motility is an important factor predicting fertilization success with ICSI.

Among cases of akinetozoospermia, two groups can be distinguished: (1) relative akinetozoospermia in which no initial motility is followed by the acquisition of nonprogressive motility by some spermatozoa after sperm preparation and incubation; and for which ICSI is feasible; (2) absolute akinetozoospermia in which there are no motile spermatozoa, even after incubation. In these cases, success with immotile spermatozoa injection is dependent on sperm origin. Nijs et al., which compares ICSI results with immotile spermatozoa obtained from the ejaculate, from the epididymis or from the testis, have shown that the fertilization rate with immotile ejaculated spermatozoa (53%) is significantly lower compared with the other two groups (epididymis: 60%; testis: 65%) (1). Ongoing pregnancies were only obtained after the injection of immotile spermatozoa of testicular origin.

TABLE 13.1. ICSI with ejaculated spermatozoa.

Cycles (C)	2277
Injected oocytes	15,406
Intact oocytes	13,984
Fertilized oocytes (2 PN/Int.Ooc)	8683 (62%)
Transferred embryos	5670
Transfers (T)	2058
Clinical pregnancies (P)	687
% P/C	30%
% P/T	33.4%

The distinction between living and dead spermatozoa is a major problem with akinetozoospermia in ICSI. A hypoosmotic swelling test (HOS-test) can be attempted to improve ICSI results with immotile ejaculated spermatozoa. This simple test makes it possible to recognize living spermatozoa that react to the hypoosmotic solution by generating flagellar swelling, which results in a characteristic looplike deformation. The application of this test in eight cases of ICSI, reported by Casper et al., has shown that it is possible to benefit from this method, obtaining better fertilization (43% vs. 26%) and pregnancy rates when compared with ICSI with no sperm selection step (2). This method was also used by Barros et al. and Liu et al., leading to the respective fertilization rates of 41.9% and 76.4% and a few pregnancies (3,4).

Our experience with repeated ICSI treatment cycles in patients whose akinetozoospermia was not permanent showed significantly different fertilization rates between those cycles in which motile spermatozoa could be injected and those in which ICSI was performed with immotile spermatozoa that did not react in the HOS-test (64.7% vs. 23.8%) (Table 13.5). These results are in agreement with those obtained by Vandervorst et al. in the same situation (5). On the other hand, the injection of immotile spermatozoa showing good vitality, performed in three patients with permanent akinetozoospermia, led to a fertilization rate of 72.7% and the establishment of one clinical pregnancy; however, it was lost spontaneously after 2 months of gestation (Table 13.6).

TABLE 13.2. ICSI with epididymal spermatozoa.

	Fresh spermatozoa	Frozen spermatozoa
Cycles (C)	127	86
Injected oocytes	920	630
Intact oocytes	844	580
Fertilized oocytes (2 PN/Int.Ooc)	554 (65.6%)	361 (62.2%)
Transferred embryos	327	219
Transfers (T)	119	82
Clinical pregnancies (P)	47	30
% P/C	37%	34.9%
% P/T	39.5%	36.6%

TABLE 13.3. ICSI with fresh testicular spermatozoa (1994–1996).

Cycles (C)	70
Cycles with spermatozoa	56
Injected oocytes	359
Intact oocytes	309
Fertilized oocytes (2 PN/Int.Ooc)	180 (58%)
Transferred embryos	134
Transfers	53
Clinical pregnancies (P)	19
% P/C	33.9%
% P/T	35.8%

TABLE 13.4. ICSI with fresh or frozen testicular spermatozoa: comparison of the results for the first 16 couples.

	Fresh spermatozoa	Frozen spermatozoa
Couples	15	16
Cycles	16	19
Injected oocytes	95	119
Intact oocytes	76 (80%)	106 (89%)
Fertilized (2 PN/Int.Ooc)	46 (60.5%)	60 (56%)
Transferred embryos	36 (2.2 E/T)	39 (2.3 E/T)
Transfers (T)	16	17
Clinical pregnancies	2 1 Miscarriage 1 Death in utero	6 1 Miscarriage 1 Therapeutic abortion for anencephalia

TABLE 13.5. ICSI with motile or immotile negative host ejaculated sperm.

	Immotile sperm + Negative host	Motile sperm
Patients	4	3
Cycles	4	6
Sperm vitality on precedent semen analysis (%)	(0–36–69–56)	—
Injected oocytes	23	42
Intact oocytes	21	34
Fertilized oocytes (2 PN/Int.ooc)	5 (23.8%)	22 (64.7%)
Cleaving embryos	5	22
Embryo transfers	4	6
Pregnancy	0	0

TABLE 13.6. ICSI with immotile ejaculated sperm and positive host.

Patients	3
Cycles	5
Sperm vitality on precedent semen analysis (%)	(44–60–67)
Injected oocytes	24
Intact oocytes	22
Fertilized oocytes (2 PN/Int.ooc)	16 (72.7%)
Cleaving embryos	15
Embryo transfers	4
Pregnancy	1 clinical pregnancy with miscarriage

In cases using testicular spermatozoa, good fertilization rates (50%) and term pregnancies can be obtained even if immotile spermatozoa are injected (Table 13.7). This finding is in agreement with the data described by Nijs et al. (1).

In the presence of total akinetozoospermia on the day of ICSI, the treatment cycle can be performed if the HOS-test is positive. Our current experience, however, does not allow us to conclude whether this simple test will permit the establishment of an acceptable percentage of ongoing pregnancies. If this is not the case, a recourse to testicular biopsy will be necessary for sperm recovery during future treatment cycles, which also applies to cases where ejaculated spermatozoa do not react to the HOS-test. The absence of motile spermatozoa in the ejaculate, however, should be determined at any ICSI treatment cycle before the recourse to testicular biopsy. In the case of repeated ICSI failure, identification of the eventual paternal factor(s) that could have an adverse effect on embryonic development (e.g., genetic and epigenetic factors, centriole abnormalities, antisperm antibodies) should be attempted, and the couple could be advised concerning either adoption or sperm donation.

TABLE 13.7. ICSI with immotile testicular sperm.

Patients	7	– 1 total asthenozoospermia – 6 nonobstructive azoospermia
Cycles	9	
Sperm vitality	ND	
Injected oocytes	59	
Intact oocytes	52	
Fertilized oocytes (2 PN/Int.ooc)	26	(50%)
Cleaving embryos	25	
Embryo transfers	8	
Ongoing pregnancy or deliverance	2	– one twin (2 boys) – one single ongoing pregnancy

Teratozoospermia

The profile of sperm abnormalities does not always have the same value. It may involve a strong predominance of a single abnormality or, in contrast, a large diversity of abnormalities. If the percentage of abnormal spermatozoa is elevated, then the question of which of the abnormal forms can be injected into oocytes without compromising fertilization and the developmental potential of the future embryo is a central dilemma for the biologist searching for those forms that show the closest possible resemblance to a normal sperm appearance. At the present time, it is already possible to exclude certain abnormal sperm forms.

Microcephalic Spermatozoa

Patients with a pure syndrome of microcephalic spermatozoa with a round head (globozoospermia) have a reduced fertilization rate after ICSI or show complete fertilization failure. Despite this, a few ongoing pregnancies have been obtained in this type of sterility. The absence of the sperm's ability to activate oocytes can be revealed with the use of heterologous human–mouse systems (6). This sperm quality is independent of the exact form and size of the injected microcephalic spermatozoon (0% oocyte activation vs. 95% with normal donor spermatozoa). In the same study, the examination of sperm karyotypes showed that microcephalic spermatozoa did not present more chromosomal abnormalities (6%) than normal spermatozoa (9%). The fertilization failure with spermatozoa from the given patient may thus be due to an oscillin deficiency.

Spermatozoa with Macrocephalic and/or Irregular Heads

There is no evidence supporting the notion that spermatozoa with an abnormal morphology are carriers of genetic abnormalities. Human sperm injection into mouse oocytes can be used to correlate sperm head morphology with its chromosomal contents. In this way, Lee et al. have demonstrated an increase in the rate of structural chromosomal abnormalities in spermatozoa with elongated heads or with a very irregular outline (26.1% of abnormal spermatozoa vs. 6.9% for spermatozoa with normal heads) (7). Even though the results of this study remain to be confirmed in a larger series of cases, they should discourage the injection of spermatozoa bearing this type of abnormality. In our experience, there does not appear to be any correlation between the percentage of atypical forms and the fertilization/pregnancy rates (Table 13.8).

We hope that a finer analysis involving the evolution of pregnancies in cases of severe teratozoospermia will allow us to decide whether this factor is responsible for an increased rate of pregnancy loss, as has been suggested (8). Some forms of severe teratozoospermia are likely to be incompatible with normal fertilization and embryonic development. In our experience, preg-

TABLE 13.8. Normal morphology and pregnancy rates in ICSI.

Typical forms %	<10	10–19	20–29	>30
Cycles	522	318	161	322
Pregnancies n	193	105	59	106
%	37.0	33.0	36.7	32.9

$p = 0.31$

nancy was not established in two cases of teratozoospermia with as few as 1% of typical forms; this was due partly to fertilization failure and partly to implantation failure after transfer of embryos that did develop in vitro. The presence of numerous macrocephalic or irregular-headed spermatozoa was detected by spermocytogram examination. Yurov et al. and In't Veld et al. have reported similar cases (teratozoospermia with 3% or 2% of typical forms and many macrocephalic spermatozoa or spermatozoa with various other head abnormalities) in which fertilization could be obtained by ICSI, but the resulting embryos failed to implant (9,10). An electron microscopic examination, as well as fluorescent in situ hybridization analysis, seem to be indispensable in such cases for understanding the cause of developmental failure.

Secretory Azoospermia

In the presence of azoospermia, spermatozoa can be obtained by epididymal or testicular sperm recovery. If azoospermia is of secretory origin, even when the FSH serum level is elevated and the testis size is small (< 15 ml by orchidometry), then it is possible to find a few spermatozoa by testicular biopsy. When no spermatozoa can be found, a search for spermatids to be injected into oocytes should be considered.

Fresh or frozen testicular spermatids have been used to fertilize oocytes and have allowed the birth of normal and fertile young in some animal species (mouse, rabbit). In these studies, the spermatids were recovered from fertile animals, whereas for the few human births that have been obtained after injection of spermatids, the spermatids were from sterile men suffering from secretory azoospermia. Despite the animal and human data showing that conception with fresh or frozen spermatids is possible, this form of treatment remains an inefficient one (11–14).

A study by Fishel et al., which compared fertilization rates after spermatid injection with those after sperm injection in 18 patients with severe oligoasthenoteratozoospermia or secretory azoospermia, showed that only 30% of spermatid-injected oocytes were fertilized as compared with 67% of the oocytes injected with spermatozoa (15).

Vanderzwalmen et al. similarly obtained higher fertilization rates after the injection of elongated spermatids (64%) as compared with the injection of round spermatids (22%); the implantation rate after the injection of round spermatids was very low (5.5%) as compared with the injection of testicular spermatozoa (10.5%) (14).

It has to be stressed, however, that the rare successful human treatment cycles using the injection of spermatids described in the literature concerned azoospermic men in whom the capacity of producing a few mature spermatozoa had been proved in the past. In some of them, testicular spermatozoa could be recovered from previous testicular biopsy attempts. A few attempts ($n = 5$) at conception using the injection of round ejaculated spermatids have been made at our center but no pregnancy has been achieved (Table 13.9). It appears that this technique is still experimental in nature and that further substantial improvements are needed if cases of nonobstructive azoospermia with spermiogenic arrest are to be treated effectively. Because elongated spermatids are easier to recognize and have a better fertilizing ability than round spermatids, *in vitro* maturation of spermatids should be attempted. It is also important to be sure that the spermatids used are genetically normal.

On the other hand, methods of artificial stimulation to promote oocyte activation can be of help in increasing the rates of normal fertilization and improving embryo cleavage. Apart from the technical problems that still have to be solved, it should not be forgotten that the techniques of spermatid conception address severe pathologies, many of which are of genetic origin. If 100% of germ cells are attained with a genetic abnormality that is incompatible with normal embryonic development, any improvement in the sper-

TABLE 13.9. ICSI with round ejaculated spermatids.

Patients	Cycle	Previous history	Serum FSH IU/ml	Round spermatids in the ejaculate	M II oocytes injected	Intact oocytes	2 PN oocytes	Cleaving embryos transferred
1	1	NO Azoospermia (with sometimes very few spz)	21	Very few	4	4	0	0
2	1	NO Azoospermia	6	Many	9	7	0	2
3	1	NO Azoospermia testicular atrophy	22	Few	8	6	0	0
4	2	Testicular cancer	6	Many	4	4	0	0
		In 1985 Destruction of frozen straws of poor quality			10	10	3	3

NO = Nonobstructive.   Fertilization rate (2 PN/int.ooc): 9.6%.

matid conception technique will hardly meet with success. Until the etiology of these cases is known and an efficient causal treatment is made available, it will be preferable to counsel these couples against any future application of ICSI.

References

1. Nijs M, Vanderzwalmen P, Vandamme B, et al. Fertilizing ability of immotile spermatozoa after intracytoplasmic sperm injection. Hum Reprod 1996;11:2180–85.
2. Casper RF, Meriano JS, Jarvi AK, Cowan L, Lucato ML. The hypoosmotic swelling test for selection of variable sperm for intracytoplasmic sperm injection in men with complete asthenozoospermia. Fertil Steril 1996;65:972–76.
3. Barros A, Sousa M, Angelopoulos T, Tesrik J. Efficient modification of intra-cytoplasmic sperm injection technique for cases with total lack of sperm movement. Hum Reprod 1997;12:1227–29.
4. Liu J, Tsai YL, Katz E, Compton E, Garcia JE, Baramki TA. High fertilization rate obtained after intracytoplasmic sperm injection with 100% non motile spermatozoa selected by using a simple modified hypoosmotic swelling test. Fertil Steril 1997; 68:373–75.
5. Vandervorst M, Tournaye H, Camus M, Nagy ZP, Van Steirteghem A, Devroey P. Patients with absolutely immotile spermatozoa and intracytoplasmic sperm injection. Hum Reprod 1997;12:2429–33.
6. Rybouchkin A, Dozortsev D, Pelinck MJ, De Sutter P, Dhont M. Analysis of the oocyte activating capacity and chromosomal complement of round-headed human spermatozoa by their injection into mouse oocytes. Hum Reprod 1996;11:2170–75.
7. Lee JD, Kamiguchi Y, Yanagimachi R. Analysis of chromosome constitution of human spermatozoa with normal or aberrant head morphology after injection into mouse oocytes. Hum Reprod 1996;11:1942–46.
8. Hamamah S, Fignon A, Lansac J. The effect of male factors in repeated spontaneous abortion: lesson from in vitro fertilization and intracytoplasmic sperm injection. Hum Reprod Update 1997;3:393–400.
9. Yurov YB, Saias MJ, Vorsanova SG, et al. Rapid chromosomal analysis of germ-line cells by FISH: an investigation of an infertile male with large headed spermatozoa. Mol Hum Reprod 1997;2:665–68.
10. In't Veld PA, Broekmans FJM, de France HF, Pearson PL, Pieters MHEC, Van Kooij RJ. Intracytoplasmic sperm injection (ICSI) and chromosomally abnormal spermatozoa. Hum Reprod 1997;12:752–54.
11. Fishel S, Green S, Bishop M, et al. Pregnancy after intracytoplasmic injection of spermatid. Lancet 1995;345:1641–42.
12. Tesarik J, Mendoza C, Testart J. Viable embryos from injection of round spermatids into oocytes. N Engl J Med 1995;333:525.
13. Tesarik J, Rolet F, Brami C, et al. Spermatid injection into human oocytes. II Clinical application in the treatment of infertility due to non obstructive azoospermia. Hum Reprod 1996;11:780–83.
14. Vanderzwalmen P, Zech H, Birkenfeld A, et al. Intracytoplasmic injection of spermatids retrieved from testicular tissue: influence of testicular pathology, type of selected spermatids and oocyte activation. Hum Reprod 1997;12:1203–13.
15. Fishel S, Green S, Hunter A, Lisi F, Rinaldi Lisi R, McDermott H. Human fertilization with round and elongated spermatids. Hum Reprod 1997;12:336–40.

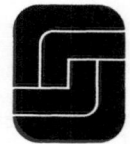

14

ICSI in Difficult Cases: Total Absence of Both Motile and Normal Spermatozoa

JEAN-FRANÇOIS GUÉRIN, MARIE-CLAUDE PINATEL, JACQUELINE LORNAGE, RACHEL LEVY, HÉLÈNE CORDONIER, GEORGES MERCIER, AND NICOLE CARLON

Intracytoplasmic sperm injection (ICSI) has become a routine technique in many IVF laboratories. The technique can give high fertilization and pregnancy rates even in cases of severe alterations in sperm characteristics (1). It has been rapidly shown that the results of ICSI are not correlated with any of the three basic parameters: total sperm count, sperm motility, and morphology (2,3). From analysis of the rare cases of total fertilization failure following ICSI procedures, however, it would appear that the total absence of sperm motility within an ejaculate represents a major cause of ICSI fertilization failure (4,5). In some but not all cases, this can be explained by a very high rate of necrozoospermia (6). In others, failure or very low rates of fertilization have been related to axonemal defects as in Kartagener's syndrome or, more recently, to anomalies in the sperm centrosome (7). Although it is generally assumed that even very low levels of spermatozoa with normal morphology do not impair fertilization rates after ICSI (2,3), some situations can mean a total absence of both normal and motile cells, as in the tail stump syndrome. One birth was reported in 1995 after transferring one embryo obtained by ICSI in this situation (8); nevertheless, in our experience the procedure is often unsuccessful, mainly when the spermatozoa contain multiple abnormalities. We report here the case of two brothers, both exhibiting a total absence of motile and normal spermatozoa in their ejaculates, with a very high index of multiple abnormalities (IMA) per sperm cell. Two ICSI attempts were made for one of these brothers, which were both unsuccessful.

Patients and Methods

Patients

Two brothers, Mr. O.N. and Mr. O.R., attended our infertility unit with a history of 10 years in both couples. The results of gynecological examinations were strictly normal and indicated the presence of male factor infertility.

Semen Analysis

Both patients provided at least three ejaculates, which were analyzed according to World Health Organization guidelines.

Sperm Ultrastructural Studies

Ejaculates were centrifuged at $600\ g$ for 15 min. The pellets were suspended in 0.2 M cacodylate buffer / 4% glutaraldehyde for 1 hour at 4°C. After washing, postfixation was carried out using 2% buffered osmium tetroxide. The samples were then dehydrated and embedded in Epon. Sections were cut with an ultramicrotome and analyzed under transmission electronic microscopy (T.E.M.).

ICSI Procedure

Ovarian stimulation was performed using purified urinary FSH (Metrodin HP®, Serono Laboratories) after GnRH desensitization (Decapeptyl®, Ipsen Laboratories). The ICSI procedure was performed according to the protocol originally described by the Brussels group (1).

Results

Sperm Characteristics

Sperm characteristics for each patient were:

Mr O.N.: sperm count: 50–60 million/ml; sperm motility: 0%; live cells: 52–72%; abnormal forms: 100%. The abnormal forms were distributed as follows: head anomalies: 5–16%; middle piece anomalies including cytoplasmic residues: 44–61%; short or absent flagellum: 77–100%; index of multiple anomalies (IMA): 1.21–1.57.

Mr O.R.: sperm count: 31–82 million/ml; sperm motility: 0%; live cells: 38–60%; abnormal forms: 100%. The abnormal forms were distributed as follows: head anomalies: 9–13%; middle piece anomalies including cytoplasmic residues: 49–65%; short or absent flagellum: 75–97%; IMA: 1.22–1.73.

TABLE 14.1. Rates of ultrastructural sperm abnormalities in two infertile brother patients.

Subjects	O.N.	O.R.	Controls
Head abnormalities	96.8%	94.5%	77.3 ± 6.4%
Middle piece	100%	100%	56.3 ± 7.2%
Principal piece	100%	100%	62.2 ± 6.1%

Ultrastructural Analysis

This analysis was carried out for each patient because of the high rate of abnormalities detected with optical microscopy, and prior to acceptance for ICSI. Ultrastructural studies (Table 14.1) confirmed the extremely high rate of anomalies, concerning all elements of the sperm cell (Figs. 14.1 and 14.2); 40 cells could be analyzed; values were identical in the two patients. Head anomaly details, as illustrated in Figure 14.1, were: anomalies in nuclear shape 38%; nuclear vacuoles 40%; abnormal acrosomes 75%; abnormal postacrosomal region 70%; and sperm heads with multiple abnormalities 70%. The region of the sperm neck was abnormal in 100% and 81% of spermatozoa, respectively (Table 14.2). In one

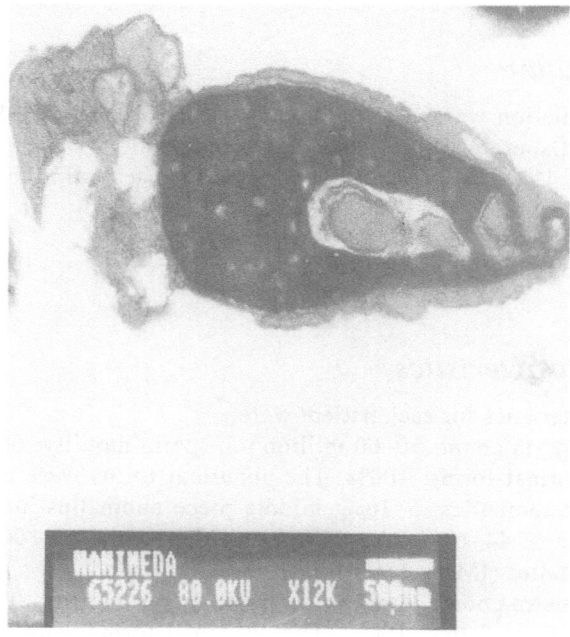

FIGURE 14.1. Longitudinal section of sperm head (Patient O.N.) showing various abnormalities: vacuolated chromatin and badly shaped acrosome in the apex area. The neck area is totally disorganized.

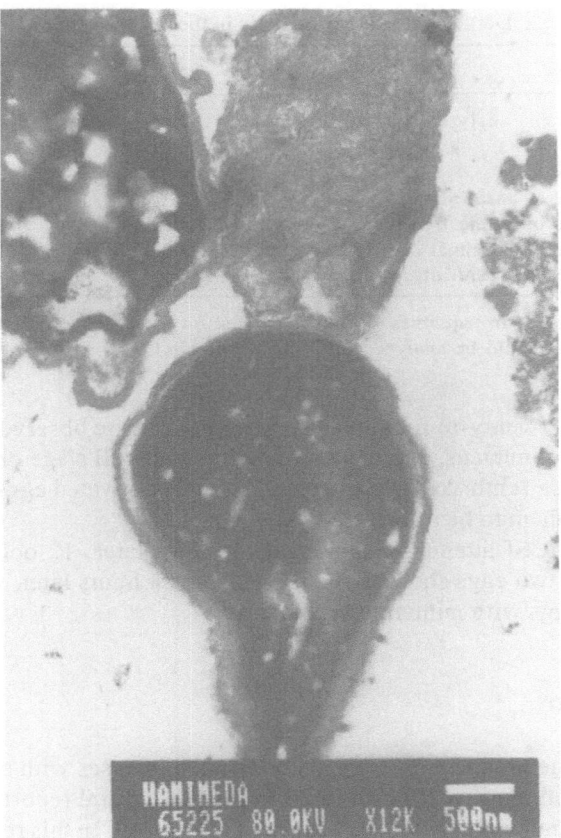

FIGURE 14.2. Details of the neck area and middle piece (longitudinal section) of one sperm cell (Patient O.N.). The basal plate, connective piece, and centriole are absent. None of the classic components of the middle piece are recognizable: mitochondria, axonemal, and periaxonemal structures.

patient (Mr. O.N.), all spermatozoa were lacking a connective piece and proximal centriole, combined with anomalies of the flagellum (Fig. 14.2). In the second patient (Mr. O.R.), 80% of spermatozoa exhibited these defects.

ICSI Procedure

Because of the multiple ultrastructural abnormalities, we informed both patients that the chances of fertilization after ICSI were small; however, one patient (Mr. O.N.) requested an ICSI attempt.

Spermatozoa were separated on a two-layer Percoll gradient; 23 metaphase II oocytes were collected, and injected with totally immobile and abnormal

TABLE 14.2. Details of the abnormalities in the region of the sperm neck.

Subjects	O.N.	O.R.
No. of cells analyzed	40	30
Normal necks	0	4 (19%)
Lysed cells	4	9
Absence of basal plate	32 (89%)	17 (80%)
Absence of connective piece	36 (100%)	17 (80%)
Absence of proximal centriole	36 (100%)	17 (80%)
Disorganized centriole	—	3 (14%)

*Percentages in parentheses were calculated on the basis of the number of cells that could be analyzed (i.e., nonlysed cells).

spermatozoa. Twenty-four hours later, no zygotes were observed, but two ova showed one pronucleus, and these were at the two-cell stage on the next day. Although these "embryos" were probably simply activated eggs, the patient's wife wanted them to be transferred.

A second ICSI attempt was made 18 months later; 12 oocytes were injected; again two eggs showed one pronucleus 24 hours later, which cleaved to two-cell eggs with numerous fragments.

Discussion

Although some pregnancies have been reported in cases with a total absence of either sperm motility (9) or normal forms (8), several reports indicate that fertilization and pregnancy rates are always low (5,9). In this report, we show that the nature of the sperm abnormalities as well as the absence of normal forms must be considered when evaluating the chances of fertilization after ICSI. In these two brothers, each spermatozoon exhibited several cell abnormalities, which were revealed by T.E.M. With optical microscopy, the main defect was related to the flagellum, which was short or absent as in the tail stump syndrome; however, T.E.M. revealed various abnormalities concerning the sperm head, particularly the neck region, as shown in Table 14.2 and Figure 14.2, which appeared totally disorganized, contrary to the ultrastructural observations in the sperm tail stump syndrome (8).

At our center, fertilization failures after ICSI are extremely rare and are mainly related to female factors, such as a lack of mature oocytes to be injected. The observation of two repeated fertilization failures, therefore clearly revealed that the patient's spermatozoa were unable to initiate a normal fertilization process. It is interesting to note that in each attempt two one-pronucleus stages were observed, indicating that these eggs were probably activated, but the sperm head was not decondensed. This may be related to the observations of head and neck abnormalities previously described. In particular, the absence of a centrosome in each sperm cell analyzed was in agreement with fertilization failure, even after ICSI (7): Injected eggs could not undergo a normal fertilization process. Thus, T.E.M. analysis is recommended for cases of total absence of normal spermatozoan forms, before deciding on whether to attempt an ICSI procedure. If T.E.M. reveals multiple abnormalities, particularly in the head and neck regions as in the present observation, ICSI should be canceled, or at the very least patients should be informed of the very low chances of success. Moreover, possible genetic risks cannot be excluded: in this study the same sperm abnormalities were observed in two brothers, which constitutes a strong argument for a "genetic" origin to these sperm defects, which could therefore be transmitted to the next generation.

References

1. Van Steirteghem A, Nagy Z, Joris H, et al. High fertilization and implantation rates after intracytoplasmic sperm injection. Hum Reprod 1993;8:1061–66.
2. Nagy Z, Liu J, Joris H, et al. The result of intracytoplasmic sperm injection is not related to any of the three basic sperm parameters. Hum Reprod 1995;10:1123–29.
3. Oehninger S, Veeck L, Lanzendorf S. Intracytoplasmic sperm injection: achievement of high pregnancy rates in couples with severe male factor infertility is dependent primarily upon female and not male factors. Fertil Steril 1995;64:977–81.
4. Liu J, Nagy Z, Joris H, et al. Analysis of 76 total fertilization failure cycles out of 2732 intracytoplasmic sperm injection cycles. Hum Reprod 1995;10:2630–36.
5. Vandervorst M, Tournaye H, Camus M, Nagy ZP, Van Steirteghem A, Devroey P. Patients with absolutely immotile spermatozoa and intracytoplasmic sperm injections. Hum Reprod 1997;2:2429–33.
6. Tournaye H, Liu J, Nagy Z, Verheyen G, Van Steirteghem AC, Devroey P. The use of testicular sperm for intracytoplasmic sperm injection in patients with necrozoospermia. Fertil Steril 1996;66:331–34.
7. Simerly C, Wu GJ, Zoran S, et al. The paternal inheritance of the centrosome, the cell's microtubule organizing center, in humans, and the implication for infertility. Nature Med 1995;1:47–53.
8. Stalf T, Sanchez R, Köhn FM, et al. Pregnancy and birth after cytoplasmic sperm injection with spermatozoa from a patient with tail stump syndrome. Hum Reprod 1995;10:2112–14.
9. Nijs M, Vanderzwalmen P, Vandamme B, et al. Fertilizing ability of immotile spermatozoa after intracytoplasmic sperm injection. Hum Reprod 1996;11:2180–85.

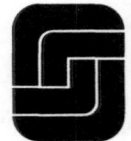

15

Difficult ICSI Cases: An Israeli Survey

Yigal Soffer, Arie Raziel, Shevach Friedler,
Deborah Strassburger, and Raphael Ron-El

Introduction

This chapter is based on a survey of published material from our center as well as from 12 other Israeli in vitro fertilization (IVF) centers during 1997. This material deals mainly with nonobstructive azoospermia, and allowed us to answer the following questions in difficult intracytoplasmic sperm injection (ICSI) cases: Is it possible to do ICSI in every nonobstructive azoospermia? How to retrieve sperm in difficult cases? Is ICSI feasible with nonmotile spermatozoa or with spermatids only? Is sperm cryopreservation contributory? Is it possible to overcome unexpected egg factor in ICSI?

Is It Possible to Do ICSI in Every Nonobstructive Azoospermia?

Madgar et al. (1) from Sheba Medical Center, Tel Hashomer analyzed the impact on ICSI outcome of surgical technique, age, FSH levels, testicular size, and histology in 54 nonobstructive azoospermia patients. They concluded that regardless of age, testicular sperm retrieval should be recommended in nonobstructive azoospermia with primary germinal failure with elevated FSH levels. In patients with high FSH and small testicular volume (< 8 ml), sperm recovery is rare. According to Friedler et al. (2) from our IVF center, histology is the best one of all of the cited criteria. Histology, however, is not advised today before testicular sperm extraction (TESE). Lewin et al. (3), from Hadassah Ein Karem IVF center, Jerusalem, did not find any exclusion criteria [FSH, testicular volume, previous extensive sperm preparation (ESP), scanning electron microscopy, histology or cytology]. For this group, all azoospermic patients should be enrolled in testicular fine needle aspiration (TEFNA) attempt; spermatozoa were recovered in 32 out of 44 patients (72%). Segal et al. (4) suggest using a testicular score based upon testicular volume, histology, FSH, previous testicular surgery, and fructose. Weiss et al. (5) advocate giving prolonged and high dosage of gonadotropin treatment in azoospermic patients with testicular spermatogenic arrest. Following such treatment, which was given for 6–8 months in 37 patients, mature spermatozoa that were not seen before appeared in 21.6% of cases either in centrifuged semen or in testicular aspirates.

How to Retrieve Sperm in Difficult Cases

Meticulous microscopic examination of the ejaculate in nonobstructive azoospermia cases scheduled for TESE may be surprising, especially when occasional spermatozoa are found and some of them are motile. Ron-El et al. (6) analyzed the value of ESP in ejaculates as a routine procedure before testicular surgery the day of ovum pick-up. Enough motile spermatozoa suitable for ICSI was found in about 30% of cases, allowing the cancellation of the surgical sperm retrieval. No predictive factor of success of this procedure was found. The authors therefore recommend this procedure in every case before beginning testicular surgery. Strassburger et al. (7) showed that very low sperm count significantly affects fertilization rate as compared with control, 42% versus 52%, in cases of nonobstructive azoospermia in whom sperm was found only after ESP. Pregnancy rate is also affected, 18% versus 30%, and more. Whether such cases do better with testicular sperm has still to be proven.

In another group, patients with anejaculation, ejaculated spermatozoa may be obtained using anejaculation. In most IVF centers, electroejaculation was sporadically done for paraplegia or psychogenic anejaculation. Hovav et al. (8), from Bikur Holim Hospital, Jerusalem, presented data in individuals with psychogenic anejaculation in 17 ICSI cycles using electroejaculation. Poor sperm quality was obtained. Fertilization rate was significantly lower than ICSI control, 27% versus 42%. One ongoing pregnancy was achieved in this group.

If ejaculated sperm is not available, testicular sperm retrieval is mandatory. Shulman et al. (9), from Sheba Medical Center, Tel Hashomer, compared ICSI outcome using testicular (40 cycles) and ejaculated spermatozoa (40 cycles). The rate of fertilization (42% vs. 55%, $p < 0.005$) was lower, but the rate of cleavage (96% vs. 93%) and ET (90% vs. 92.5%) was similar. Embryo quality, mean number of embryo per ET and pregnancy rate (22.5% vs. 20%) was similar as well (Tables 15.1 and 15.2). In our center, Friedler et al. (2) compared the results of ICSI with fresh nonejaculated spermatozoa in 24 obstructive and 25 nonobstructive azoospermia. The rate of fertilization (54 and 47%), cleavage (91 and 93%), and clinical pregnancies (31 and 26%) was not significantly different (Table 15.1). Friedler et al. (10) also compared TEFNA and TESE in nonobstructive azoospermia and showed that TESE with open biopsy is the procedure of choice in these cases (TESE 43% vs. TEFNA 11% recovery rate). Hauser et al. (11), from

TABLE 15.1. Outcome of ICSI using testicular sperm, according to the azoospermia diagnosis.

Source	Fertil	Cleavage	ET	Pregnancy	Reference
Testicular (all)	42%	96%	90%	22%	Shulman (9)
Testicular nonobstructive	47%	93%		26%	Friedler (2)
Testicular obstructive	54%	91%		31%	Friedler (2)

Liss IVF Center, Tel Aviv, agreed with this assertion. They reported in eight patients that sperm was found in TESE only, in four in both TESE and TEFNA, and in one case in TEFNA only. Sperm detection rates were 92% for TESE and 38% for TEFNA $p < 0.005$. Cryopreserved sperm aliquots following TESE, 11.4 ± 8.6, as compared with 2.4 ± 1.2 following TEFNA. According to both authors (10,11), TESE is significantly more reliable for diagnosing sperm presence in nonobstructive azoospermia and allowing more sperm aliquots to be cryopreserved. An opposite opinion was presented by Feldberg et al. (12), from Golda IVF Unit, Petach Tikva. They investigated 16 cases of obstructive azoospermia and 14 nonobstructive azoospermia. TESE, TEFNA, and PESA were done. They observed a lower fertilization and cleavage rate in nonobstructive, but the pregnancy rate was not significantly different in both groups. In 32 patients in which sperm was recovered using TEFNA, Lewin et al. (3), from Hadassah-Ein Karem IVF Center, Jerusalem, reported an implantation rate of 27.4% and a clinical pregnancy rate of 27.2%. These authors recommend TEFNA as the sperm retrieval procedure of choice in nonobstructive azoospermia and do not perform TESE.

Is ICSI Feasible with Nonmotile Spermatozoa

Another difficulty is encountered when motile sperm, either ejaculated or testicular (Table 15.2), are not available. Stein et al. (13), from Beilinson IVF Center, Petach Tikva, reported a series of 39 cycles out of 125 IVF cycles, in

TABLE 15.2. Outcome of ICSI according to sperm motility using testicular or control ejaculated sperm.

Source	Fertil	Pregnancy	Reference
Testicular motile sperm	67%	25%	Stein (13)
	62%	23.5%	Shulman (9)
Testicular immobile sperm	40%	11%	Stein (13)
	51%	5.8%	Shulman (9)
Control (ejaculate)	55%	20%	Shulman (9)
	61%	21%	Stein (13)

which ejaculated or testicular (TESE) immobile spermatozoa were used for ICSI. Fertilization of injected oocytes occurred in 35% and 40%, respectively, as compared with 61% and 67%, respectively, following ICSI with motile spermatozoa. Pregnancy rate was also low at 5% and 11%, respectively, as compared with 21% and 25% pregnancy rate, using motile ejaculated or testicular spermatozoa. For them, normal embryos suitable for transfer might occur with immobile spermatozoa, but pregnancy rate is low. Shulman et al. (9), from Sheba IVF center, Tel Hashomer, compared the outcome of ICSI with testicular sperm in 19 cycles using immobile spermatozoa to 34 cycles using poorly motile ones (Table 15.2) The fertilization rate was 51% versus 62%, implantation rate was 4.2% versus 6.6%, and ongoing pregnancy was 15.8% versus 23.5%. They concluded that immobile spermatozoa can successfully fertilize mature oocytes, resulting in viable embryos with good implantation potential. Shelef et al. (14), from Golda IVF center, Petach Tikva, compared the semen quality of repeated ejaculations for IVF or ICSI. If the first ejaculate was poor but the semen quality was known to be better in the past (81 out of 131 cycles), the repeated ejaculate was found to be of higher quality in 28.4% and used. Strassburger et al. (15), from our Center, analyzed three cases with repeated sperm immobility and absence of flagellar dynein arms at electron microscopy. Two of them had Kartagener syndrome. One ejaculate was asked in the first ICSI cycle. In the next cycles, repeated ejaculations were requested. Repeated ejaculates showed a significantly higher rate of sperm viability (68% vs. 42%) with increased ovocyte fertilization (48% vs. 3%) cleavage and ET rate in these ICSI cycles. An ongoing twin pregnancy occurred in this group. Repeated ejaculates should be requested in cases of totally immobile spermatozoa as well as necrozoospermia.

Is ICSI Feasible Using Spermatids Only

Levran et al. (16) from Wolfson IVF center, Holon, reported nine cycles with testicular round spermatids in five couples. One hundred seven oocytes were injected and ET was done in all patients. An acceptable rate of fertilization (58%) and embryo transfer (57%, 3.5 ± 1.5/embryo) was achieved in patients with spermatogenic arrest. A high incidence of damaged oocytes (9.5%), cleavage arrest (43%), and poor embryo quality (86%) were observed. No pregnancy was achieved. Barark et al. (17), from Herzlia IVF Center, Herzlia, used spermatids for ICSI in males lacking mature spermatozoa in the ejaculate or TESE material. ICSI using spermatids only was done in 21 IVF cycles in 13 couples. In 13 cycles elongated spermatids were used into 137 oocytes. In eight additional cycles round spermatids were injected into 37 oocytes. Spermatids were retrieved either from ejaculate or from testicular material. Two PN fertilizations were observed in 35% of injected oocytes and 1PN in 21%. One ongoing pregnancy occurred following ICSI with round spermatids. In this cycle, no mature spermatozoa were found in two consecutive ejaculates, although mature spermatozoa were previously found.

As testicular biopsy was refused, 12 oocytes were injected with seminal elongated spermatids and nine oocytes, with round spermatids. After 16 hours, 1PN fertilization only was observed in four out of nine oocytes injected with round spermatids. These four oocytes cleaved and were transferred in utero, which resulted in an ongoing normal singleton pregnancy and term delivery of a healthy child. In conclusion, in cases with spermatogenic arrest, ICSI procedure with round spermatids is useless.

Is Sperm Cryopreservation Contributory in Difficult Cases

Friedler et al. (18,19), from our Center, analyzed the contribution of cryopreservation in difficult ICSI cases with nonejaculated spermatozoa. In azoospermia, either obstructive, 24 cycles, with abundantly retrieved spermatozoa, or nonobstructive, 25 cycles with testicular failure, nonejaculated sperm cryopreservation was feasible and efficient. In both groups (20 and 14 cycles, respectively), the outcome of ICSI with these frozen–thawed spermatozoa was as good or even better (but not significantly different) than freshly retrieved ones: The fertilization rate was 54% versus 54%; cleavage, 86% versus 91%; pregnancy rate, 40% versus 31%, respectively, in obstructive azoospermia. The fertilization rate was 44% versus 47%, cleavage was 89% versus 93%, and the pregnancy rate was 27% versus 26%, respectively, in nonobstructive azoospermia. Moreover, the cumulative pregnancy rate per sperm retrieval is significantly increased, reaching in obstructive azoospermia a rate of 54% (10,18,19). In all cases of azoospermia, therefore, cryopreservation of all supernumerary spermatozoa is recommended to increasing the overall pregnancy rate per nonejaculated sperm retrieval procedure. BenYossef et al. (20), from Liss IVF Center, Tel Aviv, analyzed the outcome of 12 ICSI cycles using TESE or MESA motile fresh sperm recovered in 13 couples out of 19, and in eight later cycles using nonejaculated cryopreserved-thawed sperm was similar. The fertilization rate was 61% versus 67%, pregnancy rate, 30%, was similar. They therefore recommend open TESE to ensure cryopreservation for additional ICSI cycles without further surgical sperm extraction. Lewin et al. (3), from Hadassah-Ein Karem IVF center, Jerusalem, reported 11 cases of TEFNA out of 32 in which sperm was recovered, with enough spermatozoa for cryopreservation.

Soffer et al. (21), from our Center, analyzed the overall contribution of sperm banking in difficult ICSI cases. All remaining epididymal or testicular material containing spermatozoa following ICSI procedures is routinely cryopreserved, allowing further ICSI cycles without repeating surgery. In addition, in nonobstructive azoospermia, previous ejaculates with motile spermatozoa (delivered in the work-up period) were also cryopreserved. Thus, TESE could be avoided if ejaculated spermatozoa were not available the day of ovum pickup. Botchan et al. (22), from Liss Male Infertility Institute, Tel Aviv, focused its attention in cancer symptomatic patients that have a very poor sperm quality, mainly following surgery, even before chemotherapy or radiation. Before the ICSI era only few straws, if any, were kept. Many more semen straws are cryopreserved today and ICSI may be performed in such patients regardless of sperm quality (excepted necrozoospermia). Moreover, in one case, Yavetz et al. (23), from Liss Male Infertility Institute, Tel Aviv, extracted and cryopreserved healthy sperm cells from an orchidectomized seminoma-bearing testis. ICSI was successfully done later with this cryopreserved material. Thus, since the advent of ICSI, sperm bank activitity is not decreasing. On the contrary, sperm cryopreservation has become an important tool of ART that helps increase the efficacy of new reproductive technologies.

Is It Possible to Overcome Egg Factor in ICSI?

In cases with severe male factor requiring ICSI procedures, unexpected difficulties may occur due to female egg factors. Margaliot et al. (24), from Shaare Zedek IVF Center, Jerusalem, investigated this issue. There was failure of cleavage and/ or fertilization in 42 cases out of 300 couples undergoing IVF (14%). Doing ICSI in these cases in later cycles enabled them to detect egg factor in 7 of these 300 cases (2.3%); semen analyses, SPA, and HZA were normal. In these women, the oocytes were not able to develop into embryos; however, the exact pathology seems to vary from case to case and needs further evaluation. Geva et al. (25,26) found a high prevalence of various antiphospholipid and antinuclear autoantibodies in IVF failure (>3) and chemical pregnancies (>2). Farhi et al. (27), from Wolfson IVF Center, Holon, addressed the problem of immature oocytes retrieved in ICSI cycles. They reported an enhanced in vitro maturation from the germinal vesicle to the M2 stage following the addition of sperm or the removal of cumulus. Both methods combined in high rates of oocyte maturation, 80% and fertilization, up to 87%, as with normally mature oocytes

List of Israeli IVF Centers with Published Data Cited in This Survey

Assaf Harofe Medical Center, IVF Unit and Male Infertility Clinic, Zerifin
Barzilai Medical Center, IVF Unit, Ashkelon
Bikur Holim Hospital, IVF Unit, Jerusalem
Hadassah Medical Center, Ein Karem Campus IVF Unit, Jerusalem
Herzlia Medical Center, IVF units, Herzlia and Haifa
Rabin Medical Center, Beilinson Campus IVF Unit and Golda Campus IVF Unit, Petach Tikva
Shaare Zedek Medical Center, IVF Unit, Jerusalem
Sheba Medical Center, IVF Unit, Tel Hashomer and Assuta Hospital IVF Unit, Tel Aviv
Tel Aviv Medical Center, Liss Campus, IVF and Male Infertility Units, Tel Aviv
Wolfson Medical Center, IVF Unit, Holon

168   Y. Soffer et al.

References

1. Madgar I, Raviv G, Eissenberg R, Menashe Y, Levron J, Shulman A, Bider D, Maschiach S, Dor J. Testicular sperm histology and clinical characteristics predict sperm detection in azoospermic men during testicular sperm retrieval (TSR). The annual meeting of the Israel Fertility Association, April 1997, Herzlia, Israel, Abstract book, p. L1.
2. Friedler S, Raziel A, Soffer Y, Strassburger D, Komarovsky D, Bern O, Kasterstein E, Bukovsky I, Ron-El R. Intracytoplasmic injection (ICSI) of fresh and cryopreserved nonejaculated spermatozoa: a comparative study of the outcome in patients with obstructive and non-obstructive azoospermia. The annual meeting of the Israel Fertility Association, April 1997, Herzlia, Israel, Abstract book, p. L7.
3. Lewin A. Schenker JG, Reubinoff B, Benshushan A, Bar-El H, Porat-Katz A, Bartoov B, Weiss D, Safran A. The role of clinical and laboratory parameters in the diagnosis and treatment of non-obstructive azoospermia. The annual meeting of the Israel Fertility Association, April 1997, Herzlia, Israel, Abstract book, p. L7.
4. Segal S. Zohav E, Katz N, Meltzer S, Hovitz M, Gemer O, Hedvat E, Sassoon E. The testicular score for prediction of sperm production and retrieval. The annual meeting of the Israel Fertility Association, April 1997, Herzlia, Israel, Abstract book, p. P39
5. Weiss DB, Gottschalk-Sabag S, Bar-On E, Zuckerman Z, Bartoov B, Soffer Y. Prolonged and high dosage of gonadotropins treatment in patients with testicular spermatogenic arrest: a preliminary report. Harefuah 1997; in press.
6. Ron-El R, Strassburger D, Friedler S, Komarovsky D, Bern O, Soffer Y, Raziel A. Extended sperm preparation: an alternative to testicular sperm extraction in nonobstructive azoospermia. Human Reprod 1997;12(6):1222–26.
7. Strassburger D, Raziel A, Friedler S, Komarovsky D, Bern O, Kasterstein E, Soffer Y, Ron-El R. Very low sperm count effects the result of intracytoplsasmic sperm injectin (ICSI). The annual meeting of the Israel Fertility Association, April 1997, Herzlia, Israel, Abstract book, p. P50.
8. Hovav Y, Kafka I, Dan-Goor M, Shotland Y, Yaffe H, Almagor M. Lower fertilization rates after electroejaculation in combination with ICSI in patients with psychogenic anejaculation. The annual meeting of the Israel Fertility Association, April 1997, Herzlia, Israel, Abstract book, p. L54.
9. Shulman A. Feldman B, Madgar Y, Levron J, Yamini Z, Yunish M, Levin T, Bider D, Rabinovici Y, Tur-Kaspa I, Mashiach S, Dor J. The results of ICSI in patients with total immotile spermatozoa resulting from testicular sperm retrieval. The annual meeting of the Israel Fertility Association, April 1997, Herzliya, Israel, Abstract book, p. L6.
10. Friedler S, Raziel A, Strassburger D, Soffer Y, Komarovsky D, Ron-El R. Testicular sperm retrieval by percutaneous fine needle sperm aspiration (TEFNA) compared with testicular sperm extraction (TESE) by open biopsy in men with non-obstructive azoospermia. Human Reprod 1997;12(7);1488–93.
11. Hauser R. Yogev L, Botchan A, Gamzu R, Amit A, Lessing JB, Ben-Haim M, Paz G, Yavetz H. Comparison of 2 techniques for sperm retrieval in non-obstructive azoospermia: TESE vs. TESA. The annual meeting of the Israel Fertility Association, April 1997, Herzlia, Israel, Abstract book, p. L3.
12. Feldberg D, Bar-Hava I, Ashkenazi J, Segal S, Voliovitch I, Shelef M, Barak Y, Kogosowski A, Ben-Rafael Z. Results of in vitro fertilization with ICSI micromanipulation in obstructive and nonobstructive azoospermic males treated by TESE, PESA,

and TESA for surgical sperm extraction. The annual meeting of the Israel Fertility Association, April 1997, Herzlia, Israel, Abstract book, p. L2.

13. Stein A, Rufas O, Amit S, Vrech OM, Pinkas H, Goldman GA, Zuckerman Z, Ben-Rafael Z, Fisch B. Intracytoplasmic injection of ejaculated and testicular immotile spermatozoa.The annual meeting of the Israel Fertility Association, April 1997, Herzlia, Israel, Abstract book, p. L5.

14. Shelef M, Bar-Hava I, Feldberg D, Sevillia J, Schwartz A, Brengauz M, Ashkenazi J, Ferber A, Ben-Rafael Z. Second immediate ejaculate during assisted reproductive technology (ART treatment. The annual meeting of the Israel Fertility Association, April 1997, Herzlia, Israel, Abstract book, p. P41.

15. Strassburger D, Raziel A, Friedler S, Komarovski D, Bern O, Kasterstein E, Soffer Y, Ron-El R.Very low sperm count effects the result of intracytoplasmic sperm injection (ICSI). The annual meeting of the Israel Fertility Association, April 1997, Herzlia, Israel, Abstract book, p. P50.

16. Levran D, Nachum H, Kotlirov O, Benet A, Zakut H, Sidi A, Farhi J. Results of round spermatids injection (ROSI) for treatment of defective spermiogenesis. The annual meeting of the Israel Fertility Association, April 1997, Herzliya, Israel, Abstract book, p. L57.

17. Barak Y, Kogosowski A, Goldman S, Soffer Y, Gonen Y, Tesarik J. Pregnancy and birth after transfer of embryos that developed from single-nucleated zygotes obtained by injection of round spermatids into oocytes. Fertil Steril 1998;70(1):67–70.

18. Friedler S, Raziel A, Soffer Y, Strassburger D, Komarovski D, Bern O, Kasterstein E, Bukovski I, Ron-El R. Intracytoplasmic injection (ICSI) of fresh and cryopreserved non ejaculated spermatozoa: a comparative study of the outcome in patients with obstructive and non-obstructive azoospermia. The annual meeting of the Israel Fertility Association, April 1997, Herzlia, Israel, Abstract book, p. L7.

19. Friedler S, Raziel A, Soffer Y, Strassburger D, Komarovsky D, Ron-El R. The outcome of intracytoplasmic injection of fresh and cryopreserved epididymal spermatozoa in patients with obstructive azoospermia—a comparative study. Human Reprod 1998;13(7):1872–77.

20. BenYossef D, Yogev L, Schwartz T, Ben-Haim M, Hauser R, Botchan A, Yavetz H, Azem F, Yovel I, Lessing JB, Amit A. Similar fertilization and pregnancy rates following ICSI with fresh or cryopreserved testicular spermatozoa. The annual meeting of the Israel Fertility Association, April 1997, Herzlia, Israel, Abstract book, p. L8.

21. Soffer Y, Kaufman S, Friedler S, Raziel A, Ron-El R, Bukovsky I. New trends in sperm bank activity in heterologous insemination and autologous semen cryopreservation.The annual meeting of the Israel Fertility Association, April 1997, Herzlia, Israel, Abstract book, p. P27.

22. Botchan A, Hauser R, Yogev L, Gamzu R, Paz G, Yavetz H. An attitude change in sperm banking policy in the ICSI era. The annual meeting of the Israel Fertility Association, April 1997, Herzliya, Israel, Abstract book, p. L91.

23. Yavetz H, Hauser RT, Botchan A, Azem F, Yovel L, Lessing JB, Amit A, Yogev L. Pregnancy resulting from frozen-thawed embryos achieved by intracytoplasmic injection of cryopreserved sperm cells extracted from an orchidectomized seminoma-bearing testis causing obstructive azoospermia. Human Reprod 1997;12(12):101–3.

24. Margaliot EJ, Gal M, Zylber-Haran E, Brooks B, Bocker J, Abramov B, Ben Chetrit A. Diamant YZ. Egg factor infertility, a new category determined after the use of IVF and ICSI. The annual meeting of the Israel Fertility Association, April 1997, Herzlia, Israel, Abstract book, p. L76.

25. Geva E, Amit A, Lerner-Geva L, Yovel I, Azem F, David MP, Ben-Yossef D, Barkai U, Lessing JB. High prevalence of autoantibodies in infertile patients with in vitro fertilization-embryo transfer failure. The annual meeting of the Israel Fertility Association, April 1997, Herzlia, Israel, Abstract book, p. P24.
26. Geva E, Amit A, Lerner-Geva L, Lessing JB. Autoimmunity and reproduction. Fertil Steril 1997;67(4):599–611.
27. Farhi J, Nachum H, Zakut H, Levran D. Incubation with sperm enhances in vitro maturation of the oocyte from germinal vesicle to the M2 stage. Fertil Steril 1997;68(2):318–22.

Part IV

Testicular Sperm: Physiological to Pathological Aspects

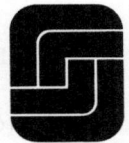

16

Growth Factors in Testis Development and Function

CLAIRE MAUDUIT, SAMIR HAMAMAH, AND MOHAMED BENAHMED

Introduction

The purpose of this chapter is to discuss the role of growth factors and cytokines in testis development and function. The testis is an organ that has two major functions: the production and secretion of steroid hormones (testosterone, dihydrotestosterone, and estradiol) and the production of competent spermatozoa. These two functions are exerted in a different manner during the fetal and the adult life of the male gonad.

Fetal Gonad

In the fetus, the male gonad develops as a local derivative of the mesonephros. Testicular somatic cells derive from surface epithelial and adjacent mesenchymal cells of the mesonephros. The germ cells differentiate in the extraembryonic mesoderm and migrate into the developing testis before histological differentiation of the gonad (1,2). Once the genital ridge is formed, the embryonic development of the gonad can be divided into two successive phases: the sexually indifferent gonad, and then the sexual differentiation of the ambiguous gonad into the testis. Both during the undifferentiated period and the differentiation into the testis, gonadal somatic and germ cells undergo different processes, including migration, proliferation, differentiation (transformation of epithelial and mesenchymal cells into Sertoli and Leydig cells), and programmed cell death.

Both during its undifferentiated period and at its differentiation into the testis, the gonad appears to be under the control of master genes. WT1, SOX9, and SF-1 are among the key genes involved in the undifferentiated gonad (3–5), whereas SRY acts to divert the developing gonad toward testicular development (6,7). Although the key role of these genes in the development of the gonad is now well recognized, the molecular and cellular mechanisms involved in their actions remain completely unknown. Indeed, these factors are known to be directly or indirectly involved in gene transcription, but their target genes remain to be identified. The target genes for WT1, SOX9, SF1, and SRY are of great importance in that they are potentially involved in the control of cellular events (i.e., migration, proliferation, death) that occur during both the formation of the undifferentiated gonad and its differentiation into testis. Although these target genes under the control of master genes involved in gonad formation are unknown, some candidates have been proposed. Among these candidates are signaling molecules such as hormones and growth factors and cytokines. These two families of signaling molecules may act separately or together. The major hormones that are in action during the development of the fetus are: (1) steroid hormones such as testosterone and its metabolites dihydrotestosterone and estradiol; (2) peptidic hormones such as FSH, LH, and hCG. The role of testosterone and its metabolite dihydrotestosterone on Wolffian duct development is well established. With regard to the other testosterone metabolite, estradiol, its role has been recently shown to also be important for testicular development and function. This chapter will focus on the potential role of growth factors and cytokines in testis development and function in the fetus.

Adult Testis

The adult male gonad consists of two compartments: interstitial tissue supporting the endocrine function through Leydig cell steroidogenesis and seminiferous tubules (containing Myoid, Sertoli, and germ cells) supporting exocrine function and gamete production.

After birth, the testes will enter a period of quiescence until puberty. At puberty, under the control of the neurohypothalamopituitary hormones (mainly LH/testosterone and FSH) spermatogenesis will be initiated and maintained through adulthood. Steroidogenesis, via testosterone production and its actions, plays a key role in the control of spermatogenesis and the development of secondary sexual characteristics. Although LH/testosterone and FSH are important for gametogenesis, no receptors for these hormones have been detected on the germ cells, which suggests that hormonal actions are exerted through somatic cells (which have hormone receptors). Under hormonal stimulation, somatic cells will produce growth factors and cytokines, which in turn modulate germ cell maturation.

Growth Factors in the Testis

Growth factors are classified into less than 10 superfamilies. After their secretion, they bind to specific membrane receptors generating intracellular signals that lead to changes in the pattern of gene expression which result in altered growth or function of the target cell. Growth factors and cytokines are distinct from the classic endocrine hormones in that their synthesis is ubiquitous and their action is local to the site of production. These factors are not only involved in the negative or positive control of cell growth but also in induction or modulation of cell differentiation and in cell death. Their action is context dependent in that the activity of each factor is dependent on the presence of the others. In addition, these factors may be secreted in an inactive form [e.g., transforming growth factor β (TGFβ) family], or together with binding proteins [e.g., insulin-like growth factor (IGF) family], or with soluble receptors (e.g., TNFα) and receptor antagonists [e.g., interleukin (IL)-1]. These different components modulate the (bio)availability of the factors for their receptors. Growth factors and cytokines act locally following different modes of action. In the autocrine mode, the factor is secreted and then binds to cell-surface receptors on the secreting cell. In the paracrine mode, the factor is secreted by one cell type and then acts on neighboring cells. With these modes of action, the actions of growth factors are potentially influenced by the environment of the target cell, which includes different extracellular factors. Indeed, before reaching their target cells the released growth factors and cytokines will interact in the cellular environment with: (1) extracellular matrix components, particularly proteoglycans, which store growth factors (such as bFGF and TGFβs), (2) proteases, and (3) agents that affect their binding to the receptors such as the binding proteins (e.g., IGFBPs, α2-macroglobulin, follistatin) and soluble receptors. In this way, the cells can sense their immediate environment (8).

During the past decade, growth factors and cytokines have been implicated in the intratesticular control. The existence of this local control was suspected some years ago (9–14). Identification of the local factors involved is mainly due to technical advances that have enabled important progress and development to be made in research into the biology of reproduction, more specifically in terms of cell and molecular biology.

Among the growth factors of interest in the development and function of the testis are TGFβ and related peptides (such as inhibins, activins, and antimullerian hormone/mullerian inhibiting substance), TGFα/epidermal growth factor (EGF), IGFs, fibroblast growth factor (FGF) family, platelet-derived growth factor (PDGF), cytokines, including the c-kit/stem cell factor, ILs 1 and 6, and tumor necrosis factor α and neurotrophines, β-nerve growth factor (βNGF).

The possibility that growth factors and cytokines may play a crucial role in testicular formation and functions is supported by at least three types of observations: (1) growth factors and their receptors are expressed in the testis at different crucial periods in the development of this organ; (2) growth factors exert potent regulatory action on the different testicular cell activities, including proliferation, differentiation, and cell death; (3) in transgenic animals in which gene expression related to growth factors and their receptors has been modified (overexpression, knock-out, mutations), infertility has been observed with certain of these factors.

This chapter will focus on the growth factors that comply with the three conditions described earlier: TGFβ and related peptides, IGFs, and NGF and stem cell factor (SCF).

TGFβs and Related Peptides

The TGFβ superfamily peptides regulate cell growth, differentiation, and death (15,16). There are three known TGFβs homologs: TGFβ1, TGFβ2, and TGFβ3. The structural analogs of TGFβ are the inhibins, the activins, the antimullerian hormone/mullerian inhibiting substance, the *vgr-1* subfamily composed of xenopus *vgr-1*, mouse *vgr-1,* the products of the Drosophila decapentaplegic complex, and bone morphogenetic factors (BMP). TGFβs act via at least two serine/threonine kinase receptors, termed TGFβ type I (53 kDa) and type II (75 kDa) (17).

As shown in Table 16.1, TGFβs and their receptors are expressed (in terms of peptides and mRNA) in both somatic and germ cells. Both the regulatory peptides and their receptor expression are under the control of hormones such as FSH, LH, T3, and prolactin (for reviews, see 11,12,18).

The data in Table 16.2 show that TGFβs modulate differentiated functions as well as the proliferation of testicular somatic cells and germ cells (for reviews, see 11,12,18). TGFβ stimulates the production of extracellular matrix components in the testicular somatic cells, which suggests that this factor may play a critical role in fetal testis formation. TGFβ antagonizes the endocrine action on the testes mainly by inhibiting LH and FSH action on Leydig cell steroidogenesis and Sertoli cell aromatase activity. Finally, TGFβ1 appears to regulate spermatogenesis in that it inhibits germ cell proliferation and it is expressed (as well as its receptors) at specific stages during the seminiferous cycle, which suggests a probable role in meiosis and/or spermiogenesis (19,20). Near similar effects are observed with TGFβ-related peptides, such as inhibins, activins, and antimullerian hormone, on testicular formation (Tables 16.3 and 16.4). Although all these effects have been observed in an in vitro system and therefore remain to be confirmed in vivo, observations particularly on transgenic animals indicate that TGFβ and its related peptides may play a crucial role both in testis formation and in spermatogenesis (Table 16.5). Indeed, in a transgenic mouse model in which mature TGFβ1 is overexpressed in the liver, several lesions have been observed in the testes, including testicular atrophy with a thickened tubular basement membrane (21). In TGFβ2 null mutant mice, cryptorchidy, and testicular atrophy have been reported (22). With regard to TGFβ-related peptides, data obtained in transgenic models point to testicular lesions. Inhibin α-deficient mice exhibit a predisposition to gonadal stromal tumors. Spermatogenesis does not seem to be directly affected, however, and the arrest of germ-cell maturation was observed only when the tumor becomes more important (23). Testicular lesions in

TABLE 16.1. Expression of TGFβs in the testis.

	mRNA	Peptide	Regulation
TGFβ	Peritubular myoid cells (TGFβ1 β2 β3) Prepubertal Sertoli cells (TGF β2) Early prepubertal Sertoli cells (TGF β3) Germ cells (TGFβ1)	Fetal Sertoli cells (TGF β1) Prepubertal Sertoli cells (TGF β2) Fetal Leydig (TGF β1) Germ cells (TGF β1)	FSH (-), T3 (+), PRL (+)
TGFβ receptor	Germ cells: receptor type I, II, III Leydig cells: receptor type I, II, III Sertoli cells: receptor type I, II, III	Germ cells: receptor type I, II, III Leydig cells: receptor type I, II, III Sertoli cells: receptor type I, II, III	LH (+), FSH (+)

TABLE 16.2. Actions of TGFβs in the testis.

	Target cells	Actions
TGFβ	Leydig cells	→ LH induced steroidogenesis → IGF I receptor
	Sertoli cells	→ FSH induced aromatase activity ↑ lactate production
	Peritubular myoid cells	↑ extracellular matrix component secretion
	Germ cells	→ proliferation

TABLE 16.3. Expression of activin/inhibin/AMH in the testis.

	MRNA	Peptide	Regulation
Inhibin and activin	Rat fetal gonad (βB chain) human fetal gonad (2nd trimester, α βB βA chains) Sertoli cells (α βA βB chains) Leydig cells (α β chains)	Sertoli cells (inhibin, activin) Leydig cells (inhibin, activin)	α chain: FSH (+) Inhibin: EGF (+), insulin (+), opioids (+) and depletion of late spermatids (-)
Activin receptor	Act RII late pachytene spermatocytes, round spermatids Act RIIB2 spermatogonies A1 and A2, Sertoli cells Act RII peritubular myoid cells		
AMH/MIS	(perinatal) Sertoli cells	Sertoli cells	SF1 (+), Testosterone (-), FSH (-)
AMH-R type I		Sertoli cells	

TABLE 16.4. Actions of activin/inhibin/AMH in the testis.

	Target cells	Actions
Activin A	Leydig cells	→ LH induced steroidogenesis
	Sertoli cells	↑ FSH induced aromatase activity
		→ androgen receptor
		↑ transferrin and inhibin production
	Germ cells	↑ proliferation
Inhibin	Leydig cells	↑ LH induced steroidogenesis
	Germ cells	→ proliferation
α chain knock out	Stromal tissue	Development of tumor after birth
AMH/MIS	Sertoli cells	→ FSH induced aromatase activity

TABLE 16.5. Transgenic animals, effects on testicular functions.

Molecule	Model	Viability	Effects on reproductive function
Act RII	KO homozygote	Normal	Reduction of plasmatic level of FSH, delay puberty
TGFβ1	Overexpression	Decreased	Testicular atrophy, thickened tubular basement membrane
TGFβ2	KO homozygote		Cryptorchidy and testicular atrophy
α inhibin	KO homozygote	Lethal at 4 weeks	Predisposition to gonadal stromal tumors, infertility
BMP8b	KO homozygote		Germ cells fail to proliferate or exhibit a marked reduction in proliferation
IGF I	KO homozygote	Normal	Infertility, testicular atrophy, reduced spermatogenesis (18% compared to the normal spermatogenesis). Low levels of testosterone production
TrkA	KO homozygote	Lethal at 4 weeks	Animals which reach adulthood are infertile

Act RII-deficient mice are probably related to a decrease in FSH production as activin is known to stimulate FSH expression. In these animals (ACTRII -/-), puberty is delayed, and the testes are small but spermatogenesis can occur (24). In mice with target mutation in bone morphogenetic protein 8b (BMP8b), both initiation and maintenance of spermatogenesis were affected. Indeed, during early puberty (2 weeks old) in homozygous mutants, the germ cells failed to proliferate or exhibited a marked reduction in proliferation. The adults were infertile due to germ cell depletion, which was a consequence of an increase in programmed cell death. Somatic cells (i.e., Leydig and Sertoli cells) appeared to be unaffected (25).

IGFs

The IGF system consists of: (1) three growth factors structurally and functionally related to insulin—IGF I, IGF II, and Leydig insulin like (Ley-IL or relaxin-related protein: RRP); (2) two receptors—type I (tyrosine kinase) and type II (similar to cation independent mannose 6 phosphate receptor); and (3) six different binding proteins. The expression of IGF I is known classically to be under the control of growth hormone (GH). All the components of this system are expressed in the testis (Table 16.6). The components of the IGF system are expressed in both somatic and germ cells. Germ cells specifically appear to express both the ligand IGF I and its receptors but not the IGF BPs.

It is interesting to note that the expression of the different components of the IGF system are more or less under the control of the endocrine system, including FSH, LH/testosterone, prolactin, retinol, T3, and GH. Some local growth factors seem to exert a regulatory action on IGF I, IGF BP, and IGF receptor expression in the testicular cells (Table 16.7). With regard to Ley-IL, this peptide is expressed solely in Leydig cells (and their female homolog thecal cells). The receptors for Ley-IL as well the biological activities of this peptide remain to be identified. The IGF system can be viewed as a positive regulator of the two testicular functions (i.e., steroidogenesis and spermatogenesis). The IGF system enhances and mediates the action of the gonadotropins (Table 16.7).

According to these data, mainly obtained in vitro, the IGF I null mutation has a dramatic impact both on the development and on the physiology of the reproductive system. Homozygous mice are infertile dwarfs. These animals exhibit testicular atrophy with reduced spermatogenesis (18% of normal spermatogenesis). Low levels of testosterone due to lesions at the level of Leydig cells may explain the infertility (26,27). Together, the data obtained in vitro suggest that IGF I may well exert a determinant action on Leydig cell development and function.

Neurotropins

NGF is among the neurotropins present in the testes. NGF was initially identified as an essential factor in the development and maintenance of sensory

TABLE 16.6. Expression in the testis of the system IGF.

	mRNA	Peptide	Regulation
IGF-I	Leydig cells Sertoli cells Germ cells	Leydig cells (porcine and rat) Sertoli cells Germ cells (pachytene spermatocytes)	GH (+), FSH (+), LH (+), PRL (-), Testosterone, (+), Retinol (+), T3 (+), EGF (+), bFGF(+), IL1α (-),TNFα (-)
IGF-II	Sertoli cells Leydig cells	Sertoli cells Leydig cells	
IGF-BP2	Leydig cells	Leydig cells	LH (+)
	Peritubular myoid cells	Peritubular myoid cells	
IGF-BP3	Sertoli cells	Sertoli cells	FSH (-), TNFα (+), IL1α (+)
IGF-I receptor type I	Sertoli cells Leydig cells	Sertoli cells Leydig cells Germ cells	LH (+) TGFβ (-)
IGF-I receptor type II	Sertoli cells Germ cells	Sertoli cells Germ cells (pachytene spermtocytes, round spermatides)	

TABLE 16.7. Actions of the system IGF in the testis.

	Target cells	Actions
IGF-I	Leydig cells Sertoli cells	↑ LH induced steroidogenesis ↑ mitogenesis ↑ lactate production ↑ glucose uptake
	Germ cells	↑ proliferation

and sympathetic peripheral neurons (28). NGF exerts its effects through inter-action with two distinct receptors: the low affinity receptor is a 75 kDa glyco-protein and the high affinity receptor (trk: 140 kDa) has been identified as a tyrosine kinase receptor (29,30). NGF mRNA and proteins have been de-tected in spermatocytes and early spermatids, but not in testicular somatic cells (31) (Table 16.8). The two types of NGF receptor are expressed in the testis and particularly in the Sertoli cells (32,33). The NGF receptor with low affinity is expressed in Sertoli cells at stages VII and VIII (32), the sites of onset of meiosis. This receptor would appear to be under the negative control of testosterone because hypophysectomy in the adult rat or EDS treatment increased NGF receptor mRNA levels 50-fold, whereas testosterone treatment restored the normal level of NGF receptor mRNA (32). The NGF receptor with high affinity (trk) did not show much variation during the seminiferous cycle (33). The NGF receptor is probably also expressed in peritubular myoid cells (34).

NGF stimulates in vitro DNA synthesis in seminiferous tubules with preleptotene spermatocytes at the onset of meiosis. This effect is probably not direct; rather, it is exerted via the Sertoli cells (33). NGF exerts a stabiliz-ing effect on cultures of human seminiferous tubules. It maintains Sertoli and myoid cell morphology and prevents thickening of the tubule wall (34,35) (Table 16.9).

NGF and TrkA target mice have been generated (36,37) Although the ma-jority of TrkA (-/-) mice die at 8 weeks old, those that reach adulthood are infertile (38). The cellular and molecular mechanisms involved in such infer-tility remain unknown.

Cytokines

SCF is a membrane-bound protein with a soluble form released by proteolytic processing of the mature protein. Differential expression of soluble or mem-brane-bound steel factor is regulated by alternative splicing of steel factor mRNA to remove the protease recognition site. Both membrane-bound and soluble steel factor are biologically active (39,40). The SCF receptor called c-kit is a tyrosine kinase receptor (39).

The SCF/c-kit system regulates primordial germ cell migration and prolif-eration (41–44). C-kit is expressed in the primordial germ cells of 12.5-day-old rat embryos (45,46), i.e., at a period that corresponds to the migration of the primordial germ cells from the yolk sac to the gonadal ridge. SCF is present from day 9 of gestation along the migratory pathway of germ cells as well as in the gonadal ridge (46). After birth, c-kit is expressed in spermatogo-nia type A (46–48) and in Leydig cells (46). The SCF is present in Sertoli cells (45,46) (see Table 16.8). Moreover, during postnatal testicular develop-ment, the expression of the SCF forms change in terms of transmembrane/soluble form ratio (49).

TABLE 16.8. Expression of NGF and SCF in the testis.

	mRNA	Peptide	Regulation
NGF	Early spermatids Pachytene spermatocyte	Early spermatids Pachytene spermatocyte	
NGF receptor	Sertoli cells (trk and low affinity receptor) Peritubular myoid cells		Testosterone (−)
SCF	Sertoli cells	Sertoli cells	FSH (+)
c-kit	Primordial germ cells Spermatogonies A Leydig cells	Primordial germ cells Spermatogonies A Leydig cells	

TABLE 16.9. Actions of NGF in the testis.

	Target cells	Actions
NGF	Sertoli cells and peritubular myoid cells	Maintains morphology Prevents thickening of the tubule wall
SCF	Germ cells Germ cells	↑ DNA synthesis Proliferation, anti-apoptotic

TABLE 16.10. Mutation of SCF and gonadal function.

Mutation	Gonadal alteration	Gene alteration
Steel	Infertility, no migration of primordial germ cells in the fetal gonad	Large deletion
Steel–Dickie	Infertility, migration of primordial germ cells in the fetal gonad, no proliferation of spermatogonia at puberty	Deletion of transmembrane domain
Steel 17H	First wave of spermatogenesis, after infertility female fertile	Deletion of cytoplasmic domain
Steel panda	Female infertility male fertile	Rearrangement in 5' regulatory region

The involvement of the SCF/c-kit system in the migration of primordial germinal cells, as well as their proliferation in the gonadal ridge, have been recognized by studying mice bearing the mutations designated Sl/Sl^d (Steel-Dickie) and W/W^v (dominant white-spotting). These mutations are characterized by the depletion of three embryonic migratory lineages: hematopoetic stem cells, neural crest-derived melanocytes and primordial germinal cells (45). Deletion of the receptor (W/W^v mice) or the ligand SCF (Sl/Sl mice) results in sterile testis depleted in germ cells, the result of a defect in the migration of primordial germinal cells to the gonadal ridge (Table 16.10). Moreover, Sl/Sl^d mice that produce only the soluble form of SCF (deletion of the transmembrane domain of the SCF gene) are infertile, although germ cells are present in the testis (50–51). When taken together, these observations would suggest that the SCF/c-kit system is mainly related to primordial germinal cell migration. The transmembrane SCF appears to support the survival (via an antiapoptotic process?) but not the proliferation of primordial germinal cells (52). By contrast, the soluble form of SCF supports the proliferation of spermatogonia A (49,52). The observation that Sertoli cells predominantly express the soluble form of SCF in the postnatal period enforces the involvement of these cells in the proliferation process that occurs at the level of spermatogonia. Together, the c-kit/SCF system may play a role during the early steps of the spermatogonia process, particularly in the mitotic progression of type A spermatogonia. The differentiation of spermatogonia B into preleptotene spermatocytes seems to be independent of c-kit (47,53).

Conclusions

Although the hormones LH/testosterone and FSH represent the major system that controlls the male gonad, it is not the only one. Local growth factors and cytokines are probably necessary to extend and adapt hormonal action to the local requirements of the complex process of spermatogenesis. Because of their pleiotropic actions on cellular proliferation, differentiation, and death, it is possible that the role of cytokines and growth factors is more important and not dependent on the hormones during fetal development of the testes. In this context, TGFβ and SCF are probably involved in germ cell migration and proliferation during fetal testis development. By contrast, in adult testicular function, the local growth factor system appears to be highly dependent on the endocrine system. Indeed, the expression of several growth factors, their receptors and/or binding proteins is controlled by the endocrine system. For example, LH increases the level of IGF-I, FSH inhibits the production of TGFβ and the gonadotropins affect the expression of IGFBPs and TGFβ receptors. Moreover, the hormonal action is modulated by local factors. Indeed, TGFβ and activin A inhibit LH-induced steroidogenesis; TGFβ and AMH inhibit FSH-induced aromatase activity. When taken together, these observations suggest that the testicular growth factors and cytokines may act as an adjusted fine local relay for the (neuro)endocrine system action in that their expression is under hormonal control and they modulate locally hormonal activities. Although in adult life testicular growth factors appear to be involved in the differentiated functions of somatic Leydig and Sertoli cells, one of the major questions that remains to be answered is whether and how testicular growth factors control germ-cell proliferation and differentiation. Local signaling molecules appear to control germ-cell functions because knockout or surexpression of growth factors induces spermatogenesis arrest (see Table 16.5), but the molecular mechanisms underlying these pathologies remain unknown.

All of these observations extend our concept of reproductive endocrinology to the level of cell–cell regulation in the gonad. The corollary is that the function of the testis is dependent on gonadotropins and the correct functioning of local growth factors. This could be illustrated by the human testicular pathology. Indeed, some etiologies are known for male infertility (oligoazoospermia), such as hormonal (Kallman-syndrome), genetic (AZF, YRRM) defects, and physical injuries (i.e., radiation), but in most cases, the etiology of male infertility is not known although hormonal blood levels are normal or subnormal. Then in certain cases of male infertility, mean that, the local hormonal relay system (i.e., testicular growth factors and cytokines) might be deficient.

Thus, the determination of important growth factors in testicular physiology, as well as their mechanisms of action and interactions, will probably help us to a better understanding of the mechanisms involved in some forms of pathological conditions that lead to infertility, particularly testicular oligoazoospermia.

Acknowledgments. Our work was supported by the Institut National de la Santé et de la Recherche Médicale (INSERM U 407), the Université Claude-Bernard (Lyon I), and the Ligue contre le cancer (comité départemental de l'Ain).

References

1. Wylie CC, Stott D, Donovan PJ. Primordial germ cell migration. In: Browder LW, editor. Developmental biology, Vol. 2. New York: Plenum Press, 1985:433–48.
2. Wartenberg H. Differentiation and development of the testes. In: Burger H, de Kretser D, editors. The testis. New York: Raven Press, 1989:67–118.
3. Kreidberg JA, Sariola H, Loring JM, Maeda M, Pelletier J, Housman DE, et al. WT-1 is required for early kidney development. Cell 1993;74:679–91.
4. Luo XR, Ikeda Y, Parker KL. A cell-specific nuclear receptor is essential for adrenal and gonadal development and sexual differentiation. Cell 1994;77:481–90.
5. Foster JW, Dominguez-Steglich MA, Guioli S, et al. Campomelic dysplasia and autosomal sex reversal caused by mutations in an SRY-related gene. Nature 1994;372:525–30.
6. Berta P, Hawkins JR, Sinclair AH, et al. Genetic evidence equating SRY and the testis determining factor. Nature 1990;348:448–50.
7. Goodfellow PN, Berkovitz G, Hawkins JR, Harley VR, Lovell-Badge R. Sex determination, sex-reversal and SRY: a review. In: Hillier SG, editor. Gonadal development and function. Serono Symposia. New York: Raven Press, 1992:6–15.
8. Wakefield L. Growth factors: an overview. In: Isidori A, Fabri A, Dufau ML, editors. Hormonal communicating events in the testis, Vol. 70. New York: Raven Press, 1990:181–90.
9. Fritz IB. Sites of action of androgens and follicle stimulating hormones on cells of the seminiferous tubule. In: Litwack G, editor. Biochemical actions of hormones, Vol. 5. New York: Academic Press, 1978:249–81.
10. Sharpe RM. Paracrine control of the testis. Clin Endocrinol Metab 1986;15:185–207.
11. Benahmed M. Growth factors and cytokines in the testis. In: Comhaire F, editor. Male infertility: clinical investigation, cause, evaluation and treatment. London: Chapman Hall, 1996:55–96.
12. Skinner MK. Cell-cell interactions in the testis. Endocrinol Rev 1991;12:45–77.
13. Mather JP, Krummen LA. Inhibin, activin and growth factors: paracrine regulators of testicular function. In: Nieschlag E, Habenicht UF, editors. Spermatogenesis, fertilization, contraception: molecular, cellular and endocrine events in male reproduction. Berlin: Springer, 1992:169–200.
14. Griswold MD. Interactions between germ cells and Sertoli cells in the testis. Biol Reprod 1995;52:211–16.
15. Roberts AB, Sporn MB. The transforming growth factor-βs. In: Sporn MB, Roberts AB, editors. Peptide growth factor and their receptors, Part I. New York: Springer, 1991:419–73.
16. Massagué J. The transforming growth factor-β family. Annu Rev Cell Biol 1990;6:597–641.
17. Massagué J, Attissano J, Wrana JL. The TGF-β family and its composite receptors. Trends Cell Biol 1994;4:172–78.
18. Gnessi L, Fabbri A, Spera G. Gonadal peptides as mediators of development and functional control of the testis: an integrated system with hormones and local environment. Endocrinol Rev 1997;18:541–609.
19. Naz RK, Kumar R. Transforming growth factor β_1 enhances expression of a 50 kDa protein related to 2'-5' oligoadenylate synthetase in human sperm cells. J Cell Physiol 1991;146:156–63.

20. Caussanel V, Tabone E, Hendrick JC, Dacheux F, Benahmed M. Cellular distribution of transforming growth factor betas 1, 2, 3 and their type I and II receptors during post natal development and spermatogenesis in the boar testis. Biol Reprod 1997;56:357–67.
21. Sanderson N, Factor V, Nagay P, et al. Hepatic expression of mature transforming growth factor β1 in transgenic mice results in multiple tissue lesions. Proc Natl Acad Sci USA 1995;92:2572–76.
22. Sandford LP, Ormsby I, Gittenberger-de Groot AC, et al. TGFβ2 knockout mice have multiple developmental defects that are non-overlappping with other TGFβ knockout phenotypes. Development 1997;124:2659–70.
23. Matzuk MM, Finegold MJ, Su JGJ, Hsueh AJW, Bradley A. α-inhibin is a tumour-suppressor gene with gonadal specificity in mice. Nature 1992;360:313–19.
24. Matzuk MM, Kumar TR, Bradley A. Different phenotypes for mice deficient in either activins or activin receptor type II. Nature 1995;374:356–60.
25. Zhao GQ, Deng K, Labosky PA, Liaw L, Hogan BL. The gene encoding bone morphogenetic protein 8B is required for the initiation and maintenance of spermatogenesis in the mouse. Genes Dev 1996;10:1657–69.
26. Baker J, Liu J-P, Robertson EJ, Efsfratiadis A. Role of insulin-like growth factors in embryonic and postnatal growth. Cell 1993;75:73–82.
27. Baker J, Hardy MP, Zhou J, et al. Effects of an igf1 gene null mutation on mouse reproduction. Mol Endocrinol 1996;10:903–16.
28. Levi-Montalcini R. The nerve growth factor 35 years later. Science 1987;237:1154–62.
29. Hempstead BL, Chao M. The nerve growth factor receptor: biochemical and structural analysis. Recent Prog Horm Res 1989;44:441–66.
30. Chao MV. Nerve growth factor. In: Sporn MB, Roberts AB, editors. Peptide growth factor and their receptors, Part II. New York: Springer, 1991:135–66.
31. Ayer-LeLievre C, Olson L, Ebendal T, Hallbrook F, Persson H. Nerve growth factor mRNA and protein in the testes and epididymis of mouse and rat. Proc Natl Acad Sci USA 1988;85:2628–32.
32. Persson H, Ayer-Lelievre C, Söder O, et al. Expression of β-nerve growth factor receptor mRNA in Sertoli cells downregulated by testosterone. Science 1990;247:704–7.
33. Parvinen M, Pelto-Huikko M, Söder O, et al. Expression of β-nerve growth factor and its receptor in rat seminiferous epithelium: specific function at the onset of meiosis. J Cell Biol 1992;117:629–41.
34. Seidl K, Holstein AF. Evidence for the presence of nerve growth factor (NGF) and NGF receptors in human testis. Cell Tissue Res 1990;261:549–54.
35. Seidl K, Holstein AF. Organ culture of human seminiferous tubules: a useful tool to study the role of nerve growth factor in the testis. Cell Tissue Res 1990;261:539–47.
36. Crowley C, Spencer SD, Nishimura MC, et al. Mice lacking nerve growth factor display perinatal loss of sensory and sympathetic neurons yet develop basal forebrain cholinergic neurons. Cell 1994;76:1001–11.
37. Smeyne RJ, Klein R, Schnapp A, et al. Severe sensory and sympathetic neuropathies in mice carrying a disrupted TrK/NGF receptor gene. Nature 1994;368:246–49.
38. Klein R. Role of neurotrophins in mouse neuronal development. FASEB J 1994;8:738–44.
39. Williams DE, Lyman SD. Characterization of the gene-product of the steel locus. Prog Growth Factor Res 1992;3:235–42.

40. Flanagan JG, Chan D, Leder P. Transmembrane form of the c-kit ligand growth factor is determined by alternative splicing and is missing in the Sl^d mutation. Cell 1991;64:1025–35.
41. De Felici M, Pesce M. Growth factors in mouse primordial germ cell migration and proliferation. Prog Growth Factor Res 1994;5:135–43.
42. Godin I, Deed R, Cooke J, Zsebo K, Dexter M, Wylie CC. Effects of the steel gene product on mouse primordial germ cells in culture. Nature 1991;352:807–9.
43. Dolci S, Williams DE, Ernst MK, et al. Requirement for mast cell growth factor for primordial germ cell survival in culture. Nature 1991;352:809–11.
44. Resnick JL, Bixler LS, Cheng L, Donovan PJ. Long-term proliferation of mouse primordial germ cells in culture. Nature 1992;359:550–51.
45. Orr-Urtreger A, Avivi A, Zimmer Y, Givol D, Yarden Y, Lonai P. Developmental expression of c-kit, a proto-oncogene encoded by the W locus. Development 1990;109:911–23.
46. Motro B, Van Der Kooy D, Rossant J, Reith A, Bernstein A. Contiguous patterns of c-kit and steel expression: analysis of mutations at the W and Sl loci. Development 1991;113:1207–21.
47. Dym M, Jia MC, Dirami G, et al. Expression of c-kit receptor and its autophosphorylation in immature rat type A spermatogonia. Biol Reprod 1995;52:8–19.
48. Yoshinaga K, Nishikawa S, Ogawa M, et al. Role of c-kit in mouse spermatogenesis: identification of spermatogonia as a specific site of c-kit expression and function. Development 1991;113:689–99.
49. Marziali G, Lazzaro D, Sorrentino V. Binding of germ cells to mutant Sld Sertoli cells is defective and is rescued by expression of the transmembrane form of the c-kit ligand. Dev Biol 1993;157:182–90.
50. Russell ES. Hereditary anemias of the mouse: a review for geneticists. Adv Genet 1979;20:357–59.
51. Brannan CI, Lyman SD, Williams DE, et al. Steel-Dickie mutation encodes a c-kit ligand lacking transmembrane and cytoplasmic domains. Proc Natl Acad Sci USA 1991;88:4671–74.
52. Tajima Y, Onoue H, Kitamura Y, Nishimune Y. Biologically active c-kit ligand growth factor is produced by mouse Sertoli cells and is defective in Sl/d mutant mice. Development 1991;113:1031–35.
53. Tajima Y, Sawada K, Morimoto T, Nishimune Y. Switching of mouse spermatogonial proliferation from the c-kit receptor-independent type to the receptor-dependent type during differentiation. J Reprod Fertil 1994;102:117–22.

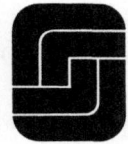

17

Microinsemination Using Spermatogenic Cells in Mammals

ATSUO OGURA AND RYUZO YANAGIMACHI

Microinsemination (MI), also called microassisted fertilization or microfertilization, has been used extensively in clinical practice and for research purposes. The first attempt to fertilize mammalian oocytes by MI was made by Uehara and Yanagimachi in 1976 (1). They demonstrated that injected sperm heads could develop into pronuclei after incorporation into homologous and heterologous oocytes. Since then MI with several mammalian species has increased our fundamental knowledge of fertilization. Full-term embryo development following intracytoplasmic sperm injection (ICSI) was first demonstrated in the rabbit (2), followed by bovines (3). Even though the efficiency of ICSI in these animal studies was disappointingly low, human ICSI proved to be very efficient and became the method of choice to overcome male factor infertility (4). The history and technical aspects of MI with mature spermatozoa have already been described elsewhere (5,6). Advancement of MI techniques has enabled us to use immature male germ cells (spermatogenic cells) as substitutes for spermatozoa. In contrast to the development of ICSI, the development of MI using spermatogenic cells was largely contributed by experiments with animals, especially mice. We will review the technical aspects of MI using spermatogenic cells and its significance for basic researches and clinical practice.

Technical Aspects of MI Using Spermatogenic Cells

Collection of Spermatogenic Cells

Spermatogenic cells need to be collected from the testicular tissue. This is in contrast to MI with mature spermatozoa, which can be isolated from ejaculated semen or the epididymis to almost 100% purity. Spermatogenic cells are collected by either pipetting (7) or enzyme treatment (8) of the seminiferous tubules. The former is simple and takes less time than does the latter, but is not suitable for collection of young spermatogenic cells, such as spermatogonia, which are located near the basement membrane. Pronase treatment of mixed cell suspension can eliminate spermatozoa and elongating spermatids, leaving only round spermatids and spermatocytes in the suspension. This makes handling of spermatogenic cells for the micromanipulation easier. This procedure also increases the efficiency of electrofusion between oocytes and spermatogenic cells at least in hamsters and mice (9).

Identification of Spermatogenic Cells

Because spermatogenic cells are round nucleated cells, as are many other testicular cells, we must accurately identify each type of spermatogenic cell before MI. Round spermatids in rodents, for example, are round, 7–10 μm in diameter (Fig. 17.1A). They have a distinct round nucleus with a relatively large amount of cytoplasm. Visual identification of spermatids can be confirmed by examining their chromosomes after injection into mature mouse oocytes (Fig. 17.1B).

Nuclear Transfer

Two different methods can be used for transfer of spermatogenic cell nuclei into oocytes: membrane fusion and intracytoplasmic injection (Fig. 17.2). Membrane fusion is one of the fundamental techniques that have been used widely in cell biology. Cell-to-cell membrane fusion is achieved in vitro by inactivated virus (e.g., HVJ), electric pulse, or chemicals (e.g., polyethylene glycol). For oocyte–spermatogenic cell fusion, only electric pulse has been successful (9). Chemicals used for membrane fusion are more or less harmful to spermatogenic cells/oocytes. Virus-mediated fusion, which is the method most frequently used in mouse blastomere fusion, is very inefficient for spermatogenic cells (probably due to lack of virus receptors). The intracytoplasmic injection of spermatogenic cells is similar to ICSI for mature spermatozoa, except that the plasma membrane of spermatogenic cells must be ruptured before injection. Table 17.1 summarizes the characteristics of intracytoplasmic injection and electrofusion. We may choose either method, depending on the characteristics of the oocytes and spermatogenic cells to be used for experiments. Germinal vesicle oocytes, for example, are very sensitive to mechanical injection. They tolerate better to electric pulse for fusion.

Centrosome Inheritance

When a prespermatozoal cell is sucked into the injection pipette, the nucleus is readily separated from the cytoplasm. The nucleus, therefore can be injected into an oocyte with minimal amount of accompanying cytoplasm. One cytoplasmic component that plays an important role in the fertilization process and in embryo development is the centrosome, an organella from which microtubule arrays develop. In most animals, the centrosome shows predomi-

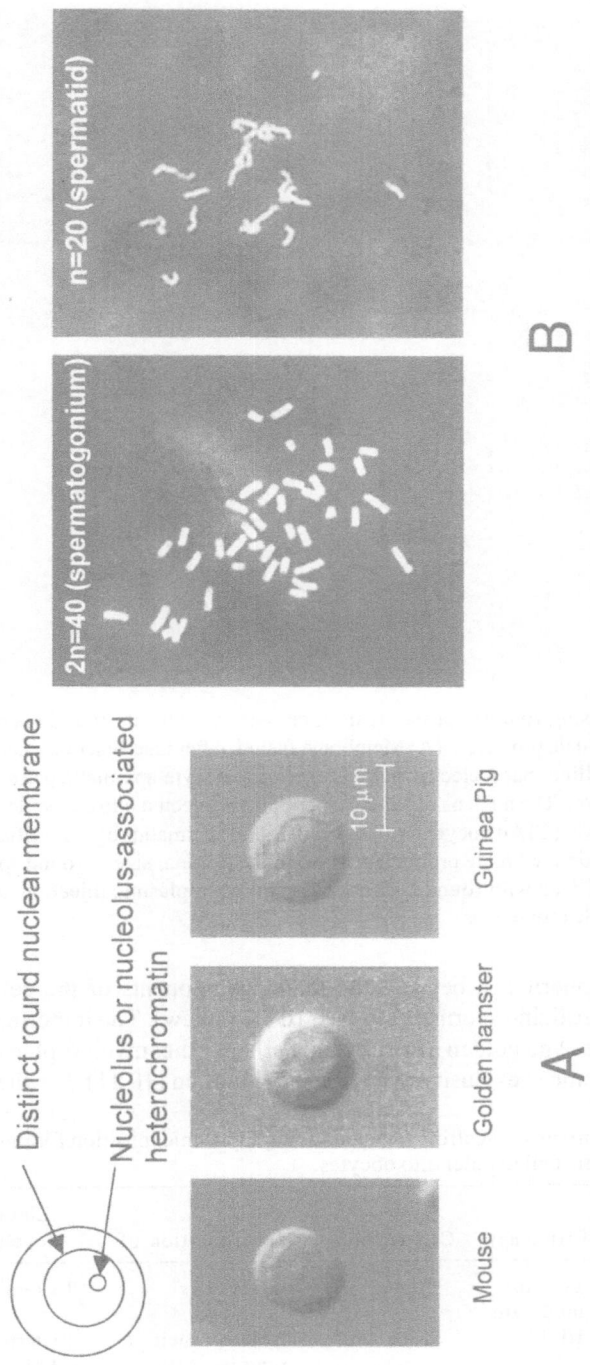

FIGURE 17.1. (A) Morphological characteristics of round spermatids. There are slight species-related differences in size. (B) Identification of round spermatids by prematurely condensed chromosomes in Met II mouse oocytes. Round spermatids show 20 (haploid) thin (single chromatid) chromosomes.

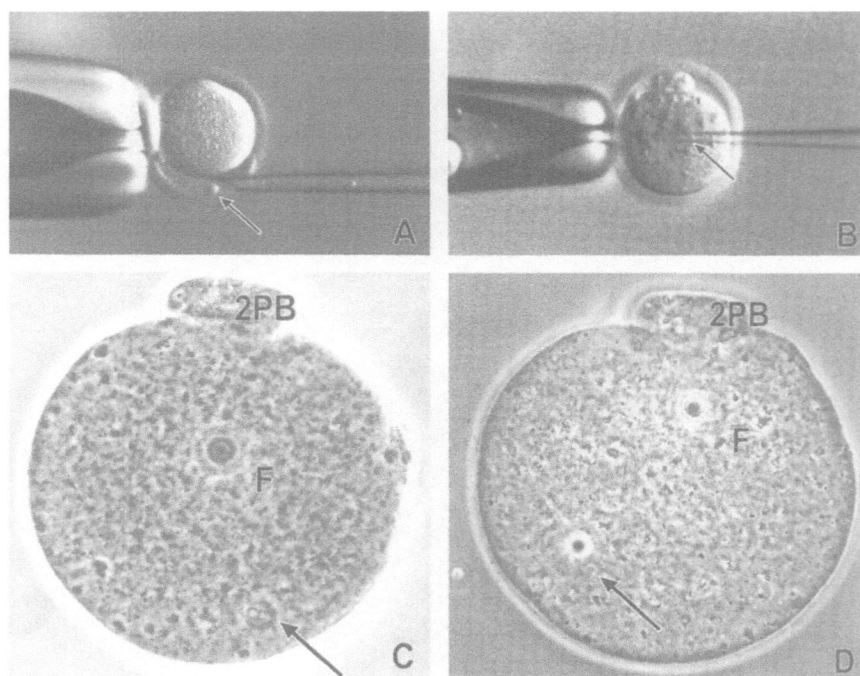

FIGURE 17.2. MI using round spermatids in mice. Arrows indicate round spermatids or spermatid-derived male pronuclei. (A) Membrane fusion. After insertion of a round spermatid into the perivitelline space, electric pulse is applied to oocyte-spermatid pairs. (B) Intracytoplasmic injection. The nucleus of a round spermatid is injected into the ooplasm with or without its cytoplasm. (C) An oocyte fertilized with round spermatids by electrofusion. Note that the spermatid-derived male pronucleus stays in the original size of round spermatids. (D) An oocyte fertilized with round spermatids by intracytoplasmic injection, showing a well-developed male pronucleus.

nantly paternal inheritance because the major components of the centrosome come from the fertilizing spermatozoa (see 10 for review). The important exceptions are the mouse and golden hamster (and perhaps other myomorphic rodents), in which centrosome is exclusively maternally inherited (10,11). In other words,

TABLE 17.1. Comparison of electrofusion and intracytoplasmic injection for introduction of the spermatogenic cell neuclei into oocytes.

Method	Efficiency	Cell viability	Incorporation of	Embryonic development
Electrofusion	Low to moderate	High	Intact cells	To term (mouse)
Intracytoplasmic injection	High	Moderate	Isolated nuclei or ruptured cells	To term (mouse, rabbit, human)

the spermatozoon does not need to bring the centrosome into the oocyte to organize the microtubular system. Microtubule-organizing centers scattered throughout the ooplasm become the center for microtubular assembly in fertilized eggs. This is true for fertilization by round spermatids (12). Thus, injection of spermatid nucleus alone is enough to produce normal offspring in the mouse (13). It is known that in human ICSI, both sperm heads and centrioles must be incorporated in the oocytes during fertilization in order for normal embryonic development to follow (14). In most mammalian species, therefore, injection of both spermatid nucleus and centrosome is recommended.

Oocyte Activation

As prespermatozoal cells are likely to be lacking/deficient in the oocyte-activating factors (at least in laboratory animals), oocytes must be activated artificially either before or after MI. In some animals (e.g., the golden hamster), oocytes may be activated by Ca^{2+} influx at the puncture site of intracytoplasmic injection, as shown spermatid injection in hamsters (7). The stimulus, however, is often insufficient to induce subsequent embryonic development (7). Oocytes receiving prespermatozoal cell nuclei, therefore, should be artificially activated before (hamster) (7) or after (human) (15) cell (e.g., spermatid) injection. Human spermatids may contain some factors that can induce Ca^{2+} oscillations in human oocytes, but spermatid injection alone cannot trigger oocyte activation (16); rather, it should be combined with other activation stimuli such as Ca^{2+} ionophore. The oscillation-inducing factor (oscillogen) in human spermatids may be too little to induce oocyte activation or different from the potent oocyte-activating factor.

Cell-Cycle Synchronization

Mature spermatozoa are in the G0 cell-cycle phase, whereas mature oocytes are in the M phase. Both enter the G1 phase simultaneously. Spermatogenic cells for MI are at the G2 phase. The cell cycle, therefore, must be synchronized between oocytes and spermatogenic cells. It is preferable, for example, to inject round spermatid nuclei into oocytes that have been activated and in the telophase II (B in Fig. 17.3). Oocytes injected with secondary spermatocytes should be activated after premature condensation of spermatocyte chromosomes (C in Fig. 17.3). Thus, a fertilized oocyte contains two haploid sets of chromosomes each from a spermatogenic cell and an oocyte.

Microinsemination Using Spermatids

Fertilizing Ability of Spermatids

The first candidates of spermatogenic cells as the substitutes for mature spermatozoa are spermatids because they have a haploid set of chromosomes as

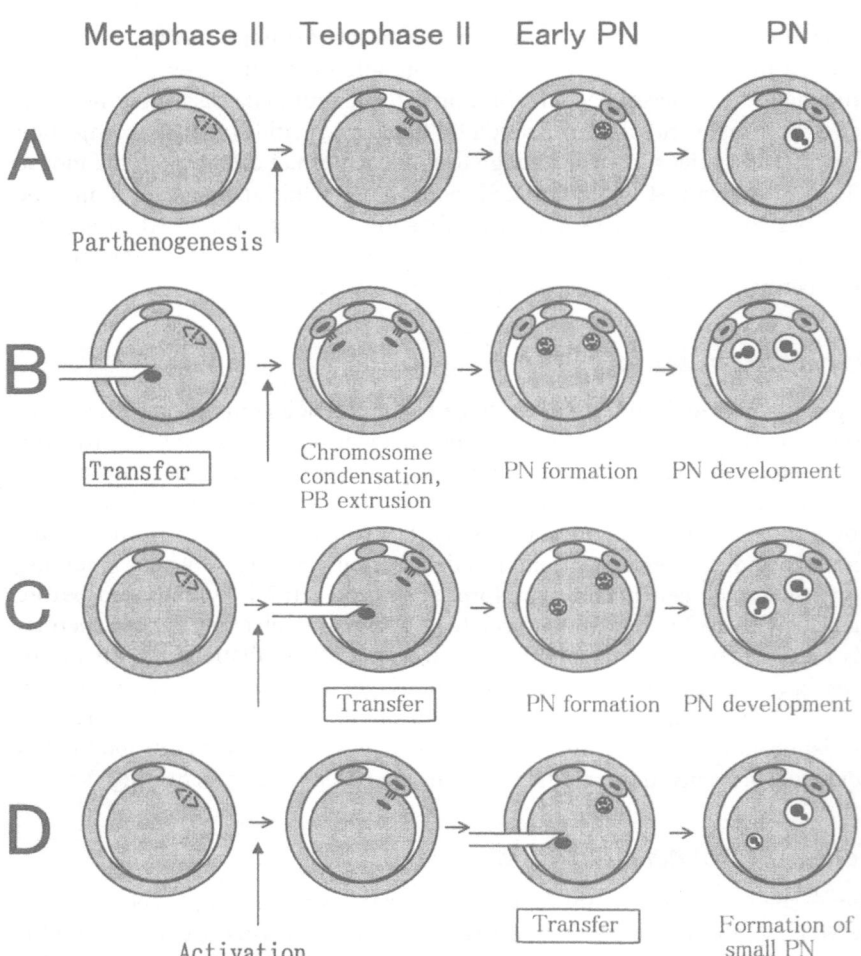

FIGURE 17.3. Pronuclear formation from spermatogenic cell nuclei following intracytoplasmic injection into matured oocytes before (B), shortly after (C), or long after (D) artificial activation.

mature spermatozoa. The first attempt to microinseminate oocytes with round spermatids was made in the golden hamster. Hamster oocytes well tolerated microsurgery as has already been reported in early hamster ICSI experiments (1). Because hamster ICSI was first performed using isolated sperm heads, round spermatids were treated with a detergent to remove cytoplasm prior to injection (7). We now know that the nucleus can be easily isolated from cytoplasm by drawing spermatids in and out of the injection pipette. After incorporation into mature oocytes, the nuclei of round spermatids participated in the pronuclear formation and the zygotes subsequently developed into two-cell embryos. Because hamster oocytes/embryos are very susceptible to in vitro micromanipulation, however, they never developed beyond the two-cell stage, even when they were transferred into the ovarian bursa, which is known as the best site for transfer of one-cell hamster embryos (17).

We therefore began to use the mouse as a model animal for MI. Intracytoplasmic injection of mouse oocytes had been extremely difficult because their plasma membrane in most oocytes rupture and lyse immediately after injection by conventional micromanipulators; therefore, we used the electrofusion technique to transfer spermatid nucleus into oocytes. Oocyte-spermatid fusion was initially very inefficient (9), but it became more efficient in later experiments (18). As the oocytes had already been activated prior to application of fusion pulse in order to increase fusion efficiency, most (> 80%) oocytes electrofused with spermatids contained a small male pronucleus (original spermatid nucleus size) (C in Fig. 17.2 and D in Fig. 17.3), which was not visible in living eggs by Nomarski optics; therefore, we transferred all of the two-cell embryos including parthenogenetic ones to recipient females. We obtained six offspring through the first series of experiments (18). Of them, at least four were proven to be fertile and had a normal longevity. This finding suggests that paternal gametic imprinting is completed in spermatids. In the senior author's laboratory, 22 offspring have been born by oocyte-spermatid electrofusion (19). It was also reported that viable rabbit embryos also developed from oocytes fertilized with round spermatids (20). Encouraged by these animal experiments, attempts were made to fertilize human oocytes using spermatids from patients with nonobstructive azoospermia. In 1995, the first successful fertilization and pregnancies were reported in humans after intracytoplasmic injection using round and elongated spermatids (15,21). A question was raised, however, as to whether or not the low MI success rates using spermatids are due to inherently low reproductive capacity of spermatids.

Kimura and Yanagimachi, who developed a simple, very reliable technique for mouse ICSI (22), showed that this is not the case; about 30% of embryos which were derived from spermatid injection developed to term after transfer into recipient females (13). We applied the spermatid injection technique as well as oocyte-spermatid electrofusion to propagate murine nephrotic genes which cause male infertility. Here again, intracytoplasmic injection worked better than electrofusion, although normal offspring can be obtained by either method (23). Unlike zygotes from oocyte–spermatid electrofusion, the majority of zygotes from spermatid injection showed a well-developed male pronucleus (D in Fig. 17.2 and C in Fig. 17.3). Intracytoplasmic injection with round spermatids has been performed in the cattle. Bull spermatids, fresh or in vitro cultured, were capable of fertilizing oocytes by MI; thus, zygotes produced developed to the blastocyst stage (24). MI using round spermatids may work when conventional in vitro fertilization and ICSI do not work well. For example, Nohara et al. found that in vitro fertilization of mastomys (*Praomys coucha*) is possible only under very stringent conditions (25). ICSI is also very difficult in this animal due to large sperm head (about

10 μm-diameter injection pipette is necessary) and fragile plasma membranes of mature oocytes. We succeeded in fertilizing mastomys oocytes, however, by injecting spermatids into oocytes using a very small injection pipette (about 3 μm). Mastomys oocytes thus fertilized could develop to the four-cell stage (Day 4) (unpublished).

Cryopreservation of Spermatids

In all studies described earlier, round spermatids were collected from testes immediately before use. If cryopreservation of spermatids is possible, then MI can be performed anytime. Moreover, this may reduce the number of animals needed for MI experiments. Repeated testicular biopsy of azoospermic patients can also be avoided. We found that mouse spermatids can easily be cryopreserved in a simple medium (PBS containing 7.5% glycerol and 7.5% fetal bovine serum). Round spermatids, thus cryopreserved and thawed, could support the full-term development after intracytoplasmic injection (26). By using cryopreserved round spermatids, viable offspring were obtained from aged (33 months old) azoospermic mice (27). The same freezing protocol can be used for cryopreservation of spermatids from the golden hamster, mastomys, guinea pig, cynomolgus monkey, and red-bellied tamarin (28). Human round spermatids were also successfully cryopreserved in a simple freezing medium (HEPES containing 15% glycerol and 0.4% human serum albumin), and one pregnancy was achieved after MI using frozen–thawed spermatids (29).

Microinsemination Using Spermatocytes

Secondary Spermatocyte

The spermatogenic cells one step younger than spermatids are secondary spermatocytes that have $2n$ haploid DNA-like mature metaphase II (Met II) oocytes. Because the mouse oocytes are seldom activated by injection of spermatogenic cell nuclei, secondary spermatocyte nuclei injected into mature oocytes can transform into Met II chromosomes within the cytoplasm of metaphase-arrested oocytes (B in Fig. 17.3). When such oocytes are activated, female and male pronuclei were formed and the zygotes thus constructed developed to term offspring (30). This finding indicates the completion of paternal gametic imprinting by the end of meiosis I as well as analogy of the mechanisms of female and male meiosis II.

Primary Spermatocyte

Primary spermatocytes are spermatogenic cells with 4n diploid DNA. In order to construct diploid zygotes using the nucleus of primary spermatocytes, their DNA must be reduced to one-fourth of the original amount. In the previous study, we introduced primary spermatocyte nuclei into maturing oocytes by electrofusion shortly before or after germinal vesicle (GV) breakdown (31). The both paternal and maternal chromosomes mingled to form a large Met II chromosome mass. The Met II chromosomes were then transferred to other enucleated fresh Met II oocytes, which were activated and cultured. Some developed to the blastocysts stage, but none was implanted (31). We thought that this poor development after embryo transfer may be due to asynchrony of chromosome cycle of the primary spermatocyte and oocyte. There are three possible ways to synchronize both paternal and maternal chromosomes within oocytes. One is to use maturing oocytes, which are arrested at the GV stage by treatment with dibutyryl cAMP (A in Fig. 17.4). The second is similar to the first one, but the oocytes are arrested at Met I by cytochalasin (B in Fig. 17.4). The last is to arrest matured oocytes at Met II, which are activated after premature condensation of primary spermatocyte chromosomes. In the last method, spermatocyte-derived pronucleus/polar body must be transferred into another Met II oocytes in order to obtain 1n haploid chromosomes (C in Fig. 17.4). When zygotes constructed by preceding methods were cultured and morulae/blastocysts were transferred to uteri of pseudopregnant recipient females, we obtained postimplantation embryos from groups A and B, but not from the group C (Table 17.2). No term offspring were obtained.

Meiosis II is very similar to mitosis in that the sister chromatids separate and migrate to the opposite poles during anaphase. In contrast, during meiosis I, sister chromatids must remain associated firmly. They segregate during anaphase II to make haploid daughter cells. Even within oocytes, the chromosomes of the primary spermatocyte must undergo meiosis I in this manner to ensure correct chromosome segregation at meiosis II. When the spermatocyte chromosomes were incorporated into GV oocytes (Method A in Fig. 17.4), a few pairs of their sister chromatids segregate at anaphase I. This premature sister–chromatid segregation was more prominent when spermatocyte nuclei were injected into Met II oocytes (Method C in Fig. 17.4) or enucleated GV oocytes. The segregation pattern of the primary spermatocyte chromosomes appeared normal when they were introduced into Met I-arrested oocytes. It was known that in Drosophila, a protein (MEI-S332), which is present in the cytoplasm before meiosis I, acts specifically at the centromere after nuclear membrane breakdown so that the sister chromatids are held together until anaphase II (32). Considering the behaviors of spermatocyte chromosomes in maturing or matured oocytes, it is conceivable that a protein like MEI-S332 is present in the cytoplasm of mouse primary spermatocytes and GV oocytes, and acts as a glue between sister chromatids after nuclear membrane breakdown.

Conclusions and Perspectives

MI using spermatogenic cells started with round spermatids in 1993 (7). Normal offspring have been born after microfertilization with round spermatids in the mouse, rabbit, and human (13,15,18,20), and with secondary spermato-

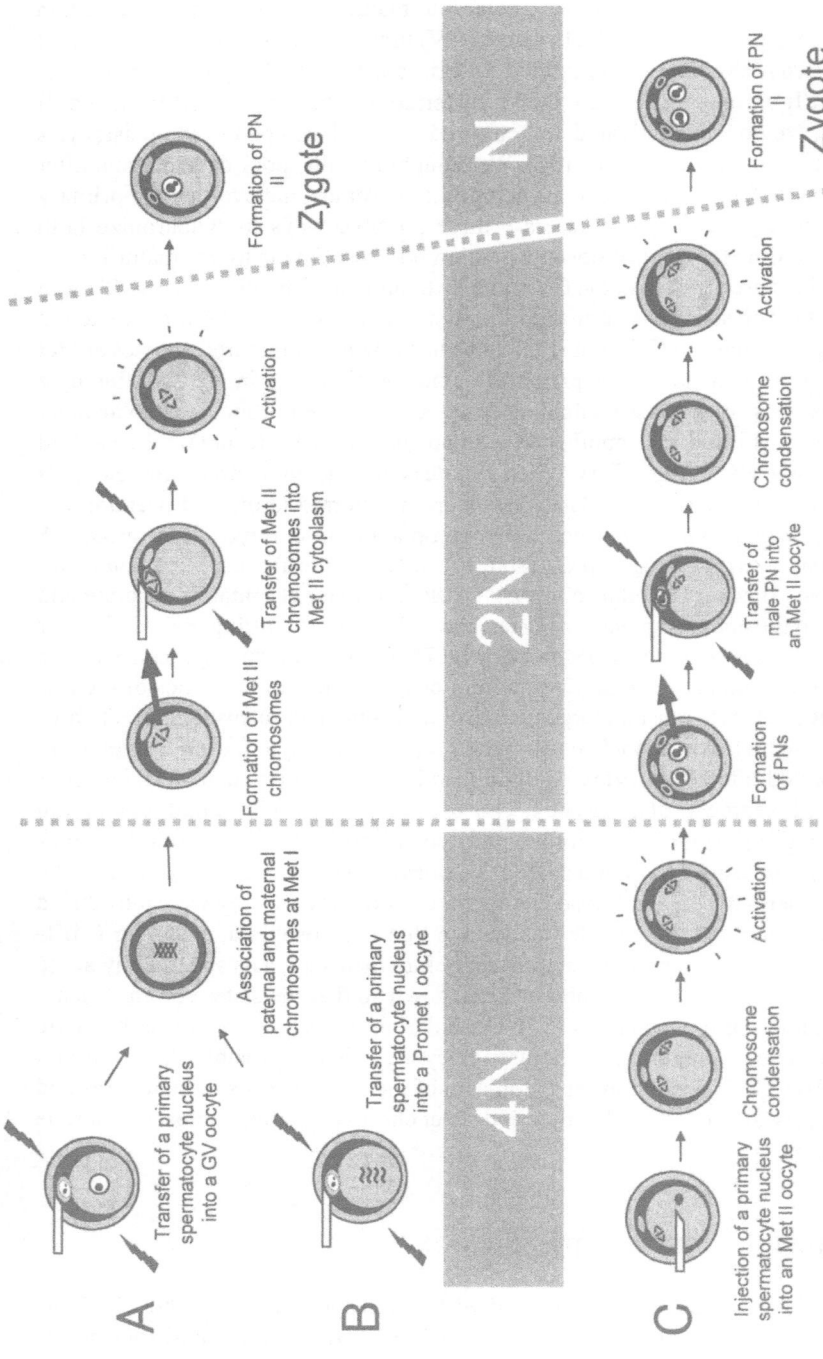

FIGURE 17.4. Production of diploid embryos from primary spermatocytes and oocytes. Spermatocyte nuclei are introduced into maturing GV oocytes (A), maturing Met I oocytes (B), matured Met II oocytes (C). "N" indicates the number of chromatid sets from spermatocytes in the oocytes.

TABLE 17.2. Development of embryos after microfertilization with primary spermatocytes.

Group	Stage of oocytes	No. of embryos cultured	No. (%) of embryos that developed to				
			1-cell	2-cell	4/8-cell	Morula/blast.	Postimplant.[*]
A	GV	103	4(4)	19(18)	39(38)	41(40)[†]	2(1/41)
B	Met I	122	2(2)	1(1)	32(26)	87(71)[‡]	9(8/87)[†]
C	Met II	247	45(18)	34(14)	98(40)	70(28)[†]	0(0/70)[‡]

Embryos were cultured for 96 hours. [*]Morulas and blastocysts were transferred into the uterus of pseudopregnant females.[†‡] $p < 0.05$ within the same column.

cytes in the mouse (30). It is now possible to use primary spermatocytes as the source of paternal chromosomes (31). Table 17.3 summarizes many attempts to fertilize oocytes with spermatogenic cells.

MI that uses spermatogenic cells increases the chance to rescue infertile patients/animals. Spermatogenic arrest could be due to either genetic factors or nongenetic factors such as infections, radiotherapy, and hormonal imbalance. Spermatogenic arrest occurs most commonly at the spermatocyte stage (33). At present, the use of spermatocytes from azoospermic patients/animals is still impractical due to the technical problems and infancy of animal experiments. It was reported that mouse premeiotic spermatogenic cells can be cultured to elongated spermatids by co-culture with Sertoli cells (34). According to other studies, however, it is very difficult to produce haploid cells from premeiotic cells in vitro, even in the presence of Sertoli cells (35,36). If the technique becomes more reliable, then spermatogenic arrest due to nongenetic factors may be overcome by culturing those cells to the postmeiotic stages that are more suitable for MI.

The fact that spermatogenic cells, as well as mature spermatozoa, can be used for MI has an implication in basic researches. Until now, several tech-

TABLE 17.3. Microinsemination with spermatogenic cells by intracytoplasmic injection (ICS) or electrofusion (EF).

Year	Species	Spermatogenic cells used	Methods	Development	Reference no.
1993	Golden hamster	Round spermatid	ICI	2-cell	7
1993	Hamster, mouse	Round spermatid	EF	2-cell	9
1994	Mouse	Round spermatid	EF	Term	18
1994	Rabbit	Round spermatid	ICI	Term	20
1995	Mouse	Round spermatid	ICI	Term	13
1995	Human	Elongated spermatid	ICI	Term	21
1995	Human	Round spermatid	ICI	Term	15
1995	Mouse	Secondary spermatocyte	ICI	Term	30
1996	Bovine	Culture-derived spermatid	ICI	Blastocyst	24
1996	Mouse	Frozen–thawed spermatid	ICI	Term	26
1997	Human	Frozen–thawed spermatid	ICI	Ongoing preg.	29
1997	Mouse	Primary spermatocyte	ICI	Blastocyst	31

niques have been used to produce transgenic animals, including microinjection of DNA into zygote pronuclei (37), adenoviral infection of fertilized eggs (38), and generation of germ-line chimeras from DNA-transfected embryonic stem cells (39). Although a number of technical improvements have been made, the efficiency of transgenesis by these methods is still low, especially in livestock animals. To circumvent the problem, male germ cell-mediated gene transfer have been tried but met with very limited success (40–43). Because mature spermatozoa have a condensed, packed nucleus, they are not suitable for DNA transfer. Spermatogenic cells have an uncondensed nucleus and may be more easily transfected; however, they are very sensitive to in vitro conditions as well as mechanical/chemical stresses. If spermatogenic cells are successfully transfected, preselected, and used for MI, then those cells can be a vector that leads to 100% efficiency. Because the technique of culturing spermatogenic cells in vitro is still far from complete, transplantation of cells into recipient testes (44) may help us to obtain spermatogenic cells in more advanced stages for MI.

References

1. Uehara T, Yanagimachi R. Microsurgical injection of spermatozoa into hamster eggs with subsequent transformation of sperm nuclei into male pronuclei. Biol Reprod 1976;15:467–70.
2. Hosoi Y, Miyake M, Utsumi K, Iritani A. Development of rabbit oocytes after microinjection of spermatozoa. Proceedings of the 11th International Congress on Animal Reproduction 1988;3:abstract 331.
3. Goto K, Kinoshita A, Takuma Y, Ogawa K. Fertilisation of bovine oocytes by the injection of immobilized, killed spermatozoa. Vet Rec 1990;127:517–20.
4. Palermo G, Joris H, Debroey P, Van Steirteghem AC. Pregnancies after intracytoplasmic injection of single spermatozoon into an oocyte. Lancet 1992;340:17–18.
5. Fishel S. Histological overview of the use of micromanipulation. In: Fishel S, Symonds EM, editors. Gamete and embryo micromanipulation in human reproduction. London: Edward Arnold, 1993:3–17.
6. Iritani A. Micromanipulation of gametes for in vitro assisted fertilization. Mol Reprod Dev 1991;28:199–207.
7. Ogura A, Yanagimachi R. Round spermatid nuclei injected into hamster oocytes form pronuclei and participate in syngamy. Biol Reprod 1993;48:219–25.
8. Tajima Y, Onoue H, Kitamura Y, Nishimune Y. Biologically active kit ligand growth factor is produced by mouse Sertoli cells and is defective in Sld mutant mice. Development 1991;113:1031–35.
9. Ogura A, Yanagimachi R, Usui N. Behavior of hamster and mouse round spermatid nuclei incorporated into mature oocytes by electrofusion. Zygote 1993;1:1–8.
10. Schatten G. The centrosome and its mode of inheritance: the reduction of the centrosome during gametogenesis and its restoration during fertilization. Dev Biol 1994;165:299–335.
11. Hewitson L, Haavisto A, Simerly C, Jones J, Schatten G. Microtubule organization and chromatin configuration in hamster oocytes during fertilization and par-

thenogenetic activation, and after insemination with human sperm. Biol Reprod 1997;57:967–75.

12. Shin T-Y, Noguchi Y, Yamamoto Y, Mochida K, Ogura A. Microtubule organization in hamster oocytes after fertilization with mature spermatozoa and round spermatids. J Reprod Dev 1998 (in press).

13. Kimura Y, Yanagimachi R. Mouse oocytes injected with testicular spermatozoa or round spermatids can develop into normal offspring. Development 1995; 121:2397–405.

14. Palermo GD, Colombero LT, Rosenwaks Z. The human sperm centrosome is responsible for normal syngamy and early embryonic development. Rev Reprod 1997;2:19–27.

15. Tesarik J, Mendoza C, Testart J. Viable embryos from injection of round spermatids into oocytes. N Engl J Med 1995;333:525.

16. Sousa M, Mendoza C, Barros A, Tesarik J. Calcium responses of human oocytes after intracytoplasmic injection of leukocytes, spermatocytes and round spermatids. Mol Hum Reprod 1996;2:853–57.

17. Ogura A, Matsuda J, Asano T, Yanagimachi R. Birth of pups after intra-ovarian bursal transfer of hamster zygotes. J Reprod Dev 1995;41:339–43.

18. Ogura A, Matsuda J, Yanagimachi R. Birth of normal young following fertilization of mouse oocytes with round spermatids by electrofusion. Proc Natl Acad Sci USA 1994;91:7460–62.

19. Ogura A, Yanagimachi R. Spermatids as male gametes. Reprod Fertil Dev 1995;7:155–59.

20. Sofikitis NV, Miyagawa I, Agapitos E, et al. Reproductive capacity of the nucleus of the male gamete after completion of meiosis. J Assist Reprod Genet 1994; 11:335–41.

21. Fishel S, Green S, Bishop M, et al. Pregnancy after intracytoplasmic injection of spermatid. Lancet 1997;345:1641–42.

22. Kimura Y, Yanagimachi R. Intracytoplasmic sperm injection in the mouse. Biol Reprod 1995;52:709–20.

23. Ogura A, Yamamoto Y, Suzuki O, et al. In vitro fertilization and microinsemination with round spermatids for propagation of nephrotic genes in mice. Theriogenology 1996;45:1141–49.

24. Goto K, Kinoshita A, Nakanishi Y, Ogawa K. Blastocyst formation following intracytoplasmic injection of in-vitro derived spermatids into bovine oocytes. Hum Reprod 1996;11:824–29.

25. Nohara M, Hirayama T, Ogura A, Hiroi M, Araki Y. Development of a successful in vitro fertilization procedure and partial characterization of the gamete in the Mastomys (Praomys coucha): a new species for laboratory research in reproductive biology. Biol Reprod 1998;58:266.

26. Ogura A, Matsuda J, Asano T, Suzuki O, Yanagimachi R. Mouse oocytes injected with cryopreserved round spermatids can develop into normal offspring. J Assist Reprod Genet 1996;13:431–34.

27. Tenemura K, Wakayama T, Kuramoto K, Hayashi Y, Sato E, Ogura A. Birth of normal young by microinsemination with frozen-thawed round spermatids collected from aged azoospermic mice. Lab Anim Sci 1997;47:203–4.

28. Ogura A, Matsuda J, Suzuki O, et al. Cryopreservation of mammalian spermatids. J Reprod Dev 1997;43:103.

29. Antinori S, Versaci C, Dani G, Antinori M, Selman HA. Successful fertilization and pregnancy after injection of frozen-thawed round spermatids into human oocytes. Hum Reprod 1997;12:554–56.
30. Kimura Y, Yanagimachi R. Development of normal mice from oocytes injected with secondary spermatocyte nuclei. Biol Reprod 1995;53:855–62.
31. Ogura A, Wakayama T, Suzuki O, Shin T-Y, Matsuda J, Kobayashi Y. Chromosomes of mouse primary spermatocytes undergo meiotic divisions after incorporation into homologous immature oocytes. Zygote 1997;5:177–82.
32. Kerrebrock AW, Moore DP, Wu JS, Orr-Weaver TL. Mei-S332, a Drosophila protein required for sister-chromatid cohesion, can localize to meiotic centromere regions. Cell 1995;83:247–56.
33. Martin-du Pan RC, Campana A. Physiology of spermatogenic arrest. Fertil Steril 1993;60:937–46.
34. Rassoulzadegan M, Paquis-Flucklinger V, Bertino B, et al. Transmeiotic differentiation of male germ cells in culture. Cell 1993;75:997–1006.
35. Goto K, Okajima K, Ookutsu S, Nakanishi Y. In vitro culture of bovine spermatocytes on murine testicular somatic cells. Theriogenology 1997;47:257.
36. Weiss M, Vigier M, Hue D, et al. Pre- and postmeiotic expression of male germ cell-specific genes throughout 2-week cocultures of rat germinal and Sertoli cells. Biol Reprod 1997;57:68–76.
37. Palmiter RD, Brinster RL, Hammer RE, et al. Dramatic growth of the mice that develop from eggs microinjected with metallothionein growth hormone fusion genes. Nature 1982;300:611–15.
38. Tsukui T, Kanegae Y, Saito I, Toyoda Y. Transgenesis by adenovirus-mediated gene transfer into mouse zona-free eggs. Nature Biotech 1996;14:982–85.
39. Capecchi MR. Altering the genome by homologous recombination. Science 1989;244:1288–92.
40. Blanchard KT, Boekelheide K. Adenovirus-mediated gene transfer to rat testis in vivo. Biol Reprod 1997;56:495–500.
41. Kim J-H, Jung-ha H-S, Lee H-T, Chung K-S. Development of a positive method for male sperm cell-mediated gene transfer in mouse and pig. Mol Reprod Dev 1997;46:515–26.
42. Lavitrano M, Camaioni A, Fazio VM, Dolci S, Farace MG, Spadafora C. Sperm cells as vectors for introducing foreign DNA into eggs: genetic transformation of mice. Cell 1989;57:717–23.
43. Ogawa S, Hayashi K, Tada N, Sato M, Kurihara T, Iwaya M. Gene expression in blastocysts following direct injection of DNA into testis. J Reprod Dev 1995;41:379–82.
44. Brinster RL, Zimmermann JW. Spermatogenesis following male germ-cell transplantation. Proc Natl Acad Sci USA 1994;91:11298–302.

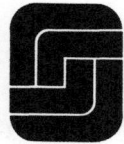

18

Cell Loss During Spermatogenesis: Apoptosis or Necrosis?

Lonnie D. Russell

Spermatogenesis is the process by which stem cell spermatogonia form sperm. In theory, one stem cell spermatogonium of the rat can produce 4096 sperm (1). The theoretical limit is never achieved in normal spermatogenesis because cells degenerate along the way. Numerous genetic, environmental, and toxicological factors can negatively influence the yield of cells. Although several papers and reviews have been written on this topic (2–5), the relatively recent description of apoptosis has prompted this author to revisit the topic.

A dictum in spermatogenesis is that once a cell has committed itself to the process of spermatogenesis it must either "go or die," which means that *cell arrest* is not a feature seen in the period that most of spermatogenesis is taking place. The dictum, even though it applies to cells other than stem and undifferentiated cells, generally holds true for most of normal spermatogenesis and under a variety of conditions that affect the testis. It has been challenged by the discovery that under certain conditions there appears to be arrested germ cells. For example, in Vitamin A deficiency (6) there appears to be arrested cells at the A_1 spermatogonia phase of development. In addition, it has been shown that spermatogonia (or young spermatocytes) may accumulate in the *bax* knockout mouse (7). Accumulation of germ cells in stages where they would not normally be present would be the feature that would be pathomneumonic for spermatogenic arrest.

For some time the literature characterized cell loss as being either cell degeneration or cell necrosis. With the description of apoptosis (8,9), however, there has been a sudden revival of interest in cell degeneration in the testis. Apoptosis was originally defined as a programmed or physiologic cell death, meaning that there is a trigger and a specific pathway for eliminating the cells during the course of normal events. Along with the definition of apoptosis, a cluster of morphological features were found in certain tissues that characterized cells in the apoptotic process. These consisted of margination of chromatin, blebbing of marginated chromatin, and fragmentation of the nucleus. Mitochondria and other organelles remained intact for some time during the apoptotic process. Cell loss was not accompanied by inflammation and cells were phagocytosed by adjacent cells rapidly. More recently, a gel electrophoresis has been used to detect internucleosome chromosome fragmentation and a histochemical test known as in situ end-labeling or TUNEL labeling (10) has served as a means to detect apoptotic cells (11). This method, or a variation thereof, has served many investigators by showing that germ cell apoptosis is common in the normal and abnormal testis.

Table 18.1 lists some of the conditions that have been described in which histochemical or biochemical apoptotic cell death has been found. Another chapter in this volume addresses the biochemical pathway(s) of apoptosis in the testis (see Chap. 19). The high number of reports of apoptosis in the testis compared with necrosis leads one to believe that either apoptosis is the primary means for cell degeneration in the testis or the methods for distinguishing apoptosis from necrosis by TUNEL histochemistry are not distinctive. The physiological definition, the morphological appearance of cells, and the

TABLE 18.1. Studies of apoptosis in the testis.

Species	Condition	Cell type undergoing apoptosis	Source
Hamster	Photoperiod	Unspecified	(32)
	look up	Spermatocytes, spermatogonia	(33)
Mouse	Low level radiation	Spermatogonia, preleptotene spermatocytes	(12)
	Hsp 70-2 knockout	Spermatogonia, spermatocytes	(35)
	CREM knockout	Unspecified	(36)
Rat	In vitro w/ testosterone	Stage specific	(34)
	GnRH antagonists	Germ cells (Stages I & XII-XIV)	(37)
	FSH agonist; hCG	Unspecified	(38)
	ionizing radiation	B spermatogonia	(2)[*]
	GnRH antagonist	Spermatocytes and spermatids in Stage VII	(28,29,39)
	Spontaneous cell death	Spermatocytes & spermatids	(14)
	Development; GnRH antagonist	Mainly spermatocytes	(37)
	Irradiation	Wide variety	(40)
	In vitro w/ FSH	Unspecified	(41)
	Cryptorchidism	Cells in stages VII-VIII and XII-XIII	(42)
	GnRH antagonist; methoxy acetic acid	Spermatocytes primarily	(43)
	Cryptorchidism	Spermatocytes	(15)
	2-methoxy-ethanol	Spermatocytes	(44,45)
	Normal	Spermatogonia	(46)
	In vitro w/ and w/o contact w/ Sertoli cells	Germ cells from 20 day-old animals	(30)
	Mild hyperthermia	Spermatocytes	(47)
	Overexpression of c-myc	Spermatocytes	(48)
	Torsion induced ischemia	Unspecified germ cells	(49)
Guinea pig	2-methoxy-ethanol	Spermatocytes	(44)

[*]Allan (2) has characterized the manner of cell degeneration by morphology in several earlier studies where specific histochemical tests of apoptosis were not evident.

histochemical/biochemical identification may not all be compatible when they apply to the testis (2,12). The morphological criteria for apoptosis may be most appropriate for the cell types (e.g., thymus) in which this phenomenon has first been characterized. Figure 18.1 shows a variety of degenerating germ cell types in the testis and their appearance.

It has been pointed out that under some conditions TUNEL labeling may label necrotic cells (13). Degenerating cells may not TUNEL label for certain phases leading to their loss. Given that necrosis is almost never found to occur in the testis, one must question if cells may degenerate by necrosis and still exhibit the histochemical features associated with apoptosis.

Most male germ cells that label histochemically for fragmented DNA do *not* show the typical morphological characteristics of apoptotic cells (personal observations; 12), although there is a claim to the contrary (14). In fact, apoptotic cells more closely resemble necrotic cells, although there are some features that may said to be characteristic of apoptosis. Spermatogonia of the type A variety usually display classical features of apoptosis no matter what causes their loss (Fig. 18.1). More advanced germ cells have variable appearances as they degenerate (Fig. 18.1). It is interesting to note that when round spermatids have been seen to degenerate under conditions that have been described as apoptotic they "reel in" their flagellum, which extends for a considerable distance into the tubular lumen, into the cell cytoplasm early in the process (5).

Labeling procedures for apoptosis may be misleading. In an examination of the micrographs of Shikone et al. (15), approximately 60% of the tubules were labeled using a 3-foot end labeling of DNA seven days after surgical operation for cryptorchidism. The large number of labeled cells were thought by the authors to be spermatocytes because numerous germ cells (presumably spermatids) were present more centrally within the tubule and remained unlabeled. In view of the rapidity of which apoptosis is known to occur, only a few possible interpretations could be made from the histochemical results: First, spermatocytes en masse suddenly may undergo apoptosis precisely at day 7 after cryptorchidism. The process of apoptosis usually takes only a few hours, so the magnitude of cell degeneration, if apoptosis were occurring, would not be expected to be visualized for any lengthy period. Second, apoptosis may take place for a longer period of time when germ cells are concerned. Third, the technique may be demonstrating something other than apoptosis; because the observation that the contralateral (sham-operated) testis is also markedly affected suggests that the testis of the contralateral testis would be virtually devoid of germ cells after 7 days if degeneration of the magnitude indicated proceeded. The literature does not reinforce massive degeneration within the contralateral testis after cryptorchidism.

In a review of cell death of germ cells, Allan (2) states that basal compartment cells invariably show apoptotic features, whereas spermatocytes and cells more advanced in development than spermatocytes show features characteristic of necrosis. My experience with agents and conditions that affect the testis generally supports this statement, with the exception that B and intermediate spermatogonia and preleptotene spermatocytes, all cells of the basal compartment, also show only occasional apoptotic features.

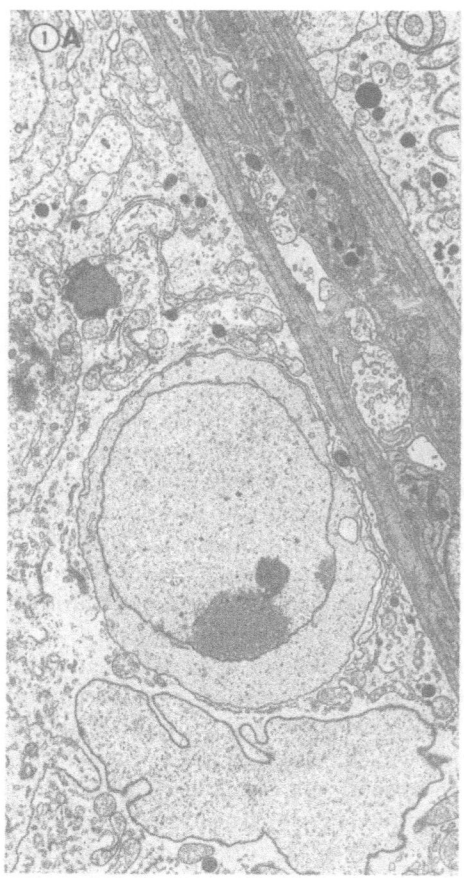

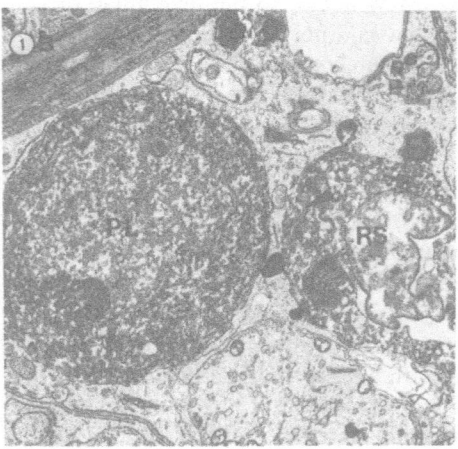

FIGURE 18.1. Appearance of some of the cell types found degenerating in the testis of the rat. (A) Spermatogonia of the type A variety invariably display chromatin margination characteristic of classically described apoptosis. This spermatogonium (centrally located cell) is in an early phase of degeneration, as evidenced by only a slight condensation of the cytoplasm. (B) The degenerating preleptotene spermatocytes (PL) shown demonstrates finely flocculated material within the nucleus and cytoplasm; only the nucleolus is visible at this phase of cell degeneration. A nearby degenerating round spermatid (RS) displays scattered marginated and centrally positioned chromatin, but lacks the typical appearance of a classically described apoptotic cell. A portion of a flagellum that has been retracted from the lumen is also seen (arrowhead). (C) The most common appearance of pachytene spermatocytes is as shown here (centrally positioned cell); they degenerate by chromatin clumping without chromatin margination; the cytoplasm also shows clumped constituents. (D) A rare form of degenerating spermatocytes (PS), which is observed only on one occasion, is more typical of classically described apoptosis; it shows chromatin margination and blebbing of the nucleus. (E) Two nuclei of condensed elongated spermatids (dense structures at left) are shown in the process of degenerating within the cytoplasm of the Sertoli cell. Their nuclei are characteristically condensed prior to undergoing degeneration and are a prime example of a specialized cell type that degenerates and, by its very nature, cannot show the classical morphological pattern of apoptosis.

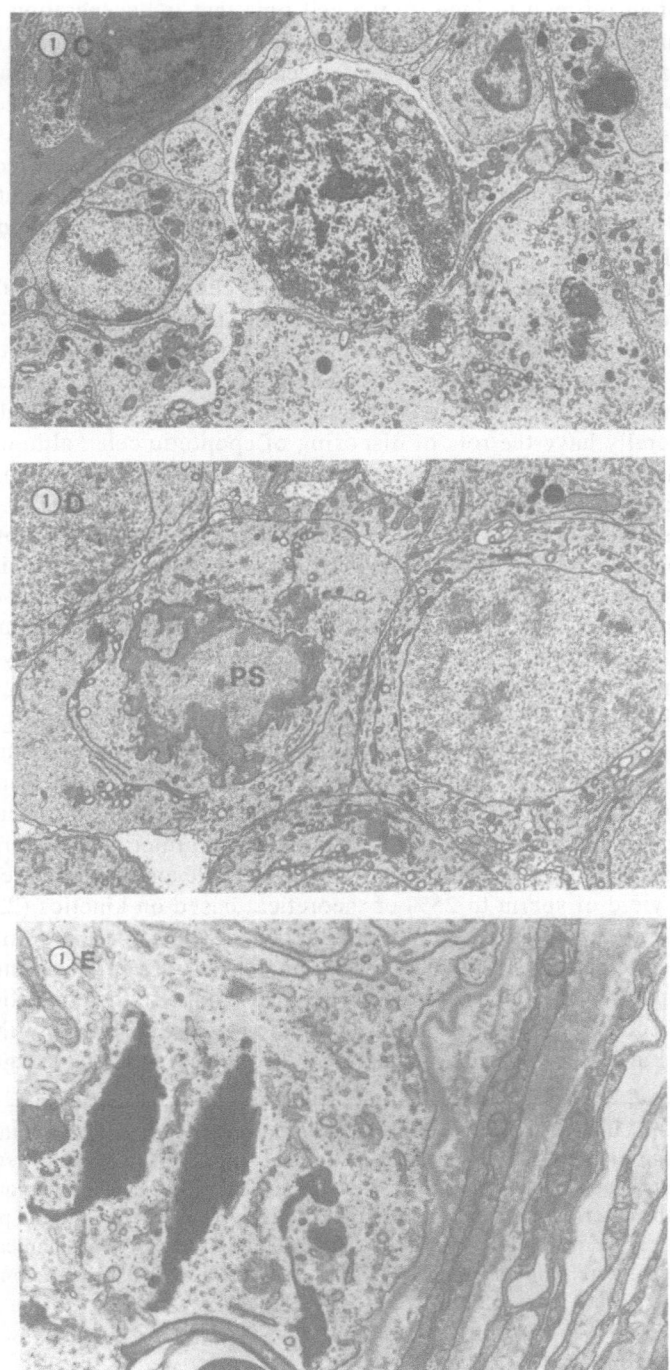

FIGURE 18.1. (*continued*).

It is often difficult to identify the cell type that is degenerating after the process has begun. It is generally the case that the degenerating germ cell type can be characterized if an early phase of degeneration is examined and compared with the viable cell of the same type. The early cytologic features of a degenerating cell and its position within the tubule give clues as to which cell is degenerating. Many degenerating cells can be characterized by light microscopy. This technique has served as an assay system for the number of particular kinds of cells that are degenerating (5). With time, it is difficult to determine the kind of cell that has degenerated as cells become dense and shrunken.

It is not known how long most degenerating cells remain within the seminiferous epithelium. Step 19 spermatids of the rat may not be fully digested by the Sertoli cell for about 4–6 days. This cell type is certainly not a representative cell from which to base the rate of degeneration of other cell types because the nucleus of the step 19 spermatid is highly condensed. Sertoli cells generally have the role of disposing of apoptotic cells, although some germ cells may be shed into the epididymis. Cultured germ cells also undergo apoptotic cell death in the presence of Sertoli cells (16).

Most studies have shown that cell degeneration in the course of normal spermatogenesis takes place at specific phases of spermatogenesis in the rat and mouse. One study shows degenerating cells virtually throughout the spermatogenic cycle (14), although cells classified as degenerating may have been mistakenly called such because of fixation artifacts. In a study by Kerr (3) degenerating cells were quantified in the normal rat. Figure 18.2 shows a quantitation of cells in each stage and the major cells this investigator and Kerr believe are contributing to cell loss. Several other reviews show germ cell loss to be marked in rat (4,17), mouse (18), rabbit (19), and human (20). In the mouse (4) and rat (21), there is cell loss in the rapid proliferation of differentiated spermatogonia from A_2 to A_3 to A_4 to intermediate forms. Cell loss at this phase of spermatogenesis is considerable and is said to reduce the potential yield of sperm to 25% of theoretical based on kinetics (22) These cells undergo apoptosis morphologically, but they are not a prominent feature of the epithelium simply because spermatogonia are not an abundant cell type compared with other germ cell types that comprise the epithelium.

Why is cell loss so great during spermatogonial divisions? Without cell loss, the kinetics of spermatogenesis would yield a much larger germ cell

→

FIGURE 18.2. Cell loss during rat spermatogenesis displayed on a cycle map of the rat. The shaded areas are representative of the major cell types found degenerating at each stage of the cycle as determined by Russell and Clermont (5) and Kerr (3). The abbreviations for cell types and the descriptions of the steps (Arabic numbers) can be found in the previously papers. Type A spermatogonia are not shown in this figure, rather, they are indicated at the bottom of the figure. [Figure from Russell et a., 1990 (1), used with permission of Cache River Press.]

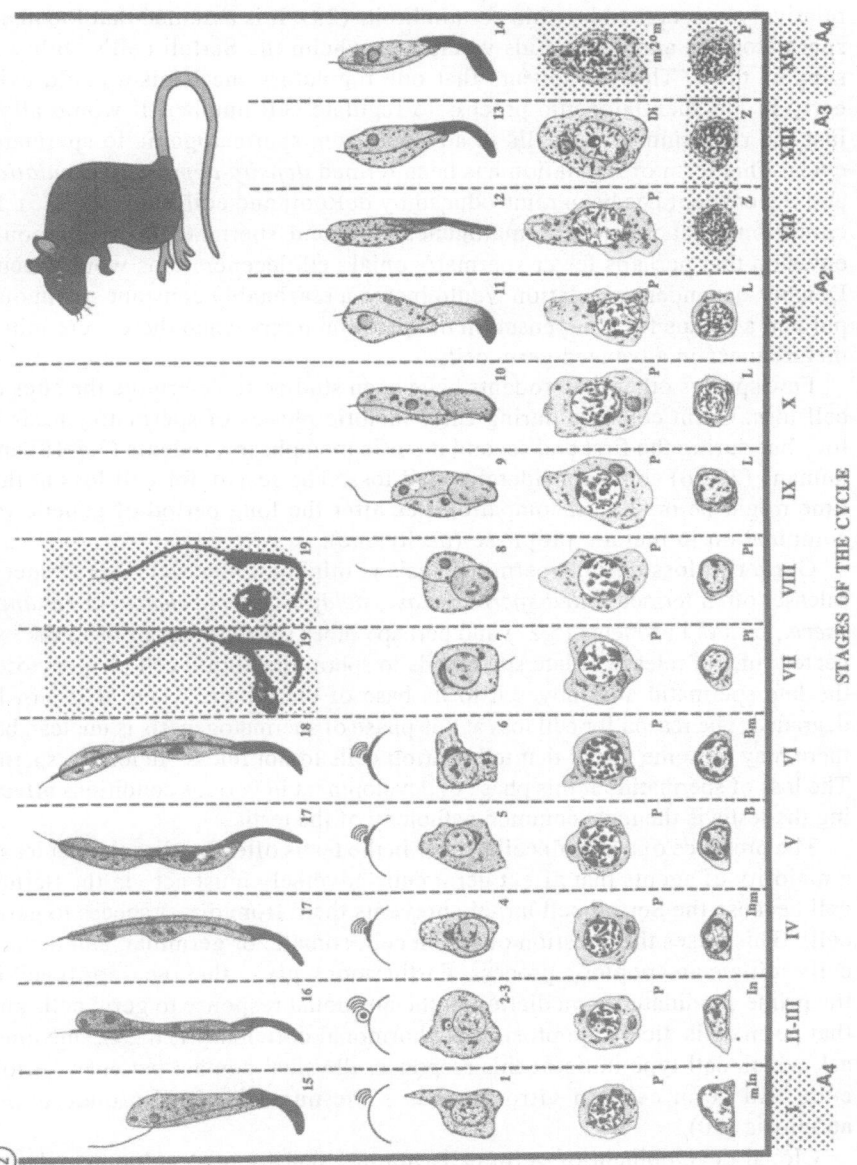

population than is currently present. There would be more than three times of the numbers of germ cells present and the testis would be about two-fold greater in size. For any given species, the ratio of germ cells to Sertoli cells is relatively constant and within certain limits (23). It is assumed that too many spermatocytes and spermatids would overwhelm the Sertoli cell's ability to support them. Thus, it appears that one regulatory mechanism could exist early in the spermatogenic process to regulate cell number. It would allow just the right number of cells to advance from spermatogonia to spermatocytes. This form of regulation has been termed *density-dependent regulation* and the concept has been reintroduced by deRooij and colleagues (24,25). In conditions that impair spermatogenesis beyond spermatogonia one could envision that perhaps fewer spermatogonial cell degenerations would occur. Density-dependent regulation would insure a reasonably constant sperm output and a means for compensation of sperm numbers when there were minor disturbances in advanced germ cells.

Few species other than rodents have been studied to determine the sites of cell loss. Germ cell loss during early meiotic phases of spermatogenesis is low, but during the first and second meiotic metaphases, rodents (3,5,18) and humans (20,26) show considerable cell loss. The reason for çell loss at this time might be meiotic incompatibilities after the long period of genetic recombination in meiotic prophase (pachytene).

Germ cell loss during spermiogenesis is minimal: however, loss at sperm release, often termed *failed sperm release, delayed sperm release,* or *retained sperm,* occurs in rodents (5,27) and perhaps other species. Just prior to the expected time of release of late spermatids to sperm the Sertoli cell phagocytoses the late spermatid and moves it to its base of the tubule, where it is slowly degraded. The reason for cell loss at this phase of spermatogenesis is unclear, but there may be some signal that tells Sertoli cells to not release defective sperm. The loss of spermatids at this phase of development in various conditions affecting the testis is the most common pathology of the testis.

The presence of a Sertoli cell barrier in the testis often implies that, at least, a majority of agents that affect germ cells adversely must act via the Sertoli cell because the Sertoli cell largely prevents them from direct access to germ cells. This raises the question of which cell, somatic or germinal, can technically initiate an apoptotic process. Furthermore, given that the Sertoli cell is the prime candidate for mediation of the hormonal response to germ cells and that germ cells die by apoptosis after hormonal deficiency (28,29), one must ask which cell type initiates this response. Physical contact between Sertoli cells and germ cells in vitro decreases the number of cells undergoing apoptosis (30).

Clonal development of germ cells implies sharing of developmental signals and messages and, thus, synchronized progression of cells. It does not however imply that when one cell of a clone dies, the whole clone is lost. In fact, a clone rarely exhibits en masse degeneration. Apoptotic spermatogonia with intact intercellular bridges have been illustrated (1,2,22,31), but this is

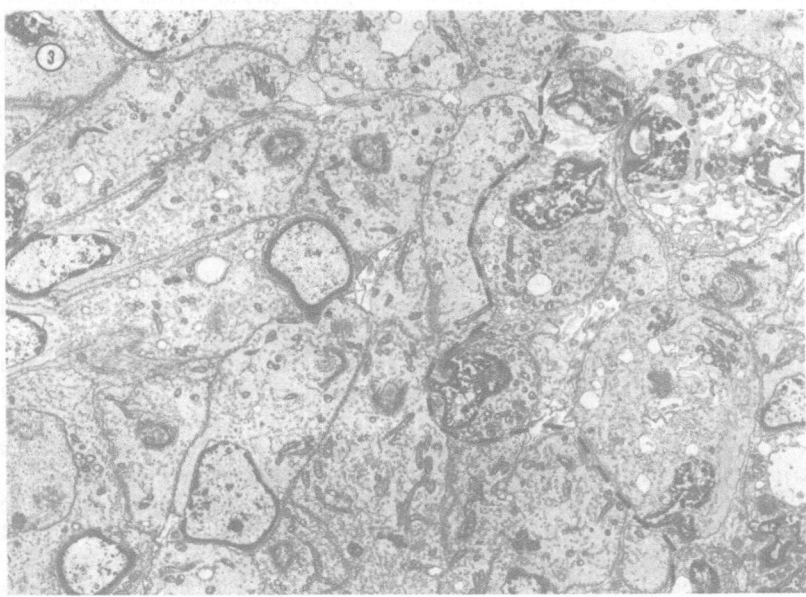

FIGURE 18.3. Degeneration of two different clones of spermatids is depicted in a transgenic animal. All cells of each clone are in the same phase of cell degeneration as they show the same morphological features. The clone on the left (separated by dotted line) is less advanced in development as compared with the clone on the right. Classically described features of apoptosis are not noted in any of the degenerating cells.

not common, especially among more advanced germ cell types. Typical cell degeneration is usually the result of pinching off of one cell of a clone and its subsequent demise among its viable neighbors. The "pinching off" phenomena has never been demonstrated, but it is presumed to occur. Demise of an entire clone(s) has been shown to occur (Fig. 18.3), giving a picture that is very different than loss of sporadic cells.

References

1. Russell LD, Ettlin RA, Sinha Hikim AP, Clegg ED. Histological and histopathological evaluation of the testis. Clearwater, FL: Cache River Press, 1990.
2. Allan HaK. Cell death in spermatogenesis. In: Potten CS, editor. Perspectives on mammalian cell death. Oxford: Oxford University Press, 1987:229–58.
3. Kerr JB. Spontaneous degeneration of germ cells in normal rat testis: assessment of cell types and frequency during the spermatogenic cycle. J Reprod Fertil 1992;95:825–30.
4. Roosen-Runge EC. Untersuchungen über die degeneration samenbildender zellen in der normalen spermatogenese der ratte. Z Zellforsch 1955;41:221–35.

5. Russell LD, Clermont Y. Degeneration of germ cells in normal, hypophysecto-mized and hormone treated hypophysectomized rats. Anat Rec 1977;187:347–66.
6. Morales C, Griswold MD. Retinol-induced stage synchronization in seminiferous tubules of the rat. Endocrinology 1987;121:432–34.
7. Knudson CM, Tung K, Tourtellotte WG, Brown G, Korsmeyer S. Bax-deficient mice with lymphoid hyperplasia and male germ cell death. Science 1995;270:96–99.
8. Kerr J, Wylie A, Currie A. Apoptosis: a basic biological phenomenon with wide-ranging implications in tissue kinetics. Br J Cancer 1972;26:239–57.
9. Wylie A, Kerr J, Currie A. Cell death: the significance of apoptosis. Int Rev Cytol 1980;68:251–306.
10. Gorczyca W, Gong J, Darzynkiewicz Z. Detection of DNA strand breaks in indi-vidual apoptotic cells by *in situ* terminal deoxynucleotidyl transferase and nick translation assays. Cancer Res 1993;53:1945–51.
11. Gavrieli Y, Sherman Y, Ben-Sasson SA. Identification of programmed cell death *in situ* via specific labeling of nuclear DNA fragmentation. J Cell Biol 1992; 119:493–501.
12. Hasegawa M, Wilson G, Russell LD, Meistrich ML. Radiation-induced cell death in the mouse testis: relationship to apoptosis. Radiat Res 1997;147:457–67.
13. Ansari B, Coates PJ, Greenstein BD, Hall PA. *In situ* end labelling detects DNA strand breaks in apoptosis and other physiological and pathological states. J Pathol 1993;170:1–8.
14. Blanco-Rodriguez J, Martinez-Garcia C. Spontaneous germ cell death in the testis of the adult rat takes the form of apoptosis: re-evaluation of cell types that exhibit the ability to die during spermatogenesis. Cell Prolif 1996;29:13–31.
15. Shikone T, Billig H, Hsueh AJW. Experimentally induced cryptorchidism increases apoptosis in rat testis. Biol Reprod 1994;51:865–72.
16. Shiratsuchi A, Umeda M, Ohaba Y, Nakanishi Y. Recognition of phosphatidylserine on the surface of apoptotic spermatogenic cells and subsequent phagocytosis by Sertoli cells of the rat. J Biol Chem 1997;272:2354–58.
17. Dym M, Clermont Y. Role of spermatogonia in the repair of the seminiferous epithelium following x-irradiation of the rat testis. J Anat 1962;128:265–82.
18. Oakberg EF. A description of spermiogenesis in the mouse and its use in analysis of the cycle of the seminiferous epithelium and germ cell renewal. Am J Anat 1956;99:391–414.
19. Swierstra EE, Foote RH. Cytology and kinetics of spermatogenesis in the rabbit. J Reprod Fertil 1963;5:309–22.
20. Barr AB, Moore DJ, Paulsen CA. Germinal cell loss during human spermatogen-esis. J Reprod Fertil 1971;25:75–80.
21. Clermont Y. Kinetics of spermatogenesis in mammals: seminiferous epithelium cycle and spermatogonial renewal. Physiologist 1972;52:198–236.
22. Huckins C. The morphology and kinetics of spermatogonial degeneration in nor-mal adult rats: an analysis using a simplified classification of the germinal epithe-lium. Anat Rec 1978;190:905–26.
23. Russell LD, Peterson RN. Determination of the elongate spermatid-Sertoli cell ratio in various mammals. J Reprod Fertil 1984;70:635–41.
24. de Rooij DG, Lok G. Regulation of the density of spermatogonia in the seminifer-ous epithelium of the Chinese hamster: II Differentiating spermatogonia. Anat Rec 1987;217:131–36.

25. de Rooij DG. Regulation of the proliferation of spermatogonial stem cells. J Cell Sci 1988;10:181–94.
26. Johnson L, Petty CS, Neaves WB. Further quantification of human spermatogenesis: germ cell loss during postprophase of meiosis and its relationship to daily sperm production. Biol Reprod 1983;29:207–15.
27. Russell LD. Role in spermiation. In: Russell LD, Griswold MD, editors. The Sertoli cell. Clearwater, FL: Cache River Press, 1993:269–303.
28. Sinha Hikim A, Wang C, Leung A, Swerdloff RS. Involvement of apoptosis in the induction of germ cell degeneration in adult rats after gonadotropin releasing hormone antagonist treatment. Endocrinology 1995;136:2770–75.
29. Sinha Hikim AP, Rajavashisth TB, Sinha Hikim I, et al. Significance of apoptosis in the temporal and stage-specific loss of germ cells in the adult rat after gonadotropin deprivation. Biol Reprod 1997;57:1193–201.
30. Mizuno K, Shiratsuchi A, Masamne Y, Hakanishi Y. The role of Sertoli cells in the differentiation and exclusion of rat testicular germ cells in primary culture. Death Differen 1996;3:119–23.
31. Gondos B, Zemjanis R. Fine structure of spermatogonia and intercellular bridges in Macaca nemestrine. J Morphol 1970;131:431–46.
32. Furuta I, Porkka-Heiskanen T, Scarbrough K, Tapanainen J, Turek FW, Hsueh AJW. Photoperiod regulates testis cells apoptosis in djungarian hamsters. Biol Reprod 1994;51:1315–21.
33. Nonclerq D, Reverse D, Toubeau G, et al. *In situ* demonstration of germinal cell apoptosis during diethylstibesterol-induced testis regression in adult male Syrian hamsters. Biol Reprod 1996;55:1368–76.
34. Henriksen K, Hakovirta H, Parvinen M. Testosterone inhibits and induces apoptosis in rat seminiferous tubules in a stage-specific manner: in situ quantification in squash preparations after administration of ethane dimethane sulfonate. Endocrinology 1995;136:3285–91.
35. Mori C, Nakamura N, Dix DJ, et al. Morphological analysis of germ cell apoptosis during postnatal testis development in normal and Hsp 70-2 knockout mice. Dev Dyn 1997;208:125–36.
36. Blendy JA, Kaestner KH, Weinbauer GF, Nieshlag E, Schultz G. Severe impairment of spermatogenesis in mice lacking the CREM gene. Nature 1996;380:162–65.
37. Billig H, Furuta I, Rivier C. Apoptosis in testis germ cells: developmental changes in gonadotropin dependence and localization to selective tubule stages. Endocrinology 1995;136:5–12.
38. Tapanainen JS, Tillyt JL, Vihko KK, Hsueh AJ. Hormonal control of apoptotic cell death in the testis: gonadotropins and androgens as testicular cell survival factors. Mol Endocrinol 1993;7:643–50.
39. Sinha Hikim AP, Lue Y, Swerdloff RS. Separation of germ cell apoptosis from toxin-induced cell death by necrosis using in situ end-labeling histochemistry after glutaraldehyde fixation. Tissue Cell 1997;29:487–93.
40. Henriksen K, Kulmala J, Toparri J, Mehrotra K, Parvinen M. Stage-specific apoptosis in the rat seminiferous epithelium: quantification of irradiation effects. J Androl 1996;17:394–401.
41. Henriksen K, Kangasniemi M, Parvinen M, Kaipia A, Hakovirta H. *In vitro*, follicle-stimulating hormone prevents apoptosis and stimulates DNA synthesis in the rat seminiferous epithelium in a stage-specific fashion. Endocrinology 1996;137:2141–49.

42. Henrickson K, Hakovirta H, Parvinen M. *In situ* quantification of stage-specific apoptosis in the rat seminiferous epithelium: effects of short-time experimental cryptorchidism. Int J Androl 1995;18:256–62.
43. Brinkworth MH, Weinbauer GF, Schlatt S, Nieschlag E. Identification of male germ cell undergoing apoptosis in adult rats. J Reprod Fertil 1995;105:25–33.
44. Ku W, Wine R, Chae B, Ghanayem B, Chapin R. Spermatocyte toxicity of 2-methoxyethanol (2-ME) in rats and guinea pigs: evidence for the induction of apoptosis. Toxicol Appl Pharmacol 1995;134:100–10.
45. Wine RN, Ku WW, Li L-H, Chapin RE. Cyclophilin A is present in rat germ cells and is associated with spermatocyte apoptosis. Biol Reprod 1997;56:439–46.
46. Allan DJ, Harmon B, Roberts S. Spermatogonial apoptosis has three morphologically recognizable phases and shows no circadian rhythm during normal spermatogenesis in the rat. Cell Prolif 1992;25:241–50.
47. Blanco-Rodriguez J, Martinez-Garcia C. Mild hypothermia induces apoptosis in rat testis at specific stages of the seminiferous epithelium. J Androl 1997;18:535–39.
48. Kodaira K, Takahashi R-I, Hirabayashi M, Suzuki T, Obinata M, Ueda M. Overexpression of *c-myc* induces apoptosis at the prophase of meiosis of rat primary spermatocytes. Mol Cell Reprod 1996;405:403–10.
49. Turner TT, Tung KSK, Tomomasa H, Wilson LW. Acute testicular ischemia results in germ cell-specific apoptosis in the rat. Biol Reprod 1997;57:1267–74.

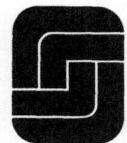

19

Regulation of Apoptosis in the Testis

TIM L. BEUMER AND DIRK G. DE ROOIJ

Introduction

It has become clear that germ cell death in the testis, inducible by a variety of rather diverse factors and circumstances, invariably proceeds via a process resembling that of active cell death, called *apoptosis* as described for other cell types (for review, see 1). Apoptosis may take place following several pathways, probably dependent on the kind of apoptotic stimulus the cells get. The regulation of apoptosis has appeared to be of increasing complexity. Apoptosis can be divided into phases (2), with the various apoptosis regulators acting during different phases of the apoptotic pathway. In the first phase, the cell becomes affected by an apoptotic stimulus. For germ cells, many factors have been shown to directly or indirectly act as an apoptotic stimulus, such as temperature, hormone levels, and xenobiotic agents like radiation and cytostatic drugs (1). In the second phase, the cell detects the apoptotic stimulus, whereafter, in phase three, the cell responds. Finally, at phase four, the cell completely degrades. Proteins involved in apoptosis regulation in each of these phases were shown to be expressed in the testis, leading to an initial understanding of which apoptotic pathways are present in germ cells. As the factors involved in the first phase of apoptosis induction have already been described in this volume (1), only the factors that regulate other phases of apoptosis will be described in this chapter, with the emphasis on those already known to be expressed in the testis (Table 19.1).

Genes Involved in the Regulation of Germ-Cell Apoptosis

P53

The stability of the genome is very important during germ-cell development; however, hypoxia, mutagens, cytostatic drugs, and X-irradiation can lead to

TABLE 19.1. Genes shown to be expressed in the testis involved in the regulation of apoptosis.

Gene	Cell type in which expressed	Species	Reference
p53	Spermatogonia (after DNA damage) spermatocytes	Mouse, rat, Human	(11–13; Beumer TL et al., unpublished observations)
Bcl-x$_{S/L}$	Spermatogonia	Human	This chapter
Bcl-x$_L$	Immature testis	Mouse	(22)
Bax	Spermatogonia (2.5-wk-old testis) spermatogonia (mature testis, weak signal)	Mouse	(22) (26)
Bcl-2	Not detectable	Mouse	(22,26)
Mcl-1	Spermatocytes, Leydig cells	Human	(26)
FasL	Sertoli cells	Mouse, human	(39–41)
FasR	Spermatocyte	Mouse	(39)
TGFβ1	Sertoli cells, spermatocytes, and early spermatids Primordial Sertoli cells (E14.5-E18.5), neonatal Leydig cells	Mouse, rat Rat	(28,29) (48)

DNA damage. One of the genes that is induced early after infliction of DNA damage and which may be involved in the detection of the damage is p53. P53 is also referred to as the guardian of the cell cycle and has important functions in cell growth and differentiation (for review, see 3). After DNA damage (e.g., one caused by ionizing irradiation) an upregulation of p53 is often seen in mammalian cell lines that results in the initiation of apoptosis, repair pathways (4), and a G_1/S (5,6) or G_2/M cell cycle arrest (7). As a transcription factor, p53 is able to upregulate a series of proteins involved in the regulation of apoptosis (Bax; 8), DNA damage repair (Gadd45; 9), or of the cell cycle (Cyclin dependent kinase inhibitor p21[Cip1/WAF1]; 10).

During normal spermatogenesis, p53 mRNA was only detected in early spermatocytes (11). In both mouse and rat, the p53 protein was found to be expressed in spermatocytes, as determined by using CAT reporter transgenic mice and immunohistochemistry (12,13). In agreement with the p53 expression in spermatocytes, in p53 knock out mice or transgenic p53 mice, increased degeneration of spermatocytes was described (14). From these results it was concluded that p53 has a role during the meiotic prophase.

In the normal mouse testis, using immunohistochemistry, no p53 protein expression could be detected in spermatogonia. After a dose of 4 Gy of X-rays, however, high levels of p53 staining were observed in spermatogonia (Beumer TL et al., unpublished observations). Because virtually all spermatogonia are doomed to go into apoptosis after a dose of 4 Gy of X-rays (15), here p53 expression correlates with apoptosis induction. This suggestion could be confirmed by studying p53 knock out mice. P53 knock out mice develop normally, although the tumor incidence is higher than it is in wild-type mice (16). Spermatogenesis in p53-deficient mice appears normal, but the number of A spermatogonia was found to be higher than in wild-type mice. Ten days after irradiation, in p53 knock out mice much higher numbers of giant spermatogonial cells were found than in wild-type mice (Beumer TL et al., unpublished observations). As these giant cells are lethally damaged spermatogonial stem cells having difficulties in entering apoptosis (17), it can be concluded that p53 is involved in stem cell apoptosis. P53 deficiency, however, does not change the radiosensitivity of spermatogonial stem cells (18; Beumer TL et al., unpublished observations). Furthermore, Burgoyne (personal communication) observed a delayed apoptosis of differentiating type spermatogonia after a dose of 5 Gy. In addition, more differentiating type spermatogonia were found to survive a dose of 5 Gy of X-rays in p53 knock out mice than in wild-type mice (Beumer TL et al., unpublished observations). P53 clearly plays an important role in the removal of damaged differentiating-type spermatogonia; however, as apoptosis of all lethally damaged stem cells and of most of the damaged differentiating type spermatogonia eventually does take place, it can be concluded that there are reserve apoptotic pathways that, can take over the role of p53,even if less efficiently.

One of the genes that is under transcriptional control of p53 is p21. P21 is a cell-cycle inhibitor that can induce arrest of cells in the G1 phase of the cell cycle. In many cell types apoptosis is induced by p53 through the action of p21. The p21 protein, however, was not found to be expressed in spermatogonia before or after irradiation (15,19). Hence, the irradiation-induced, p53-mediated apoptosis of spermatogonia does not involve p21. P21 expression was found in spermatocytes, where it probably has a role in the meiotic process (15,19).

Bcl-2 Family

A well-studied group of apoptosis effectors is the Bcl-2 family of proteins, which can either induce or protect from apoptosis. New proteins are regularly discovered that belong to this family, which is characterized by the presence of Bcl-2 homology 1 and 2 (BH1 and BH2) domains. These domains allow the Bcl family members to form homodimers or heterodimers with each other. The balance between homo- and heterodimers is crucial for the decision whether or not a cell will enter the apoptotic pathway (20).

Bcl-2 was discovered at a reoccurring breakpoint at a translocation in follicular B-cell-lymphoma. This 25 kDa protein is often correlated with both physiological apoptosis (e.g., by growth factors, cytokines) and genotoxic apoptosis (e.g., by UV irradiation, X-irradiation, free radicals). Anchored to the nuclear, mitochondrial, and endoplasmatic membranes by a hydrophobic carboxy terminal end, Bcl-2 may regulate the Ca^{2+} flux and protein translocation (for review, see 21). Bcl-2, however, is not present in the mammalian testis (22; own immunohistochemical observations in the mouse). Nevertheless, Bcl-2 overexpression in spermatogenic cells has dramatic effects on spermatogenesis. During normal spermatogenesis, considerable numbers of spermatogonia go into apoptosis as a consequence of a density regulatory mechanism (23). When Bcl-2 is overexpressed this density regulation does not take place, a massive accumulation of spermatogonia occurs and subsequently both spermatogonia and the spermatocytes formed, go into apoptosis (22,24). These results showed that the Bcl-2 family is important in spermatogenesis, although the Bcl-2 protein itself does not seem to be involved.

Another member of the Bcl-2 family is the Bcl-x gene that produces at least two splice variants, Bcl-x$_S$ and Bcl-x$_L$. Whereas Bcl-x$_L$ suppresses apoptosis, Bcl-x$_S$ has opposing effects. Using an antibody directed to an epitope present in both Bcl-x$_L$ and Bcl-x$_S$, spermatogonia in the human testis were found to stain immunohistochemically (Fig. 19.1). This indicates that the Bcl-x gene plays a role in spermatogenesis. Indeed, in mice overexpressing Bcl-x$_L$ the same phenomena were seen as with overexpression of Bcl-2 (22).

Bax is a 21 kDa protein, belongs to the Bcl-2 family and is a potent inducer of apoptosis. Even though Bax is barely detectable using immunohistochemistry (25), Bax knock out mice were found to be sterile (22,26). The histological features of the testes from Bax knock out mice resembled that of the Bcl-2 and Bcl-x$_L$ transgenic testes (i.e., accumulation of spermatogonia). Although Bax is an apoptosis inducer, apoptosis is massively present in the Bax knock out mouse testis. Hence, spermatogonia and early spermatocytes can also go into apoptosis via a pathway that does not involve the Bax protein.

Mcl-1, a 37 kDa protein, is a family member that inhibits apoptosis, like Bcl-2. Whereas Bcl-x is expressed in spermatogonia and primary spermatocytes, Mcl-1 is only expressed in spermatocytes, which suggests distinct roles for the different Bcl family members in apoptosis regulation in different cell types (25).

In conclusion, the Bcl-2 family clearly has a role in the regulation of apoptosis in germ cells. To date, only few of the many members of this family have been studied with respect to a possible role in the testis, but Bcl-x and Bax are certainly involved in regulating germ-cell numbers and the removal of damaged cells.

TGFβ Family

The TGFβs are disulphide-linked polypeptide, dimeric growth factors that are multifunctional regulators of both growth and development in many different tissues. Three TGFβs have been described for mammalian tissues. All three TGFβs have been reported to be expressed in the testis. In the mouse and the rat testis, TGFβ1 and TGFβ3 mRNAs have been localized in Sertoli cells and peritubular/myoid cells throughout testicular development. TGFβ2 mRNA appears to be predominantly present in the prepubertal testis (27). In the adult testis, TGFβ1 mRNA has been detected in germ cells (28). The TGFβ1 protein was found in Sertoli cells and in spermatocytes and early round spermatids, whereas TGFβ2 protein was localized in late round and elongating spermatids (29). TGFβ1 has especially been shown to induce apoptosis in various cell types [e.g. fetal hepatocytes (30), fibroblasts (31), and microglia (32)].

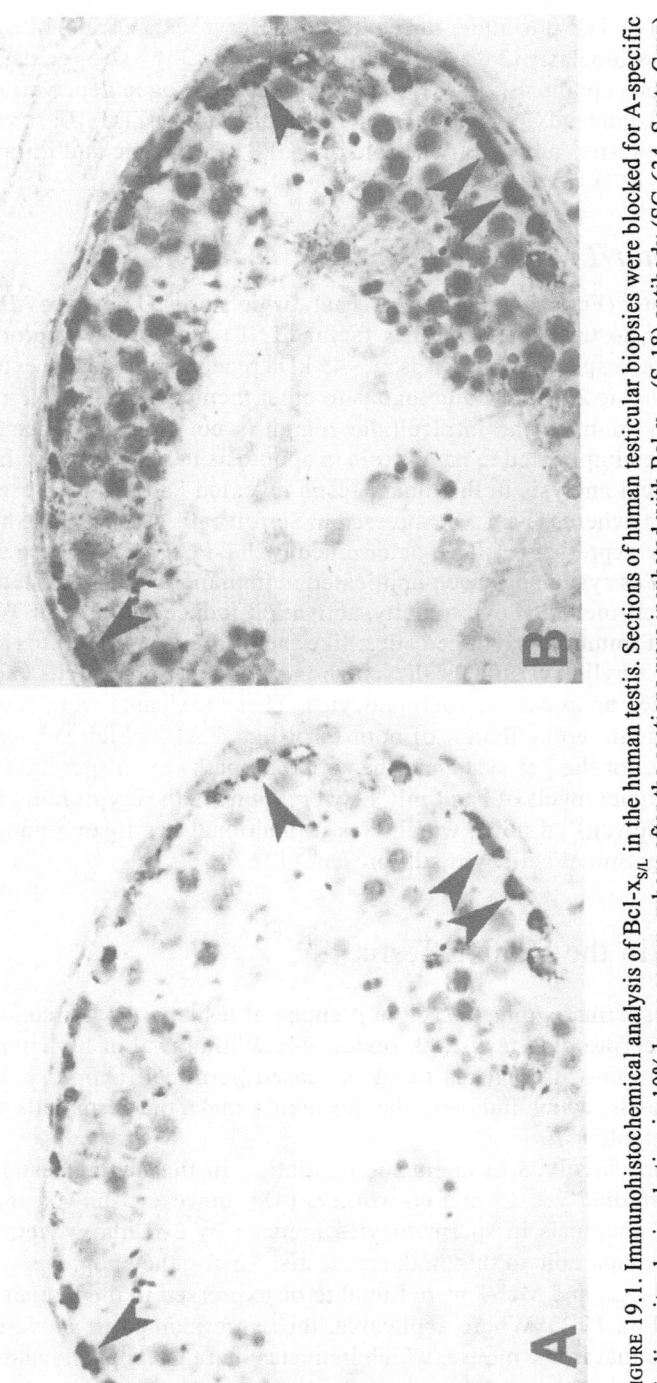

FIGURE 19.1. Immunohistochemical analysis of Bcl-$x_{S/L}$ in the human testis. Sections of human testicular biopsies were blocked for A-specific binding sites by incubation in 10% horse serum, where after the sections were incubated with Bcl-$x_{S/L}$ (S-18) antibody (SC-634, Santa Cruz) overnight at 4°C. A biotin conjugated antirabbit antibody was coupled to the primary antibody, where after the bound antibodies were visualized by using the Vector Elite Staining Kit (Vector Laboratories). In the human testis, spermatogonia (arrowheads) are stained for Bcl-$x_{S/L}$. (A) Immunohistochemical Bcl-$x_{S/L}$ staining. (B) Haematoxylin and Bcl-$x_{S/L}$ staining.

Regulation of TGFβ is under the control of at least sex steroids, like estrogens (33). In osteoclasts (34) or prostatic carcinoma (35), estrogen has been shown to induce apoptosis via TGFβ, although also estrogen deprivation can lead to TGFβ-induced apoptosis (36). Overexpression of TGFβ1 results in atrophy of the testis, supporting the role of TGFβ1 in fibrotic and inflammatory disorders (37).

Fas Receptor/Ligand System

The Fas receptor (FasR) and Fas ligand (FasL, which is also known as APO1 or CD95) belong to the tumor necrosis factor (TNF) family of receptors and growth factors, respectively. FasR is an ~45 kDa receptor and has an extracellular region that is 20–25% homologous to other members of the TNF receptor family. In contrast, the intracellular region is not conserved. FasL and FasR have been implicated to have a role in apoptosis in many tissues. Immunohistochemical analysis in the mouse testis revealed FasR to be present on spermatocytes, whereas FasL is expressed in Sertoli cells (38–40). The human testis strongly expresses FasL, as determined by RT-PCR and Western analysis (41). The Fas system has been implicated in immune regulation, including cytotoxic T-cell-mediated cytotoxicity, activation-induced suicide of T-cells, and control of immune-privileged sites, like the testis. Sertoli-cell toxicants, like mono-(2-ethylhexyl) and 2,5-hexanedione, damage Sertoli cells and secondarily induce apoptosis of spermatocytes. These toxicants were found to induce a dramatic upregulation of both FasR and FasL, which suggests an important role for the Fas system in the apoptotic pathway in spermatocytes. In addition, higher levels of FasR mRNA were found in the cryptorchid testis. In lpr(cg) or lpr(cg)-gd mice, which lack a functional Fas ligand, apoptosis induction in germinal cells was still present (42).

Apoptosis in the Human Testis

Apoptosis of spermatogonia is seen in prepuberal testis in the human, and is decreased in cryptorchid testis (43, review 44). Withdrawal of human chorionic gonadotropin (hCG) leads to an increased germ-cell apoptosis in the cryptorchid testis, which indicates that hormones make the germ cells viable to undergo apoptosis.

The proteins involved in apoptosis regulation in the human testis have hardly been studied yet. Li and co-workers (45), however, showed that the regulation of apoptosis in spermatocytes induced by 2-methoxyacetic acid (2-MAA) is comparable to that in the rat testis. Among the apoptosis regulators, p53, Bcl-$x_{S/L}$, and Mcl-1 were found to be expressed in the human testis (Table 19.1; Fig. 19.1). Where applicable, the expression patterns were also comparable to that in the mouse, which indicates that the apoptosis pathways in the human and in mouse and rat may be similar.

Discussion and Conclusions

Apoptosis is an important process in spermatogenesis. The regulation of apoptosis in the testis is clearly complicated and is as yet far from clear. Several pathways that seem to differ for each cell type are involved. Nevertheless, some key factors have already been identified. First, after infliction of DNA damage the p53 protein is a key factor in the removal of the spermatogonia in which this damage can not be repaired. Second, when apoptosis that normally occurs in spermatogonia in the framework of cell density regulation is suppressed (by knocking out Bcl-xL or Bax), these cells massively accumulate and ultimately die via another apoptotic pathway. The Bcl-2 family of apoptosis that induces and inhibits proteins is apparently of vital importance in the density regulation of spermatogonia. Third, all germ cells, but especially spermatocytes and spermatids depend on proper functioning of the Sertoli cells that sustain these cells. After infliction of damage to Sertoli cells, spermatocytes die by way of apoptosis induced via the FasR/FasL pathway, Sertoli cells that produce FasL and spermatocytes expressing the FasR.

Even though the regulation of apoptosis is already complex, as different apoptosis regulators are important in different germ-cell types, the complexity increases even more because the different apoptosis regulators interact with each other. For example, the transcription factor p53 downregulates the expression of bcl-2 and is able to induce bax. Members of the Bcl-2 family, on their turn, affect either p53, Fas, or TGFβ-induced apoptosis programs. In addition, many of the factors involved also have a role in the regulation of normal proliferation and differentiation and the meiotic process. Downstream in the apoptotic process, the various pathways may converge into a common path. Either TGFβ-, p53-, or Fas-induced apoptosis may involve the activation of specific caspases, which is a family of proteolytic enzymes that are indispensable for apoptosis induction (46). The activity of the different caspases results in specific degradation of cellular proteins. One of the most investigated of these enzymes is caspase 1 or interleukin 1β converting enzyme (ICE) (46). So far, only ICE mRNA expression in the testis has been shown, using Northern analysis (47). We are clearly only at the beginning of understanding the regulation of apoptosis in spermatogenesis because most of the factors found in other tissues to regulate apoptosis have not been studied as yet for a possible role in apoptosis in spermatogenesis.

Acknowledgments. Tim L. Beumer is supported by the J.A. Cohen Institute for Radiopathology and Radiation Protection, Leiden.

References

1. Russell LD. Cell loss during spermatogenesis: apoptosis or necrosis? In: Hamamah S, Mieusset R, Olivenes F, Jouannet P, Frydman R, editors. Male sterility for motility disorders: etiological factors and treatment. New York: Springer, 1998.

2. Vaux DL, Strasser A. The molecular biology of apoptosis. Proc Natl Acad Sci USA 1996;93:2239–44.
3. Levine AJ. P53, the cellular gatekeeper for growth and division. Cell 1997;88: 323–31.
4. Chernova OB, Chernov MV, Agarwal ML, Taylor WR, Stark GR. The role of p53 in regulating genomic stability when DNA and RNA synthesis are inhibited. Trends Biochem Sci 1995;20:431–34.
5. Kuerbitz SJ, Plunkett BS, Walsh WV, Kastan MB. Wild-type p53 is a cell cycle checkpoint determinant following irradiation. Proc Natl Acad Sci USA 1992;89:7491–95.
6. Zölzer F, Hillebrandt S, Streffer C. Radiation induced G1-block and p53 status in six human cell-lines. Radiother Oncol 1995;37:20–28.
7. Guillouf C, Rosselli F, Krishnaraju K, Moustacchi E, Hoffman B, Liebermann DA. P53 involvement in control of G2 exit of the cell cycle: role in DNA damage-induced apoptosis. Oncogene 1995;10:2263–70.
8. Miyashita T, Reed JC. Tumor suppressor p53 is a direct transcriptional activator of the human bax gene. Cell 1995;80:293–99.
9. Kastan MB, Onyekwer O, Sidransky D, Vogelstein B, Craig RW. Participation of p53 protein in the cellular response. Cancer Res 1992;51;6304–11.
10. El-Deiry WS, Tokino T, Velculescu VE, et al. WAF1, a potential mediator of p53 tumor suppression. Cell 1993;75:817–25.
11. Almon E, Goldfinger N, Kapon A, Schwartz D, Levine AJ, Rotter V. Testicular tissue-specific expression of the p53 suppressor gene. Dev Biol 1993;156: 107–16.
12. Schwartz D, Goldfinger N, Rotter V. Expression of p53 protein in spermatogenesis is confined to the tetraploid pachytene primary spermatocytes. Oncogene 1993;8:1487–94.
13. Sjöblom T, Lähdetie J. Expression of p53 in normal and gamma-irradiated rat testis suggests a role for p53 in meiotic recombination and repair. Oncogene 1996;12:2499–505.
14. Rotter V, Schwartz D, Almon E, et al. Mice with reduced levels of p53 protein exhibit the testicular giant-cell degenerative syndrome. Proc Natl Acad Sci USA 1993;90:9075–79.
15. Beumer TL, Roepers-Gajadien HL, Gademan IS, Rutgers DH, de Rooij DG. P21[(Cip1/Waf1)] expression in the mouse testis before and after X-irradiation. Mol Reprod Dev 1997;47:240–47.
16. Donehower LA, Harvey M, Slagle BL, et al. Mice deficient for p53 are developmentally normal but susceptible to spontaneous tumours. Nature 1992;356:215–21
17. Van Beek MEAB, Davids JAG, van de Kant HJG, de Rooij DG. Response to fission neutron irradiation of spermatogonial stem cells in different stages of the cycle of the seminiferous epithelium. Radiat Res 1984;97:556–69.
18. Hendry JH, Adeeko A, Potten CS, Morris ID. P53 deficiency produces fewer regenerating spermatogenic tubules after irradiation. Int J Radiat Biol 1996;70:677–82.
19. West A, Lähdetie J. P21WAF1 expression during spermatogenesis of the normal and X-irradiated rat. Int J Radiat Biol 1997;73:283–91.
20. Korsmeyer SJ. Bax-deficient mice with lymphoid hyperplasia and male germ cell death. Science 1995;270:96–99.
21. Kroemer G. The proto-oncogene Bcl-2 and its role in regulating apoptosis. Nature Med 1997;3:614–20.

22. Rodriguez I, Ody C, Araki K, Garcia I, Vassalli P. An early and massive wave of germinal cell apoptosis is required for the development of functional spermatogenesis. EMBO J 1997;16:2262–70.
23. De Rooij DG, Lok D. The regulation of the density of spermatogonia in the seminiferous epithelium of the Chinese hamster. II. Differentiating spermatogonia. Anat Rec 1987;217:131–36.
24. Furuchi T, Masuko K, Nishimune Y, Obinata M, Matsui Y. Inhibition of testicular germ cell apoptosis and differentiation in mice misexpressing Bcl-2 in spermatogonia. Development 1996;122:1703–9.
25. Krajewski S, Bodrug S, Krajewska M, et al. Immunohistochemical analysis of Mcl-1 protein in human tissues. Differential regulation of Mcl-1 and Bcl-2 production suggests a unique role for Mcl-1 in control of programmed cell death in vivo. Am J Pathol 1995;146:1309–19.
26. Knudson CM, Tung KSK, Tourtelotte WG, Brown GAJ, Korsmeyer SJ. Bax-deficient mice with lymphoid hyperplasia and male germ cell death. Science 1996;270:96–99.
27. Skinner MK, Moses HL. Transforming growth factor beta gene expression and action in the seminiferous tubule: peritubular cell-Sertoli cell interaction. Mol Endocrinol 1989;3:625–34.
28. Watrin F, Scotto L, Assoian RK, Wolgemuth DJ. Cell lineage specificity of expression of the murine transforming growth factor beta 3 and transforming growth factor beta 1 genes. Cell Growth Differ 1991;2:77–83.
29. Teerds KJ, Dorrington JH. Localization of transforming growth factor beta 1 and beta 2 during testicular development in the rat. Biol Reprod 1993;48:40–45.
30. Chen RH, Chang TY. Involvement of caspase family proteases in transforming growth factor-factor-beta-induced apoptosis. Cell Growth Differ 1997;8:821–27.
31. Hipp ML, Bauer G. Intercellular induction of apoptosis in transformed cells does not depend on p53. Oncogene 1997;15:791–97.
32. Xiao BG, Bai XF, Zhang GX, Link H. Transforming growth factor-beta1 induces apoptosis of rat microglia without relation to bcl-2 oncoprotein expression. Neurosci Lett 1997;226:71–74.
33. Oursler MJ, Cortese C, Keeting P, et al. Modulation of transforming growth factor-beta production in normal human osteoblast-like cells by 17 beta-estradiol and parathyroid hormone. Endocrinology 1991;129:3313–20.
34. Hughes DE, Dai A, Tiffee JC, Li HH, Mundy GR, Boyce BF. Estrogen promotes apoptosis of murine osteoclasts mediated by TGF-beta. Nature Med 1996; 2:1132–36.
35. Landstrom M, Eklov S, Colosetti P, et al. Estrogen induces apoptosis in a rat prostatic adenocarcinoma: association with an increased expression of TGF-beta 1 and its type-I and type-II receptors. Int J Cancer 1996;67:573–79.
36. Chen H, Tritton TR, Kenny N, Asher M, Chiu JF. Tamoxifen induces TGF-beta 1 activity and apoptosis of human MCF-7 breast cancer cells in vitro. J Cell Biochem 1996;61:9–17.
37. Sanderson N, Factor V, Nagy P, et al. Hepatic expression of mature transforming growth factor beta-1 in transgenic mice results in multiple tissue lesions. Proc Natl Acad Sci USA 1995;92:2572–76.
38. Sanberg PR, Saporta S, Borlongan CV, Othberg AI, Allen RC, Cameron DF. The testis-derived cultured Sertoli cell as a natural Fas-L secreting cell for immunosuppressive cellular therapy. Cell Transplant 1997;6:191–93.

39. Lee J, Richburg JH, Younkin SC, Boekelheide K. The Fas system is a key regulator of germ cell apoptosis in the testis. Endocrinology 1997;138:2081–88.
40. Bellgrau D, Gold D, Selawry H, Moore J, Franzusoff A, Duke RC. A role for CD95 ligand in preventing graft rejection. Nature 1995;377:630–32.
41. Xerri L, Devilard E, Hassoun J, Mawas C, Birg F. Fas ligand is not only expressed in immune privileged human organs but is also coexpressed with Fas in various epithelial tissues. Mol Pathol 1997;50:87–91.
42. Ohta Y, Nishikawa A, Fukazawa Y, et al. Apoptosis in adult mouse testis induced by experimental cryptorchidism. Acta Anat 1996;157:195–204.
43. Heiskanen P, Billig H, Toppari J, et al. Apoptotic cell death in the normal and the cryptorchid human testis: the effect of human chorionic gonadotropin on testicular cell survival. Pediatr Res 1996;40:351–56.
44. Dunkel L, Hirvonen V, Erkkilä K. Clinical aspects of male germ cell apoptosis during testis development and spermatogenesis. Cell Death Differ 1997;4:171–79.
45. Li LH, Wine RN, Chapin RE. 2-Methoxyacetic acid (MAA)-induced spermatocyte apoptosis in human and rat testes: an in vitro comparison. J Androl 1996;17:538–49.
46. Salvesen GS, Dixit VM. Caspases: intracellular signaling by proteolysis. Cell 1997;91:443–46.
47. Keane KM, Giegel DA, Lipinski WJ, Callahan MJ, Shivers BD. Cloning, tissue expression and regulation of rat interleukin 1 beta converting enzyme. Cytokine 1995;7:105–10.
48. Gaultier C, Levacher C, Avallet O, et al. Immunohistochemical localization of transforming growth factor-beta 1 in the fetal and neonatal rat testis. Mol Cell Endocrinol 1994;99:55–61.

Part V

Testicular Sperm Retrieval

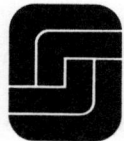

20

Thermic and Metabolic Microsensors for Testicular Sperm Extraction (TESE) Before ICSI

JOSEPH TRITTO, ANDRÉ DITTMAR, MARIE-ODILE NORTH, AND GABRIEL ARVIS

Introduction

The expanding field of in vitro fertilization (IVF) and assisted reproduction technologies (ART) takes advantage of advanced microtechnologies and microoptics for laboratory microscopy as micromanipulators and microlasers for cell photoactivation and drilling (1).

In the andrological field surgical microscopes with powerful vision capabilities are introduced in microsurgery of male infertility, specifically for microsurgical correction of varicocele, for vasoepididymostomy (end-to-end or side-to-end tubulodeferential and/or ductulodeferential anastomoses), and for microepididymal sperm aspiration (MESA) in the bilateral congenital absence of vas deferens (CAV) (2). The introduction of testicular sperm extraction (TESE) opens new insights on the functional organization of the human testes. The application of new advanced microtechnologies in vivo in the surgical theater permits the improvement of sperm retrieval procedures (3).

Microsensors and Microsystems in Andrology

The foundation of Laboratories for integrated Micro-Mechatronic Systems (as LIMMS from CNRS-France and IIS-Japan) and the development of microsensors and microsystems in the biomedical applications have opened new perspectives in the functional exploration and manipulation of human organs in vivo with minimally invasive procedures and microsurgical tools (MEMS: Micro-Electro-Mechanical Systems; MIMS: Micro-Mechatronic

Systems, MIMET: Micro-Mechatronic Tools; MIMETOR: Micro-Mechatronic Robots) (4).

Integrated microsensors have been developed for biomedical applications: A single microsensor is able to measure multiple parameters (as the thermic microsensor Betatherm 10K3MCD2) or a single hybrid microsensor in which multiple microprobes are micro-encapsulated or micropackaged (as the Micromed µTAS: C-D.R. Microsystèmes C.N.R.S.) (5).

Thermic microsensors have been applied for the first time in male infertility for the study of the thermoregulation of the human testes: The tissue temperature, the tissue thermic conductivity (mW/cm.°C), and the tissue blood flow (ml/min.100g) are evaluated in real-time with continuous measurements (6).

Metabolic microsensors (MICROMED µTAS) are used to measure 10 parameters: microcirculation, temperature, tissue thermic conductivity, glucose, lactate, pyruvate, $pO2$, NO, tissue properties with optrode, and thermic methods (7). They are applied in the microcirculation analysis of the intratesticular environment and in the thermic mapping of the testicular lobules during microsurgery (8) and for the metabolic score of the erectile tissue in corpora cavernosa for erectile dysfunctions. The micromeasurements are compared with more classical even if sophisticated procedures as laser-Doppler flow probe studies on vasomotion (9) and video-micro-capillaroscopy for in vivo morphological studies of the microvascular pattern (10).

New perspectives will open on the application of metabolic microsensors in brain studies of monkeys and humans for emotional and conditioned sexual behaviors compared with angio-MRI dynamic images in male andrology and sexology (11). Microsensors in andrology represent a part of two large projects of the Biomedical European Community on Mechatronic and Micromechatronic Integrated Tools for Surgery (MITS Biomed Project 2C/A BMH4-CT96-0317), respectively, in which microsurgery and microrobotics are among the three basic areas of interest, and on the Euro-BME Project on Technology and Socio-Economic Mutations in Biomedical Engineering (a Leonardo da Vinci Program).

Thermoregulation of the Human Testes

From the countercurrent heat-exchange mechanism (CCHE) to the intrinsic-core thermoregulation of the human testis the specific application of thermic and metabolic microsensors in the human testes in vivo is based on the innovative studies on the thermoregulation in the human and nonhuman spermatogenesis in vitro and in vivo and on the environmental and hazardous effects of physical (thermic and not-thermic) sources on human reproduction. The pioneeristic works of Waites and Setchell on experimental animals on one side and of Zorgniotti and Sealfon on clinical studies on the other side permitted the establishment of the state of the art at the First International Symposium on Temperature and Environmental Factors and the Testis, held in 1989 in New York (12). In his message Zorgniotti wrote: "These proceedings will persuade . . . that intrinsic and extrinsic temperature alterations do play a major role in testis physiology and male fertility and are worthy of study. Areas which still remain largely unexplored are the possible implications for genetic alterations, fetal wastage, and possible testicular cancer."

The theoretical model, developed by Sealfon and Zorgniotti, is based on the countercurrent heat exchange (CCHE) mechanism in the pampiniform plexus and predicts, with an open loop analysis, that there is no feedback or regulation. The open loop (nonfeedback) model seems to agree with data obtained from humans in pathological conditions, but it is not in agreement with data from men with normal temperature; therefore, a closed loop model can be hypothesized, if intrinsic mechanisms that control testicular temperature exist and can be demonstrated (13).

The thermodynamic model of the testis developed by Tritto is based on the computer-assisted finite-element modeling and simulation of the CCHE system and on the analysis of the fractal organization of the microanatomical (vascular and microtubular) network of the human testis.

The Testis as a Fractal Organ

Using the analog electrical model of Sealfon (14) or the F.E.M. thermodynamic model of Tritto on the CCHE pampiniform plexus mechanism (15), the hypothesis of a testis as an ovoid with isotropic and homogenous properties is not congruent with the simulation data and the experimental measurements in animals because no significant mechanism to stabilize or control testis temperature is evident. The countercurrent heat-exchange mechanisms only seem able to set the entry temperature of the testis, but not to assure its uniformity into the organ. New insights on the organization of animal and human testes come from the studies on the microvascular organization of the vasculature of the testis (16,17), on the intertubular lymphatics' distribution, and on the interstitial organization of the available spaces (18), on the studies of the spiral pattern of the spermatogenetic waves of the seminiferous tubules in humans (19) and on the spatial distribution of spermatogenetic stages in topological sets of tubule segments in animal testes. On these anatomical and microanatomical bases a fractal, compartmentalized model of the human testis is developed on computer-assisted modeling using volumetric, thermic, and morphometric analyses from animal and human testes.

The "Intellectual Feedback Model" of the thermoregulation of the human testis presented in 1990 (20) represents the first computer-assisted thermic model of the testis, illustrating equivalences and analogies between heat transfer modalities and anatomofunctional mechanisms in relation to the local control of male fertility: the extrinsic thermoregulatory mechanism of convective heat transfer (the countercurrent heat exchange system of the spermatic cord) is coupled to the intrinsic mechanisms of conductive heat transfer into the testis with dynamic feedback (20). The particular three-dimensional organization of the microvasculature inside the testis seems appropriate to modulate the thermic gradient, assuring a like-uniform distribution of the temperature or a more specific, topological thermic distribution in relation to the main branching streaming flows' compartmentalization, and, at a more sophisticated level, to the elicoïdal intratubular mapping of the spermatogenesis classes. In the realization of a thermic-oriented, simulation model of the microarchitecture of the human testis, the generation of specific microvascular patterns to fill the testis volume completely in well-defined anatomic boundaries is accomplished with fractal techniques and geometries (21,22).

The first-step bidimensional generation of the microvascular network on arterial and venous sides is based on studies with scanning electron microscopy (SEM) of the microvascular architecture of human and nonhuman testis: Vascular geometry of intertubular and peritubular vessels surrounding the seminiferous tubules is described in a bidimensional view as a polygonal in mouse, hexagonal in rat, and circular in human testis. The application of both von Kock curves as a polygonal generator and Apollinian circles' packing procedure as fractal primitives permits the generation of the corresponding geometries at the appropriate level with a precise fractal dimension. A recursive initiator-generator is applied to obtain fractal images for both microvascular and tubular patterns; the resulting self-similarity dimension is the same as the fractal and Hausdorff-Besicovitch. Scaling the bidimensional array of the microvascular and tubular pattern on a three-dimensional organization, on the resulting three-dimensional thermic-oriented model of the testis, the thermic analysis of the flow distribution is carried out separately on the arterial inflow and the venous outflow pathways in order to individualize the thermic equilibrium zones and boundaries in relation to the intratestis lobular partition and to the intratubular spiral organization of the process of spermatogenesis. Temperature-dependent fractal images of the microarchitecture of the testis are obtained in relation to the pitches of the microvascular (arterial and venous) arcades and to the divergence angle of the distributional spiral pattern of primary spermatocytes into the seminiferous tubules. The introduction of biodynamic situations: # variations of inflow and outflow rates # scaling of the fractal level of vascular organization # perturbation of the regular distribution of the complex vascular-tubular array, # simulating physiological and pathological anatomofunctional situations, permits (1) the development for the first time of a fractal analysis of the topological T-gradient distribution into the testis and its relation to the spatial organization of the microvascular network and of the intratubular–spermatogenetic process, and (2) the verification of the presence of normal or distorted regional flow heterogeneity (23).

For the first time the fractal model of the human testis is able to justify how the testis can assure a like-uniform distribution of the temperature and a more specific topological thermic distribution in relation to the interlobular branches and to the elicoïdal intralobular branches and to the elicoïdal intratubular mapping of the spermatogenetic classes.

The studies on the angioarchitecture of the lobular organization of the human testis introduce new elements to the multifractal model in the sense that they get into the parameters of regionalization of the volumetric space available for the intrinsic thermoregulation, the at-risk focal zones for parenchyma atrophy, and new insights for testicular biopsy (24).

The clinical utilization of enhanced ultrasound with power doppler capabilities permits the visualization of the interlobular and the intralobular patterns of the vasculature of the human testis in vivo in preoperative evaluation and the proposition of a semi-quantitative score for homogenous and nonhomogenous distributed lobular patterns (25).

Azoospermia and Bilateral Varicocele

Azoospermia and bilateral varicocele is a new clinical profile in which thermoregulatory impairment of both testes sustained by varicocele is associated with azoospermia and severe perturbation of the spermatogenetic cycle on testicular biopsy (26).

On a series of 127 bilateral varicocele submitted to microsurgery, azoospermia represents 23% of cases. Systematic odd-couple testicular biopsies on opposite quadrants in both testes in azoospermia and bilateral varicocele show significant differences in the quantitative score between both testes and, moreover, between quadrants into the same testis: This means that the impairment of the microcirculation in the testis in the presence of varicocele realizes a spotted pattern in the lobular organization, jeopardizing the meiotic cycle and the entire spermatogenetic process (27).

The cytogenetic studies of the meiotic process on the testicular biopsies from azoopsermic patients with bilateral varicocele shows an incidence of 28.6% of meiotic abnormalities with a high representation of pure toxic abnormalities (28). After the microsurgical correction the reversibility of these toxic abnormalities is demonstrated for the first time (29).

Thermic Microsensors in Azoospermia and Varicocele

Clinical measurements are carried out in azoospermic patients with unilateral or bilateral varicocele, implanting thermic microsensors (Betatherm 10K3MCD2), as active probes, in opposite poles of both testes in order to evaluate the intrinsic microvascular and microcirculatory impairments before performing testicular biopsies and TESE. A classical thermic distribution is presented in which the azoospermic patient shows an epididymal obstruction on one side and a third-degree varicocele on the other (Fig. 20.1).

The relationship between the time blood flow (ml/min.100 gr) and the temperature (°C) from the on-line recordings in the surgical theater in standardized conditions with closed and open scrotum shows that in the absence

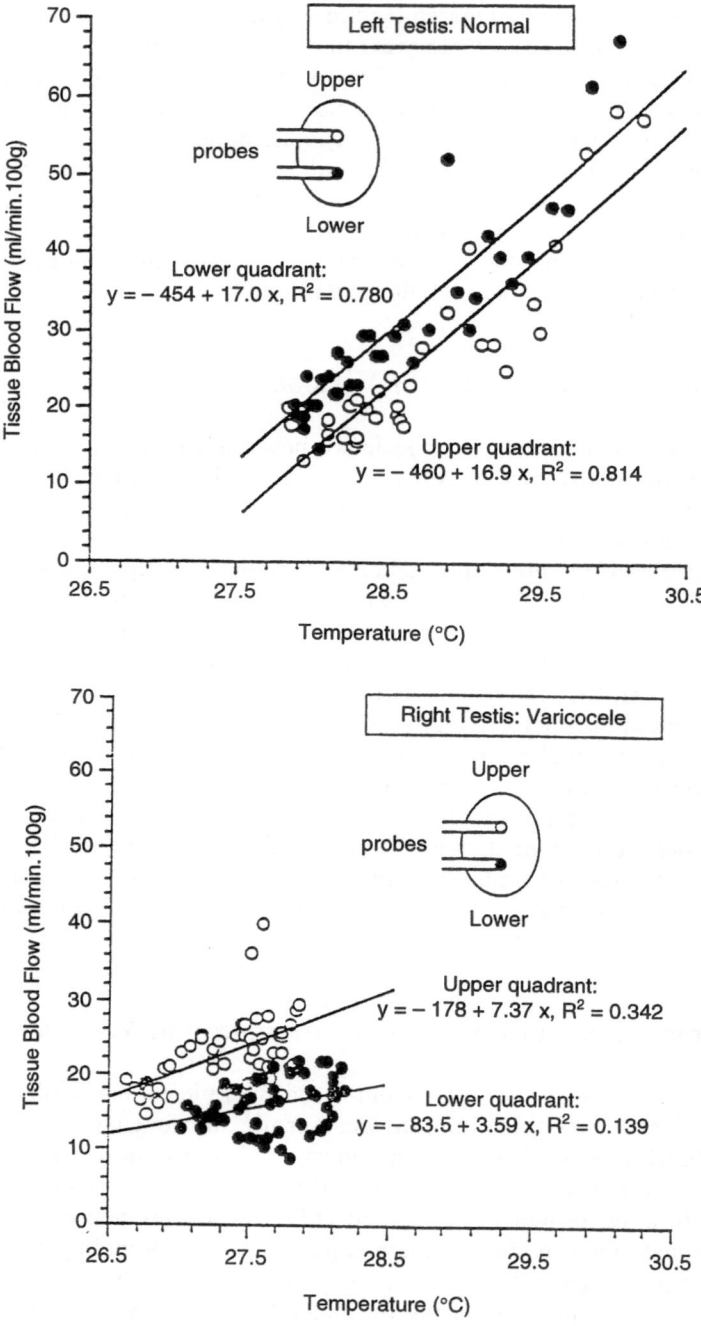

FIGURE 20.1. Thermic distribution across the testes of an azoospermic patient.

of vascular impairment the thermodynamic mechanism of the testis is preserved on opposite poles with a normal score on the spermatogenetic cycle on
the biopsy samples; on the contrary, in the presence of vascular pathology, as
varicocele, the mean values of the thermic parameters are modified and a
large difference exists between opposite poles: The biopsy scores on opposite poles are also different and express severe histopathological findings. In
the attempt to establish the degree of impairment of the testicular microvascular network in order to perform the microsurgical correction of bilateral
varicocele, in azoospermia, a pharmacological vasoactive test is realized by
injecting a microquantity of vasoactive drug (PGE1: 0.1µg/0.1ml; or
Fonzilane®) and the thermodynamic response is evaluated.

In cases with vasoactive response the classical thermodynamic pattern is
encountered, showing a reactive biphasic response of the microcirculation in
situ (Fig. 20.2). The local biopsy confirms that the spermatogenetic process is
still present; therefore, the possibility of testicular recovery after microsurgery can be sustained.

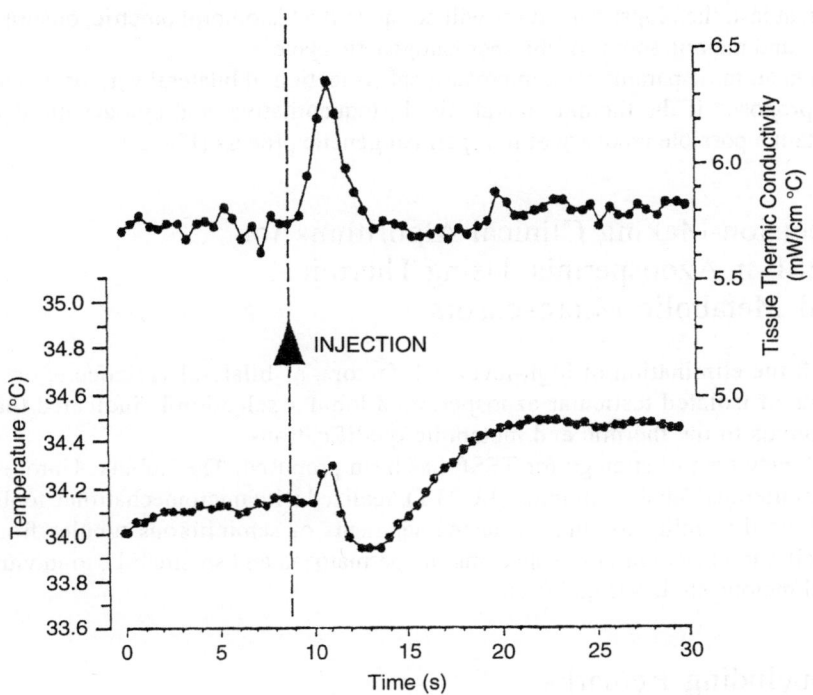

FIGURE 20.2. The thermodynamic pattern associated with a reactive biphasic response
of the testicular microcirculation in situ.

In the absence of thermodynamic response the disappearance of the biphasic pattern occurs, and the arrest of maturation is encountered on the bioptic sample or a complete fibrotic involution is found.

In the responders' cases a large increase on tissue blood flow (~12 ml/min.100gr) and a temperature decrease (~0.4°C) of the testis are measured; in the nonresponders, a low thermal conductivity value (~5.5 mW/cm.°C) is calculated.

Decision-Making Clinical Algorithms for TESE in Azoospermia and Varicocele, Using Thermic and Metabolic Microsensors

In azoospermic patients with bilateral varicocele the color-coded duplex ultrasound studies with power doppler energies will confirm the varicocele and exclude the epididymal obstruction. The power doppler studies of the testes will detect heterogeneous lobular areas and will permit the classification of the pattern in a quantitative and qualitative way.

The intraoperative studies with thermic-probes on opposite poles will evaluate the thermic difference, the vasoactive tests in situ, the microvascular response, and, at last, the biopsies analyses will compute the histomorphometric, quantitative, and meiotic scores of the spermatogenetic cycle.

On all these parameters a microsurgical correction of bilateral varicocele will be proposed if the thermic, metabolic, histoquantitative, and cytogenetic data sustain a possible recovery of the spermatogenetic process (Fig. 20.3).

Decision-Making Clinical Algorithms for TESE in Azoospermia, Using Thermic and Metabolic Microsensors

With the elimination of high-level risk factors, as bilateral varicocele, or in cases of isolated testicular azoospermia a lobular selection is indicated that responds to the thermic and metabolic qualifications.

A new type of strategy for TESE has been proposed: The Lobular Unrolled Seminiferous Tubule Trimming (LUSTT), realized with micromechatronic tools, permits the ability to obtain selected segments of seminiferous tubules from specific lobules to in vitro squeezing of spermatozoa and spermatids, to in vitro vital meiotic studies (Fig. 20.4).

Concluding Remarks

Microtechnologies applied to the human testis in male infertility support a new comprehension and an expanding vision of the intrinsic thermodynamic

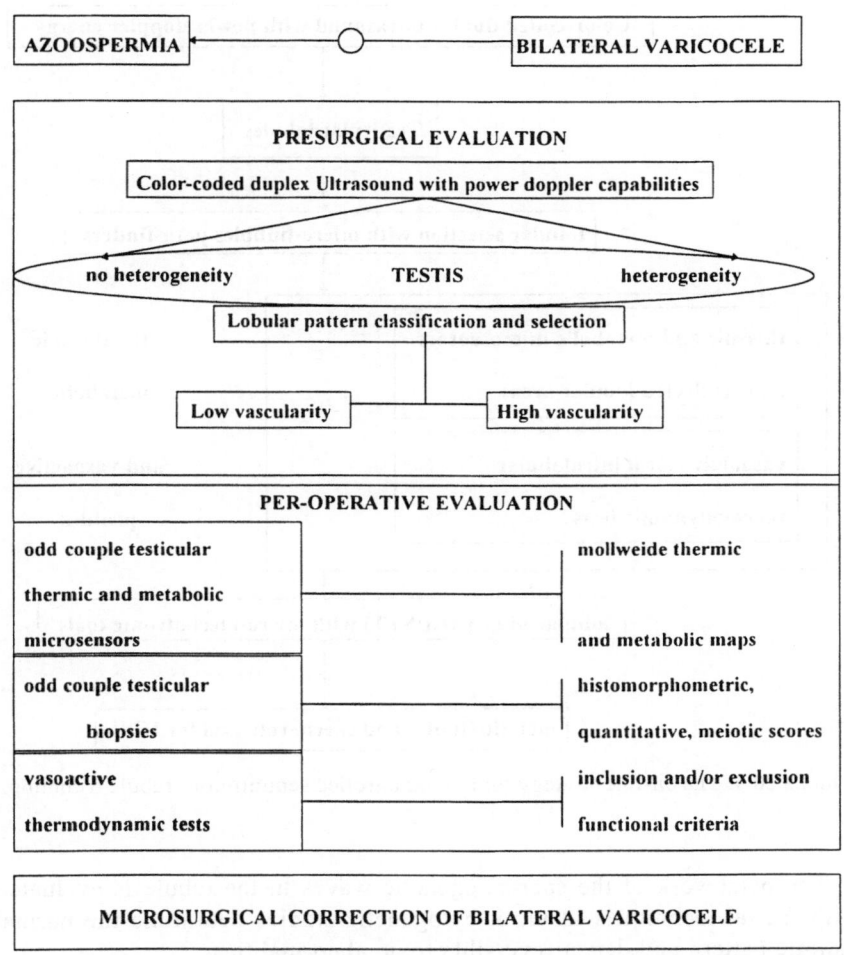

FIGURE 20.3. Parameters assessed prior to microsurgical correction of bilateral varicocele.

and microdynamic regulation of the testes. The application of thermic and metabolic microsensors is able to detect specific areas into the testis with normal microcirculatory and microthermic parameters that can sustain a normal spermatogenetic cycle. The comparative and parallel morphological and meiotic studies confirm the strict relationship between microvascular network and tubular organization, supported by the computer-assisted simulation models of a virtual fractal testis.

Enhanced imaging techniques in vivo permit the selection of the well-vascularized lobular compartments, and micromechatronics tools (MIMET) help the surgeon to perform the intralobular seminiferous tubule retrieval (LUSTT).

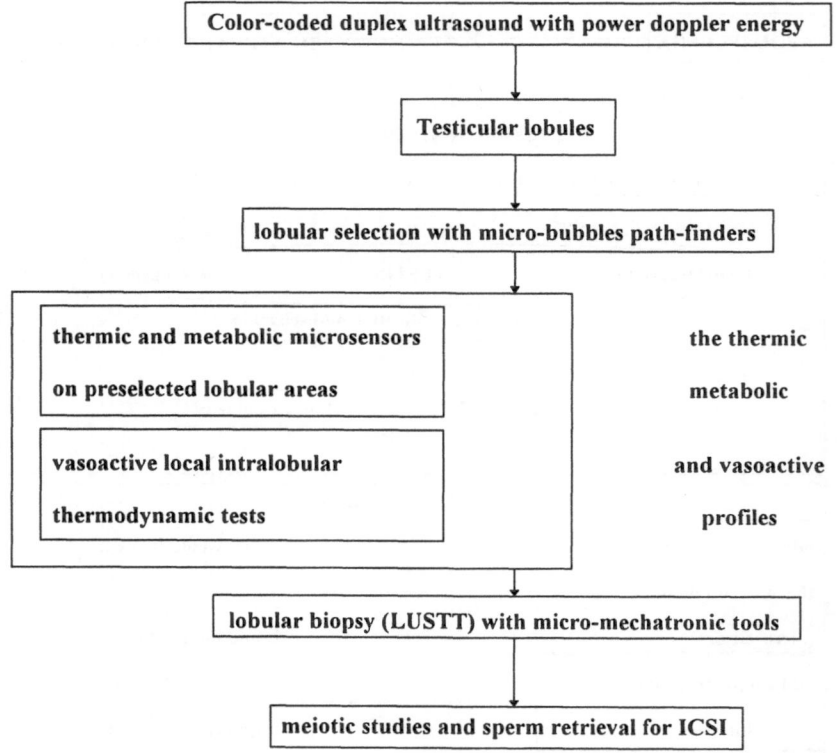

FIGURE 20.4. The on-line strategy for lobular unrolled seminiferous tubule trimming.

The patchwork of the spermatogenetic waves in the tubule is evaluated with fractal techniques in vitro; cytogenetic studies determine the normal meiotic pattern and detect reversible toxic abnormalities.

A new methodological and scientific support can now be offered to the andrologist using microtechnologies and bioengineering approaches to retrieve sperm from the testis for ICSI in azoospermic patients with high-level risk factors, such as bilateral varicocele.

References

1. Cohen J, Malter HE, Talansky BE, Grifo J. Micromanipulation of human gametes and embryos. New York: Raven Press, 1992.
2. Goldstein M. Surgery of male infertility. Philadelphia: WB Saunders, 1995.
3. Tritto J. Bioengineering and microsurgical practice in operative andrology. Workshop on Andrology and Mechatronics (Section: Mechatronics and Robotics in Operative Andrology), IEEE EMBS, 30 October–2 November, Chicago, 1997. In: Tritto J, Brett P. Andrology and mechatronics.

4. Dittmar A, Depeursinge C. Microtechnics, microsensors and actuators in biomedical engineering. AMBER, 5–7 July 1995, 119–23.
5. Dittmar A, Delhomme G, Roussel Ph, Barbier D. Les microcapteurs et microsystèmes biomédicaux. Revue de l'Electricité et de l'Electronique, Numéro spécial du Congrès Mondial de Génie Biomédical, Nice, 14–19 September 1997, 1–16.
6. Dittmar A, Delhomme G, Tritto G, Newman WH, Bowman HF. Continuous measurement of testicular tissue blood flow by a micro-probe using thermal diffusion. IEEE EMBS 1993;15:992–93.
7. Roussel Ph, Dujuis V, Delhomme G, et al. Implantable hybrid multimicrosensor for the metabolic characterization of living tissue. World Congress on Medical Physics and Biomedical Engineering. Med Biol Eng Comput 1997;35(Suppl, Part 2):1281.
8. Dittmar A, Tritto G, Delhomme G, Martelet C, Esteve D, Depeursinge C. Microcirculation and thermoregulation of the human testis in male infertility. Real time measurements using thermal diffusion microsensors. World Congress on Medical Physics and Biomedical Engineering. Med Biol Eng Comput 1997;35(Suppl, Part 2):597.
9. Setchell BP, Bergh A, Widmark A, Damber JE. Effect of testicular temperature on vasomotion and blood flow. Int J Androl 1995;18:120–26.
10. Damber JE, Bergh A, Fagrell B, Lindahl O, Rooth P. Testicular microcirculation in the rat studied by videophotometric capillaroscopy, fluorescence microscopy and laser doppler flowmetry. Acta Physiol Scand 1986;126:371–76.
11. Tritto J. Neuroandrology: a new field in clinical andrology. Proceedings of the VII International Symposium on Andrology, Palma de Mallorca, Spain, 30 April-2 May 1998, 81–85.
12. Zorgniotti AW. Temperature and environmental effects on the testis. In: Zorgniotti AW, editor. Advances in experimental medicine and biology, Vol. 286. New York: Plenum Press, 1991.
13. Sealfon AI, Zorgniotti AW. A theoretical model for testis thermoregulation. In: Zorgniotti AW, editor. Advances in experimental medicine and biology, Vol. 286. New York: Plenum Press, 1991:123–35.
14. Tritto J, Pirlo G. Computer modelling and simulation of temperature-dependent fractal organization of the microcirculation of the testis. Proceedings of the 8th International Conference on Mathematical and Computer Modelling, College Park, Maryland, 1–4 April 1991, 153.
15. Tritto J. The multi-level compartmentation of the simulation models of the countercurrent heat exchange (CCHE) mechanism of the testis. In: Zorgniotti AW, editor. Advances in experimental medicine and biology, Vol. 286. New York: Plenum Press, 1991: 137–51.
16. Suzuki F, Nagano T. Microvasculature of the human testis and excurrent duct system. Cell Tissue Res 1986;243:79–86.
17. Weerasooiya TR, Yamamoto T. Three-dimensional organization of the vasculature of the rat spermatic cord and testis. Cell Tissue Res 1985;241:317–23.
18. Fawcett DW, Neaves WD, Flores MN. Comparative observations on intertubular lymphatics and the organization of the interstitial tissue of the mammalian testis. Biol Reprod 1993;9:500–6.
19. Schulze W, Riemer M, Rehder U, Hohne KH. Computer-assisted three-dimensional reconstructions of the arrangement of primary spermatocytes in human seminiferous tubules. Cell Tissue Res 1986;244:1–8.

20. Tritto J. Computer-assisted modelling and simulation of the intrinsic thermo-regulation of the testis: the multi-level compartmentation. Proceedings of the IASTED Conference on Computers and Advanced Technology in Medicine, Health Care and Bioengineering, Honolulu, 15–17 August 1990:88–90.

21. Bassinghwaighte J. Physiological heterogeneity: fractal link determinism and randomness in structures and functions. News Physiol Sci 1988;3:5–10.

22. Kiani MF, Hudetz AG. Computer simulation of growth of anastomosing microvascular networks. J Theor Biol 1991;150:547–60.

23. Tritto G, North MO, Pirlo G. Computer modelling and simulation of temperature-dependent fractal organization of the microcirculation of the testis; World Congress on Medical Physics and Biomedical Engineering. Med Biol Eng Comput 1997;35(Suppl, Part 1):598.

24. Ergun S, Stingl J, Holstein AF. Segmental angioarchitecture of the testicular lobule in man. Andrologia 1994;26:143–50.

25. Tritto J. Explorations échographiques dans le diagnostic de l'azoospermie sécrétoire. 2ème journées FFER, Clermont-Ferrand, 24–26 Septembre 1997 (in press).

26. Tritto J, Erdei E, Giargia E, Marandola C, Arvis G. Microsurgical correction of bilateral varicocele in severe male infertility factor. Eur Urol 1996;30(Suppl 2):450.

27. Tritto J, Giargia E, Crozes C, Erdei E, Morlier D. The role of testicular biopsy in microsurgical correction of bilateral varicocele. Proceedings of the First International Congress on Andrology, Biomedical Engineering and Sexual Rehabilitation 1995; 274–78.

28. Tritto J, Erdei E, North MO. Azoospermia, maturation arrest and bilateral varicocele: the role of the microsurgery. Proceedings of the 10th World Congress on in Vitro Fertilization and Assisted Reproduction, Vancouver, 24–28 May 1997. Bologna: Monduzzi Ed, 1997:615–18.

29. North MO, Bourgeois CA, Dadoune JP, Arvis G, Tritto J. Reversal meiotic abnormalities in human infertile male with bilateral varicocele after microsurgical correction. 5ème Réunion de la Société Française de Génétique Humaine, 2–3 Décembre 1997, Paris. Ann Genet (in press).

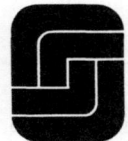

21

ICSI with Epididymal and Testicular Sperm Retrieval

SHERMAN J. SILBER

Introduction

Silber et al. and Tournaye et al. initially developed the use of intracytoplasmic sperm injection (ICSI) to treat obstructive azoospermia due to congenital absence of the vas deferens (CAV), failed vasopepididymostomy (V-E), and otherwise irreparable obstruction, using microsurgically retrieved *epididymal* sperm (1,2). We coined this procedure "MESA" (i.e., *m*icrosurgical *e*pididymal *s*perm *a*spiration). Devroey et al., Silber et al., and Schoysman et al. then demonstrated the systematic use of ICSI with *testicular* sperm in cases where there is either no epididymis or no motile sperm in the epididymis (3–5). Several months later, Devroey et al. and Silber et al. demonstrated that intracytoplasmic sperm injection using frozen–thawed epididymal spermatozoa retrieved from a previous attempt at fresh MESA was as successful as using freshly retrieved sperm (4,6). The present state-of-the-art appears to be that there are very few cases of obstructive azoospermia that cannot be successfully treated with sperm retrieval methods and ICSI, as long as the wife has adequate eggs (7). This may involve the use of epididymal sperm, or, if epididymal sperm cannot be retrieved, the use of testicular sperm.

Sperm Retrieval Methods

There have been many trivial debates over how best to collect epididymal or testicular sperm from azoospermic patients for ICSI. The reader can decide what works best in a particular setting. Our preference is as described in the following.

For cases of obstructive azoospermia, there is usually some epididymis present. If so, then we prefer to perform MESA via a very small "window"

239

incision in the scrotum under local anesthesia using 0.5% marcaine. By injecting both the spermatic cord as well as the anterior scrotal skin, we can easily expose the epididymis, and with an operating microscope, complete the procedure in about 15 min. The advantage of epididymal sperm retrieval performed in this fashion is that huge numbers of the most motile sperm can readily be obtained from the most proximal ducts, and then frozen for an unlimited number of future ICSI cycles. There is often only one specific area of the proximal epididymis where the most motile sperm can be retrieved, and this can be found more easily through microsurgery than through a blind needle stick. The disadvantage, particularly for the gynecologist, is that it requires skills the infertility physician may not possess.

For cases of obstructive azoospermia where there is no epididymis (most unusual), a simple needle stick into the testis will usually retrieve enough sperm for ICSI, but not enough for reliable freezing for future cycles. Because our open biopsies are so simple, quick, and painless, we still prefer it to a needle stick in these cases. For nonobstructive azoospermia, an open biopsy under local anesthesia is clearly the preferred approach.

Nonobstructive Azoospermia

Men with the most severe spermatogenic defects causing complete azoospermia often have a minute number of sperm, or mature spermatids, very sparsely present in an extensive testicular biopsy (which could then be used for ICSI) (8). This approach was based on quantitative studies of spermatogenesis dating back to the late 1970s (9–11). Testicular histology of azoospermic, oligospermic, and normospermic men has shown that the number of sperm in the ejaculate is directly correlated to the number of mature spermatids found quantitatively in the testis. Although there is a wide variation in each tubule, the average mature spermatid count in a large number of tubules was very clearly always predictive of the sperm count in the ejaculate. It is intriguing that many patients with complete azoospermia in the ejaculate were found to have extremely low numbers of mature spermatids per seminiferous tubule. These studies of quantitative spermatogenesis in the late 1970s and early 1980s gave the impetus for our efforts to extract sperm, however few, from men with azoospermia caused by Sertoli cell only or maturation arrest, and to use these few sperm for intracytoplasmic sperm injection (ICSI).

Applying the technique of testicular sperm extraction (TESE), which was developed originally for obstructive azoospermia, it was found that even in azoospermic men with apparently absent spermatogenesis (diagnosed as "Sertoli cell-only syndrome"), there is very frequently a tiny focus of sperm production still to be found somewhere in the testicles (6,12,13). This went undiscussed in those early papers, but it is now apparent that an extremely diminished quantity of sperm production in the testes will result in absolute azoospermia in the ejaculate, even though there is some sperm being produced. A certain tiny threshold of sperm production is necessary before any sperm can actually appear in the ejaculate. It was quite possible, therefore, that very small, tiny numbers of spermatozoa might exist in the testes sufficient for an ICSI procedure, seen in patients who are azoospermic apparently from "absence" of spermatogenesis. This observation led us to perform successful TESE for patients with azoospermia due to Sertoli cell-only syndrome, or those with cryptorchid testicular atrophy, who had high FSH levels, very small testes, apparently absent spermatogenesis, and no obstruction (6).

Thus, severe oligospermia (which is readily treated with ICSI) is just a quantitative variant of azoospermia in that there is some minute presence of spermatogenesis in 60% of azoospermic men, but the amount of spermatogenesis is below that threshold necessary for a few sperm to "spill over" into the ejaculate. For the purpose of comparing Y chromosomal deletions to the degree of spermatogenic defect, azoospermic men with at least a few sperm retrievable from the testes may be in a similar category to very severely oligospermic men. Azoospermic men in whom there was absolutely no sperm retrievable either from the ejaculate or from testicular sperm extraction turn out to be in a different category from azoospermic men who have a minute amount of sperm production (14–16).

In those infertile men who are Y-deleted, larger deletions appear to be associated with a total absence of testicular sperm; however, smaller deletions, limited simply to DAZ, are associated with the presence of small numbers of sperm that are sufficient for ICSI. This implies that there are other modifying genes on the Y that can further affect the severity of the spermatogenic defect in DAZ-deleted infertile men.

References

1. Silber SJ, Nagy ZP, Liu J, Godoy H, Devroey P, Van Steirteghem AC. Conventional in-vitro fertilization versus intracytoplasmic sperm injection for patients requiring microsurgical sperm aspiration. Hum Reprod 1994;9:705–9.
2. Tournaye H, Devroey P, Liu J, Nagy Z, Lissens W, Van Steirteghem A. Microsurgical epididymal sperm aspiration and intracytoplasmic sperm injection: a new effective approach to infertility as a result of congenital absence of the vas deferens. Fertil Steril 1994;61:1045–51
3. Devroey P, Liu J, Nagy P, Tournaye H, Silber SJ, Van Steirteghem AC. Normal fertilization of oocytes after testicular sperm extraction and intracytoplasmic sperm injection (TESE and ICSI). Fertil Steril 1994;62:639–41
4. Silber SJ, Van Steirteghem AC, Liu J, Nagy Z, Tournaye H, Devroey P. High fertilization and pregnancy rate after intracytoplasmic sperm injection with sperm obtained from testicle biopsy. Hum Reprod 1995;10;148–52.
5. Schoysman R, Vanderzwalmen P, Nijs M, et al. Pregnancy after fertilisation with human testicular spermatozoa. Lancet 1993;342:1237.
6. Devroey P, Silber S, Nagy Z, et al. Ongoing pregnancies and birth after intracytoplasmic sperm injection (ICSI) with frozen-thawed epididymal spermatozoa. Hum Reprod 1994;10:903–6.

7. Silber SJ, Nagy Z, Liu J, et al. The use of epididymal and testicular spermatozoa for intracytoplasmic sperm injection: the genetic implications for male infertility. Hum Reprod 1995;10:2031–43.

8. Silber SJ, Nagy Z, Devroey P, Tournaye H, Van Steirteghem AC. Distribution of spermatogenesis in the testicles of azoospermic men: the presence or absence of spermatids in the testes of men with germinal failure. Hum Reprod 1997;12:2422–28.

9. Steinberger E, Tjioe DY. A method for quantitative analysis of human seminiferous epithelium. Fertil Steril 1968;19:960–70.

10. Zuckerman Z, Rodriguez-Rigau L, Weiss DB, Chowdhury LJ, Smith KD, Steinberger E. Quantitative analysis of the seminiferous epithelium in human testicle biopsies and the relation of spermatogenesis to sperm density. Fertil Steril 1978;30:448–55.

11. Silber SJ, Rodriguez-Rigau L. Quantitative analysis of testicle biopsy: determination of partial obstruction and prediction of sperm count after surgery for obstruction. Fertil Steril 1981;36:480–85.

12. Silber SJ. What forms of male infertility are there left to cure? Hum Reprod 1995;10:503–4.

13. Silber SJ, Van Steirteghem AC, Devroey P. Sertoli cell only revisited. Hum Reprod 1995;10:1031–32.

14. Lahn BT, Page DC. Functional coherence of the human Y chromosome. Science 1997;278:675–80.

15. Reijo R, Lee T-Y, Salo P, et al. Diverse spermatogenic defects in humans caused by Y chromosome deletions encompassing a novel RNA-binding protein gene. Nat Genet 1995;10:383–93.

16. Tiepelo L, Zuffardi O. Localization of factors controlling spermatogenesis in the nonfluorescent portion of the human Y chromosome long arm. Hum Genet 1976;34:119–24.

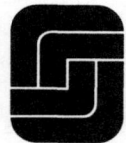

22

Pathophysiologic Changes after Testicular Sperm Extraction: Patterns and Avoidance of Testicular Injury

Peter N. Schlegel, Li-Ming Su, and Philip Shihua Li

Introduction

Intracytoplasmic sperm injection (ICSI) has allowed improved sperm fertilization and pregnancy rates for men with sperm in the ejaculate despite severely defective sperm production (1). Sperm retrieval in conjunction with ICSI was initially performed for men with normal sperm production and reproductive tract obstruction (2,3). Preliminary studies demonstrated that rare sperm may be present within the testicles of men with nonobstructive azoospermia—despite severely defective sperm production (4). Using extensive testicular biopsies, spermatozoa can be retrieved for ICSI from at least some men with non-obstructive azoospermia (5–7). Unlike standard diagnostic biopsies, testicular sperm extraction (TESE) is a noninvasive procedure that may involve multiple sites of biopsy from one or both testes to find the very few spermatozoa that are present only within the testis of these men with severely defective sperm production.

In order to understand the potential effects of testicular biopsy on the testis and spermatogenesis, it is necessary to consider the normal structure and function of the testis. The testicular blood supply is derived primarily from branches of the internal spermatic artery, with collateral branches off of the cremasteric and vasal arteries (8). Regardless of the original source of testicular blood flow, the arteries enter the testis as a series of end-arteries by penetrating the tunica albuginea and traveling subjacent to the tunica albuginea in a variable course, branching into further end-arteries that cover a large area of the surface of the testis. The vessels will typically travel along the posterior surface of the testis, protected by the epididymis, traveling to the lower pole of the testis, and eventually entering the testicular parenchyma after coursing in a serpiginous and variable pattern under the tunica albuginea over the surface of the seminiferous tubules (9).

The vessels then penetrate the testicular parenchyma in the septae between spermatogenic tubules. Because all arteries within the testis are end-arteries, devascularization of large regions of the testis can result from division or ligation of individual major arteries or multiple smaller arteries under the surface of the tunica albuginea. Elegant human autopsy studies of the testicular blood supply have shown that no single area of the testis can be blindly opened without potential injury to a major vessel of the testis (9).

Simple diagnostic testis biopsies may directly affect the testis. Harrington et al. have reported that 29% of single open diagnostic testicular biopsies resulted in intratesticular hematoma formation, with development of a hypoechoic lesion on scrotal ultrasound (10). Hematoma formation also occurs after percutaneous testis biopsy. The multiple biopsies or removal of a larger sample of testis required for TESE appear to result in more inflammation and greater disruption of spermatogenesis than that reported for a simple diagnostic biopsy. For men with quantitatively impaired sperm production, including men with nonobstructive azoospermia, significant transient or permanent damage to the testis could occur after TESE, affecting future attempts at sperm production or testicular function. The effects of multiple biopsies on testicular function have not been previously well described. We present a series of 64 men who were evaluated after TESE procedures and, based on these observations, suggest techniques for TESE that limit the potential for testicular injury and optimize the chances for sperm retrieval.

Patient Evaluation

A total of 64 patients underwent TESE for nonobstructive azoospermia at our Center or elsewhere. Subsequent evaluation of patients was then performed at The New York Hospital-Cornell Medical Center. Recommended evaluation included eliciting any symptoms related to the TESE procedure and physical examination. All patients were recommended to have scrotal ultrasound evaluation and serum hormonal evaluation, including measurement of serum FSH and testosterone levels. Men who underwent multiple TESE procedures were evaluated for the ability to extract spermatozoa in the second TESE procedure, as well as the interval between TESE procedures. The results of these analyses have been previously published in *Human Reproduction* (11). Additional information on the effects of TESE was obtained using histologic analysis of prior TESE/biopsy sites after fixation of excised prior biopsy sites in Bouin's solution, embedding in paraffin, and hematoxylin-eosin staining.

Findings after TESE

History/Physical

Two patients noted progressive unilateral testicular atrophy after bilateral TESE procedures. Mild pain associated with normal postoperative processes was reported by all evaluated patients. Only minimal induration of the tunica albuginea and/or incision(s) was typically present on physical examination within 1 month of TESE procedures. No acute perioperative complications, such as a clinically evident hematoma or wound infection, were noted.

Ultrasonographic Findings

Of the 17 patients who underwent scrotal ultrasound evaluation at 3 months after TESE, 14 out of 17 (82%) had acute findings, described as either a discrete hypoechoic region or diffuse heterogeneity of the testicular parenchyma (Fig. 22.1). These ultrasonographic abnormalities have been previously reported as reflecting regions of hematoma formation, inflammation, or diffuse intraparenchymal testicular bleeding associated with testicular trauma (12–14). Of the four patients with acute findings on sonography at 3 months post-TESE who had subsequent ultrasound evaluation, all acute findings had resolved by 6 months after TESE.

Overall, 14 patients had scrotal ultrasonography performed six or more months after their TESE procedure. Three patients (21%) had findings still consistent with acute inflammation or had a hematoma detectable. Chronic

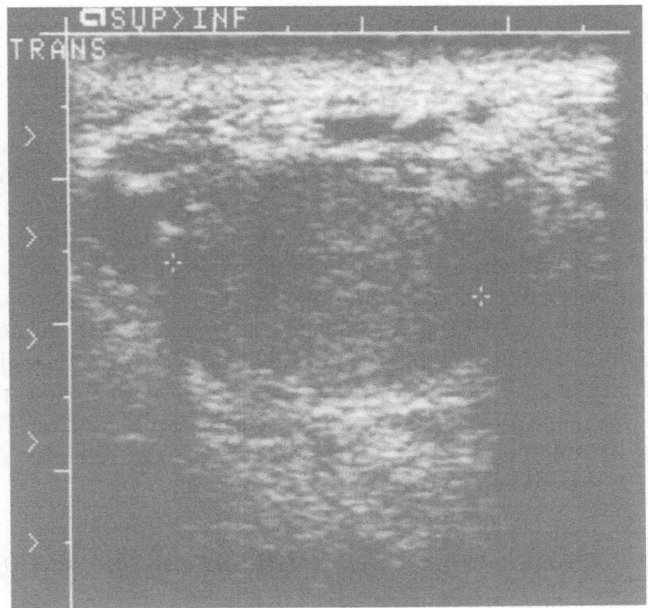

FIGURE 22.1. Classic appearance of hypoechoic lesions within the testis after TESE procedure, reflective of hematoma formation, is depicted in this longitudinal view of a testis on scrotal ultrasonography.

ultrasound findings more than 6 months after TESE were present for 9 out of 14 (64%) of patients in this group. Typical chronic findings included parenchymal calcification, or the presence of a linear hyperechoic scar. Evidence that these findings are truly chronic was provided by the observation that at least five of the nine patients had chronic findings present more than 1 year after the TESE procedure. The remaining two patients evaluated more than 6 months after TESE had normal scrotal ultrasound evaluation.

Testicular Blood Flow Analysis

The two patients who reported unilateral testicular atrophy after TESE were evaluated further with color Doppler ultrasound. In the first patient, ultrasound of the atrophic testis revealed a large region without blood flow within the parenchyma of the symptomatically atrophied right testis, confirming devascularization of the testis during the TESE procedure. This was the second TESE attempt for this patient; each attempt, performed at another institution, had reportedly involved multiple biopsies from the subsequently atrophic (right) testis. The second patient also had multiple sites of the testis biopsied during a TESE attempt, and arterial flow on doppler ultrasound was globally decreased as compared with the contralateral testis. In addition, the surface of the testicular parenchyma was noted to have surface changes consistent with the fibrosis and retraction that commonly accompanies testicular ischemia.

Effects of Multiple TESE Procedures

A total of 19 patients underwent multiple TESE attempts. All had viable spermatozoa obtained for ICSI at the initial TESE procedure. Four of the patients had a second TESE procedure after the initial TESE, with an interval of 2, 3, 3, and 4 months after the initial successful TESE. For three patients (3 out of 4; 75%) no spermatozoa were found, whereas the fourth patient had rare spermatozoa retrieved with cytologic evidence of extensive numbers of inflammatory cells and debris. The retrieved spermatozoa had shortened tails. No normal fertilizations nor pregnancy was achieved. For 15 patients who underwent multiple TESE attempts at retrieval of spermatozoa, the repeat procedure was made more than 6 months after the initial attempt. For 12 out of 15 (80%) of attempts, testicular spermatozoa were also retrieved during the second TESE procedure.

Histologic Evaluation of TESE Effects on Spermatogenesis

Routine evaluation of TESE sites was performed for six patients after an initial testis biopsy procedure for TESE or diagnostic purposes. Whereas maturation arrest or hypospermatogenesis was present in the initial biopsy, interstitial fibrosis and a Sertoli cell-only pattern was present at the site of earlier TESE procedures. These findings suggest that local effects of healing after TESE procedures may have significant adverse effects on adjacent, apparently previously functioning spermatogenic testicular tissue.

Effects on Androgen Secretion

Evaluation of serum testosterone levels before and after TESE has been prospectively performed for seven men. Clinically significant alterations in serum testosterone levels were seen for only one man. Removal of up to 75% of initial testicular volume was performed for several patients with residual volume per testis of as little as 1 ml without clinically significant alterations in serum testosterone levels. These findings suggest that residual Leydig cell function is able to compensate for resection of dramatic proportions of the original hormonally active testicular volume without significant effects on circulating androgen levels.

Discussion

TESE retrieval of spermatozoa from some men with nonobstructive azoospermia (NOA) is now possible for use with ICSI. The TESE procedure has provided a new treatment option for men with testicular failure, where sperm production is quantitatively very limited, if it is present at all. Without this option, only substitutive treatments such as donor insemination or adoption would be the only means for these men to become fathers. Because TESE is a new procedure, an understanding of the physiological effects of TESE on the testis and spermatogenesis is important. This knowledge may help to improve the perception of the risks of TESE and to help in planning repeat TESE procedures to optimize the chances of successful sperm retrieval.

Spermatogenesis is very sensitive to subtle influences such as heat, chemical exposures, and drug use, as well as varicoceles, cryptorchidism, and genitourinary infections. Patients with unilateral testicular processes will frequently show contralateral testicular dysfunction. Contralateral testes of men with unilateral epididymoorchitis will typically demonstrate a reduction of the population of germ cells and quantitatively reduced spermatogenesis (15). Testicular surgery can also produce inflammation that may impair sperm production. In an animal model, Del Vento et al. found hypoechoic regions within the testis and histologic alterations after testis biopsy up to 1 month after testicular biopsy in stallions (16).

The results reported in this study indicate that the physiologic consequences of TESE procedures are more significant than can be superficially appreciated on routine clinical evaluation for men with NOA. Ultrasonographically detectable testicular abnormalities are present in most men after TESE, whereas physical exam is normal. Given the 74-day duration of spermatogenesis in humans, effects on sperm output may persist for up to 3 months after local effects from

TESE can be documented on ultrasound. Given the quantitatively limited sperm production that is, by definition, present in men with NOA, any adverse effect on spermatogenesis may ablate the limited opportunity for sperm extraction from the testis for these men. Based on the nearly 3-month duration of spermatogenesis, we chose to evaluate patients at 3 and 6 month intervals after TESE. The high (82%) frequency of testicular abnormalities after TESE on scrotal ultrasonography suggested that sperm production may be impaired for most men with NOA for at least 6 months after TESE.

Our findings of frequent abnormalities on 3 month post-TESE ultrasound with normal ultrasound evaluations at 6 months, with a nearly 3-month duration of spermatogenesis, suggested that sperm retrieval rates may be adversely affected for up to 6 months after TESE, when compared with sperm retrieval attempts more than 6 months after an initial TESE procedure. This expectation was supported by a high TESE success rate more than 6 months after TESE, with a poor retrieval rate when sperm retrieval was re-attempted within the first 6 months. We always delay attempts, therefore, until after acute ultrasonographic findings have resolved for at least 3 months, and at least 6 months after an initial successful TESE procedure. Use of frozen testicular tissue is always considered prior to repeating an invasive procedure for sperm retrieval.

We did not evaluate the effects of TESE on subsequent sperm retrieval for men with normal spermatogenesis and obstructive azoospermia, in part because epididymal sperm retrieval is a far more efficient site for sperm retrieval in this condition. We would speculate that sperm production is normal and therefore quantitatively high in men with obstructive azoospermia, so the ability to retrieve sperm for ICSI even early after a prior TESE procedure will not be affected because only limited numbers of sperm are needed for ICSI; therefore, we would predict different qualitative effects of TESE on men with obstructive versus NOA. Although some adverse effects are probably present after TESE for all patients, the sperm production in men with obstructive azoospermia are so high to start with that some sperm production will still be present despite a partial impairment in spermatogenesis. For men with NOA, however, any impairment in spermatogenesis (from TESE) is more likely to ablate the limited chances for sperm retrieval unless optimal sperm production is restored after a TESE procedure.

In addition to the known transient effects of biopsy on spermatogenesis, our observations also indicate that permanent devascularization of the testis may occur after TESE procedures. Based on prior studies by Jarow, we have postulated that multiple incisions in the tunica albuginea, as suggested by others as the technique for TESE, may result in interruption of a sufficient proportion of the testicular blood supply to result in devascularization of the testis. This observation suggests that limiting the number or amount of incision on the surface of the tunica albuginea may help to prevent the devastating complication of testicular injury.

TESE: Recommended Clinical Approach—Cornell Experience

Based on the observations summarized in this chapter, we have refined our approach to TESE. TESE procedures on men with NOA require that sampling of testicular tissue be performed in an attempt to find the limited, heterogeneous area(s) of sperm production in the testis. The sperm-producing areas of testicular parenchyma may be limited in number and are often randomly dispersed throughout the testis. The initially proposed approach of multiple, limited biopsy samples through different incisions in the tunica albuginea allows sampling of only small, peripheral regions of the testis. This approach does not sample deeper or central regions of the testis. In addition, this approach can have the highest risk of testicular injury because multiple blind incisions in the tunica albuginea have a higher chance of injury to testicular end-arteries. Based on these observations, we have applied three major changes in the TESE technique.

First, the choice of an incisional site into the testis is determined after observation of subtunical blood vessels with optical magnification at 10–15× power under an operating microscope. This allows selection of an area with a minimum of testicular vessels, minimizing risks of injury to the testicular blood supply. Second, we perform sperm retrieval procedures using a single, larger incision in the selected avascular region of the tunica albuginea. A wide incision allows access to superficial/peripheral regions of the testis as well as to deeper, more central areas of testicular parenchyma. Finally, we have observed that seminiferous tubules containing better sperm production can be directly identified and differentiated from fibrotic tubules or those with Sertoli cell-only pattern using optical magnification at 20× power under an operating microscope. This approach is supported by the simple knowledge that normal spermatogenic tubules are primarily composed of germ cells. Seminiferous tubules with optimal sperm production will therefore be larger than seminiferous tubules with Sertoli cell-only pattern or otherwise impaired spermatogenesis. Optimal tubules for removal are larger, and typically have a whitish appearance (Fig. 22.2). Because very few tubules may have sperm production within the testis of men with NOA, removal of only very small volumes of testicular tissue is needed to affect a successful TESE procedure (Fig. 22.3). Controlled studies at our center support the effectiveness of removal of only limited, highly selected areas of the testis, with greater spermatozoal yield when compared with excision of 1000-fold higher volumes of excised testicular parenchyma.

Because excised tissue cannot be replaced and is lost for subsequent potential testicular function, it only makes sense to limit the amount of testicular tissue excised. Extraction of spermatozoa from a small volume of testicular tissue is also far less technically demanding than excision of a large chunk of testicular tissue that then must be microdissected, red blood cells lysed, and

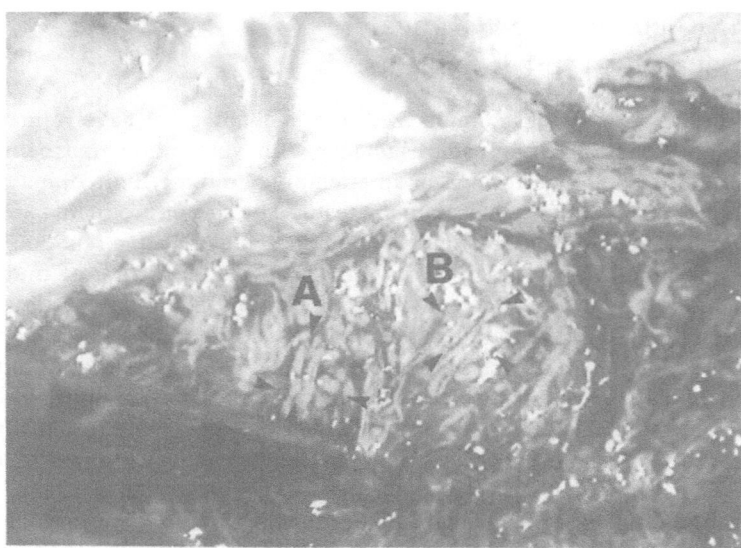

FIGURE 22.2. Intraoperative view of testis, as viewed with optical magnification during TESE procedure. Enlarged tubules, reflective of normal regions of spermatogenesis are outlined by arrowheads (Region A). Thin, fibrotic tubules, containing histologic Sertoli cell-only pattern, are outlined by arrowheads as region B.

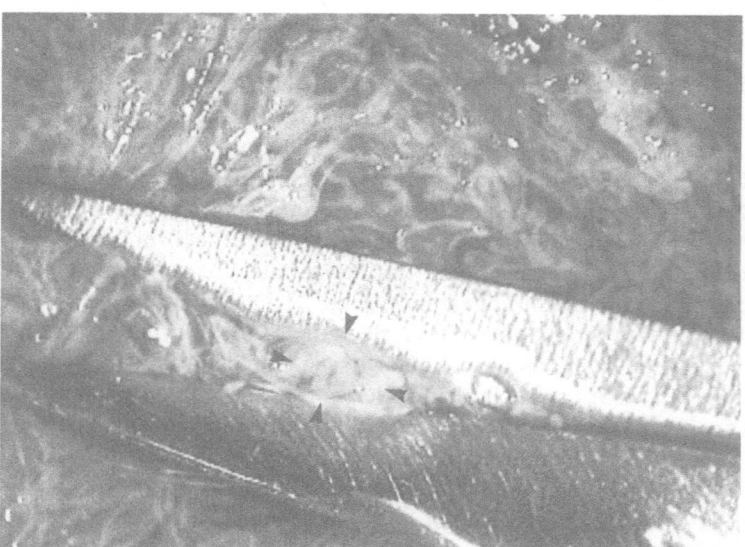

FIGURE 22.3. Excision of approximately 1 mm³ region of spermatogenic tubules, depicted in Figure 22.2 as region A, is demonstrated during a TESE procedure. This small area of resected tissue will typically have as many sperm extractable as a much larger, standard excisional biopsy.

the rare spermatozoa searched for in a tedious fashion under a dissecting microscope. Selection of spermatozoa from a smaller population of contaminating testicular cells is faster and far more efficient.

Prospective application of this approach to testicular sperm retrieval for men with NOA at The New York Hospital-Cornell Medical Center in the last 27 TESE procedures has improved sperm retrieval efficiency without any evidence of adverse effects on testicular function.

Summary/Conclusions

TESE is an effective potential treatment to effect sperm extraction from men with NOA. TESE may cause significant transient effects on spermatogenic function. Effects on androgen production appear to be limited. Permanent effects of extensive TESE procedures may, occasionally, cause complete loss of the testis through vascular compromise. Potential subjects for TESE should be informed of this potential risk. Transient adverse effects after TESE may last up to 6 months.

Repeat TESE procedures should be withheld until at least 6 months after an initial TESE procedure, and the use of frozen testicular tissue known to contain spermatozoa should always be used prior to a repeat biopsy procedure. Healing within the testis after TESE may lag far behind external findings on physical examination. Patients after TESE should be followed with serial scrotal ultrasounds every 3 months to determine when resolution of the expected inflammation and bleeding from the initial biopsy procedure has occurred, prior to preparation for any subsequent TESE attempts.

Use of optical magnification during a TESE procedure can limit the risk of TESE by identifying testicular vessels under the tunica albuginea prior to placement of an incision into the testis. Optical magnification with an operating microscope can also allow direct identification of tubules with sperm production to facilitate efficient sperm extraction from men with NOA. Application of these techniques limits the risk of TESE procedures and dramatically improves the efficacy of sperm extraction with significantly less testicular tissue removed from patients.

Acknowledgments. This chapter was adapted, with permission of the authors, from Schlegel and Su, "Physiologic consequences of testicular sperm extraction," *Human Reproduction* 12:1688–1692, 1997 (11).

The clinical observations presented in this chapter would not have been possible without the collaborative efforts of the entire staff of the Cornell Center for Reproductive Medicine, Dr. Zev Rosenwaks, and especially laboratory team members Deborah Liotta, Zhen Ye, Silvia Menendez, Dr. Lucinda Veeck, and Dr. Gianpiero Palermo. Special acknowledgment is also extended to Dr. Marc Goldstein for contributing his advise regarding microsurgical procedures.

References

1. Nagy Z, Liu J, Jansenwillen C, Silber S, Devroey P, Van Steirteghem A. Using ejaculated, fresh and frozen-thawed epididymal and testicular spermatozoa gives rise to comparable results after intracytoplasmic sperm injection. Fertil Steril 1995;63:808–15.

2. Tournaye H, Devroey P, Liu J, Nagy Z, Lissens W, Van Steirteghem A. Microsurgical epididymal sperm aspiration and intracytoplasmic injection: a new effective approach to infertility as a result of congenital bilateral absence of the vas deferens. Fertil Steril 1994;61:1045–51.

3. Schlegel PN, Palermo GD, Alikani M, et al. Micropuncture retrieval of epididymal sperm with IVF: importance of in vitro micromanipulation techniques. Urology 1995;46:238–41.

4. Jow WW, Steckel J, Schlegel PN, Magid MS, Goldstein M. Motile sperm in human testis biopsy specimens. J Androl 1993;14:194–98.

5. Devroey P, Liu J, Nagy Z, et al. Pregnancies after testicular sperm extraction and intracytoplasmic sperm injection in non-obstructive azoospermia. Hum Reprod 1995;10:1457–60.

6. Kahraman S, Ozgur S, Alatas C, et al. Fertility with testicular sperm extraction and intracytoplasmic sperm injection in non-obstructive azoospermic men. Hum Reprod 1996;11:756–60.

7. Schlegel PN, Palermo GD, Goldstein M, et al. Testicular sperm extraction with intracytoplasmic sperm injection for non-obstructive azoospermia. Urology 1997;49:435–40.

8. Schlegel PN, Chang TSK. Physiology of male reproduction: the testis, epididymis and ductus deferens. In: Walsh PC, Retik AB, Vaughan ED, Wein AJ, editors. Campbell's urology, Seventh edition, Chapter 42. Philadelphia, PA: WB Saunders, 1998:1254–86.

9. Jarow JP. Clinical significance of intratesticular arterial anatomy. J Urol 1991;145:777–79.

10. Harrington TG, Schauer D, Gilbert BR. Percutaneous testis biopsy: an alternative to open testicular biopsy in the evaluation of the subfertile man. J Urol 1996;156:1647–51.

11. Schlegel PN, Su L-M. Physiologic consequences of testicular sperm extraction. Hum Reprod 1997;12:1688–92.

12. Anderson KA, McAninch JW, Brooke Jeffrey R, Laing FC. Ultrasonography for the diagnosis and staging of blunt scrotal trauma. J Urol 1983;130:933–35.

13. Corrales JG, Corbel L, Cipolla B, et al. Accuracy of ultrasound diagnosis after blunt testicular trauma. J Urol 1993;150:1834–36.

14. Fournier GR, Jr, Laing FC, Brooke Jeffrey R, McAninch JW. High resolution scrotal ultrasonography: a highly sensitive but nonspecific diagnostic technique. J Urol 1985;134:490–93.

15. Osegbe DN. Testicular function after unilateral bacterial epididymo-orchitis. Eur Urol 1991;19:204–8.

16. Del Vento VR, Amann RP, Trotter GW, Veeramachaneni DN, Squires EL. Ultrasonographic and quantitative histologic assessment of sequelae to testicular biopsy in stallions. Am J Vet Res 1992;53:2094–101.

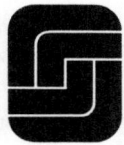

23

Cytological Evaluation of Germinal Populations as Part of a Testicular Sperm Retrieval Strategy

VINCENT IZARD, DOMINIQUE MARMOR, ANNE PERON,
VALÉRIE PARADIS, GÉRARD BENOÎT,
JEAN-CLAUDE SOUFIR, AND ALAIN JARDIN

Introduction

An immediate estimation of spermatogenesis supplies precious data for determining a surgical therapeutic strategy. Extemporaneous examination of testicular tissue remains difficult, however, even for well-trained cytologists. Hence, a fast staining method appropriate for visualizing germinal cells harvested from the testis may be useful in cases of nonobstructive pathology. Such a biological peroperative approach reduces the potential for scattered punctures and avoids causing trauma to the testicular tissue.

Surgical Approach to the Testis

Surgery is generally performed under general or locoregional anaesthesia (rachianaesthesia with lidocaine or bupivacaine). After medial incision of the scrotal sac, and incision of the tunica vaginalis, the consistency of the testis is assessed. The white (or blue-white) tunica albuginea is then incized. The vascularization may sometimes be well individualized and seen under the tunica.

Albugineal incision reveals the testicular tissue. The seminiferous tubules are clearly visible macroscopically or under an operating microscope as the pulp is gently squeezed out. The size, consistency, and color of the tubules can be assessed. The color of the seminiferous tubules ranges from ivory-white to gold-yellow. The thickness of the tubule walls can be measured as the pulp spreads out. A small specimen should be deposited on a sterile glass slide. Consistency and the cohesion of the tubes is determined after dissection with microsciscors. The fragment must be given immediately to the biologist. Arterial or venous leakage at the site of incision is variable. Hemostasis may require the use of bipolar forceps beneath the tunica albuginea.

Biological Analysis of the Testis

Testicular Biopsy

Histological study can yield an accurate but delayed analysis of testicular tissue, but it is informative only when the technique is optimally performed (1). The testicular sample must be large enough to allow at least 40–50 intact sections of the seminiferous tubules to be examined. Immediate fixation is mandatory in the operating room: Tubes containing aqueous Bouin's liquor must be prepared in advance and labeled with the patient's name, biopsy site, and whether it is the left or right side.

Formalin fixative solution is not appropriate for testicular tissue that is to be paraffin embedded. In fact, immersive fixation in buffered formalin results in poor penetration of the fixative, giving rise to many artefacts caused by shrinkage and swelling, and marked deterioration of tissue and cell structure and preservation (2–4). The lamina propria of the seminiferous tubules shrinks and the intercellular connections are lost, producing displacement of the germinal cells and many apparent intercellular vacuoles.

The histological technique is efficient, but it needs updating because iterative observation of the slides is possible using modern techniques when the quality of the tissue fixation remains good.

If the number of analyzable seminiferous sections is sufficient, with perfect fixation and coloration procedures, then testicular histology is very informative and deserves to be used more widely; however, examination of human spermatogenesis is associated with several specific problems. Spermatogenesis in humans is poor compared with other mammals, and analysis is much more difficult because few cells are at the same stage at the same time. No testicular staging can be performed as in the rat due to reductional production of germinal lines: 16 spermatozoa derive from a spermatogonia in human beings compared with 112 in the rat and 256 in the monkey. The mature cell population, therefore, is reduced. Techniques need to fit with this poor production and spermatogenic staging.

Peroperative Cytology of Germinal Cell Population

In cases of seminal tract obstruction, a drop of fluid obtained by puncturing the vas deferens, the epididymal tubule, or the vasa efferentia region is informative enough simply using a biological examination with slide and coverslip, and it gives information for both retrieval and reconstructive strategies.

When a peroperative evaluation of spermatogenesis is necessary, however, a fast staining method to examine the germinal cells harvested from the testis is mandatory.

Classical surgical biopsy of testicular tissue is performed under locoregional or general anaesthesia rather than local anaesthesia through short scrototomy. Clean autoclave sterilized glass slides are prepared in advance. The slides are rinsed with sterile distilled water and wiped dry. A testicular fragment is deposited on the sterile glass slide in a drop of saline, avoiding contamination with blood cells, and gently dissected with sterile microscissors by the surgeon. Slow extensive dissection is mandatory for the following procedures. A very small fragment (less than that required for a histological sample) containing a limited number of tubules is needed. The pulp dissection seems easier in cases of hypospermatogenesis. The slide is air-dried and then stained with a staining procedure derived from May Grunwald Giemsa (DiffQuik® Dade Laboratory, France), which consists of three ready-made solutions: fast green, eosine, and thiazidic dye. The slide is then rinsed in plain water, air-dried, and examined under an optical microscope. The whole procedure takes no more than 5 minutes. Germinal cells can be recognized at the maturation stage.

Slides prepared in this fashion allow cytological analysis of the sperm cells, which is often difficult with a testicular biopsy. The different stages of the germinal cells are easily recognized. Necrotic cells can be identified, as can partial meiotic arrest or total meiotic arrest and its stages.

Sertoli cells, as well as immature and mature germinal cells, can be easily identified. Spermatids and spermatozoa are counted, and even their morphology can be analyzed optically. The intensity of spermatogenesis and the homogeneity of the repartition of mature sperm on the slide can be assessed.

Multinuclear cells and degenerating spermatids are sometimes observed. This is of particular interest as they are very difficult to see on a human testicular biopsy (5). In animal experimentation, multinuclear cells represent a classic, early sign of spermatogenic impairment, particularly after drug administration.

Nitrofurans cause extensive reversible damage to the germinal epithelium of the rat. After 1 week of treatment, spermatids and secondary spermatocytes are absent or abnormal, and the primary spermatocytes are undergoing necrosis. Within a week of cessation of the treatment, regenerative changes are observed. The specific site of nitrofuran action appears to be meiotic division, with arrest of the primary spermatocytes at the leptotene stage (6).

Testicular cytology using slides gives no information on testicular architecture and the interstitium: Testicular cytology and histology can be seen as two complementary procedures, just as bone myelogram and medullar biopsy are in hematology.

In the estimation of spermatogenic quality, the correlation between immediate cytological examination and delayed testicular biopsy is very good. Discordance is only observed in cases of severely impaired spermatogenesis with very scarce germinal cells (much less than one spermatid per seminiferous tube section on testicular biopsy). For these patients, mature spermatozoa are sometimes observed with only one of the two techniques.

This technique is now routinely used in our urological operating room and leads to immediate assessment of testicular tissue status at the precise site of biopsy. It allows immediate diagnosis, choice of the best site for sperm retrieval, and an immediate surgical decision on whether to continue or end the andrological surgical procedure.

The slides can be stored for prolonged periods for further analysis.

Peroperative Cytology in Assisted Reproductive Technology (ART)

Testicular sperm extraction (TESE) in humans involves the removal of sperm from testicular tissue (7,8). TESE is currently performed as a routine procedure for infertile males with presumed hypospermatogenesis (cryptozoospermia, secretory azoospermia). TESE can only lead to pregnancy through the micromanipulation of gametes (9,10) and intracytoplasmic oocyte sperm injection (ICSI). There is no current place in our experience for the percutaneous sperm aspiration method (11) through this cytological technique.

Obstructive Pathology: Where to Retrieve?

Peroperative biological assessment of sperm in the seminal tract is easy and helpful in cases of obstructive pathology (12,13). The decision to procede with reconstructive surgery can indeed be decided extemporaneously. Appropriate sites for sperm retrieval and bypass operations are determined through macroscopic (ivory-white fluid) and microscopic biological data (motile cells). In fact, a drop of fluid obtained by puncturing the vas deferens, the epididymal tubule, or the vasa efferentia is informative using a simple biological examination with phase contrast light microscope between slide and coverslip. Such a simple procedure provides immediate information on the spermatozoa in terms of count estimation, mobility, and forward motility, but it requires microincisions of the epididymal tubule under an operative microscope when the level of epididymal markers is decreased in the preoperative ejaculate. Multiple microsurgical and biological examinations are required. Spermatozoa without flagella, broken isolated flagella, and amorphous spermatozoa associated with macrophages are located at various levels in the seminal tract upstream to the site of obstruction. Since 1991, we have been able to cryopreserve motile epididymal spermatozoa for both curative and palliative opportunities at the time of reconstructive microsurgery (14). In fact, most sites appropriate for vasoepididymostomy are located proximally to the head of the epididymis.

The question remains as to whether proximal retrieval is necessary in cases of distal epididymal blockage or vasectomy reversal at a location where microsurgical bypass is easy and surgical retrieval of sperm for appropriate cryopreservation may fail (distal vasoepididymostomy, proximal tip of the vas).

Hence, testicular sperm retrieval might provide a new palliative strategy for sperm autoconservation associated with a distal bypass far downstream of the rete testis in selected cases. Testicular sperm retrieval may be planned to occur at the same time as, or prior to, the ICSI procedure. A direct iterative testicular approach does not disturb vasoepididymostomy patency follow-up.

Nonobstructive Pathology: When to Give Up?

Cytological peroperative evaluation allows appropriate assessment and harvesting of male gametes from one or both testes without having to go back and forth between the operating room and the laboratory.

Spermatogenesis can be affected by numerous factors such as fever (15) or drugs (6). Testicular biopsy rarely gives a definitive verdict and may vary with time just as the spermogram does. In some cases, biopsy does yield a diagnosis of irreversible infertility through a complete Sertoli cell-only syndrome or total fibrohyalinosis of the seminiferous tubules; however, meiotic arrest, for example, can be due to a genetic anomaly (asynapsis, premature desynapsis) or to an iatrogenic temporary factor. In these cases, further examinations are necessary, such as caryotype, meiosis analysis, or the fluorescent in situ hybridation (FISH) procedure. Drug-induced anomalies in testicular histology are well known in pharmacotoxicology. Testicular histology assessment is one of the required tests of toxicity before starting clinical experimentation with new therapeutic drugs. Necrozoospermia associated with a decreased level of epididymal markers in ejaculate may require operative testicular sperm retrieval.

This bioclinical management is of particular help in cases of nonobstructive pathology where ART is being considered.

Therapeutic Schedule: Synchronous or Prior to Oocyte Retrieval . . . ?

Testicular biopsy may be scheduled at the same time as, or prior to, oocyte retrieval in the female. Male scrototomy can easily be put off in cases of intercurrent disease as the female is not involved in ovarian stimulation. Unilateral testicular pulp evaluation prior to female stimulation may assess the opportunity for ovarian stimulation procedure.

As we lack the biological data comparing results in quality of the conceptus between frozen–thawed and fresh testicular sperm, it seems imperative to collect as much cytological and histological information as possible through a very short peripheral and gentle testicular biopsy.

Conclusion

We have described a simple rapid method for cytological evaluation of spermatogenesis, which can be performed in the operating room. This bioclinical approach to nonobstructive infertility is particularly useful when ART is being considered, and when operative sperm retrieval is planned for ICSI at the same time as, or previous to, oocyte retrieval. The technique needs further study to allow discussion between research groups and correlation with the TESE strategy, as testicular tissue may not benefit from inadequate scattering iterative pulp extraction.

References

1. Magis MS, Cash KL, Goldstein M. The testicular biopsy in the evaluation of infertility. Semin Urol 1990;8:51–64.
2. Rowley MJ, Heller CG. The testicular biopsy: surgical procedure, fixation, and staining techniques. Fertil Steril 1966;17:177–86.
3. Lamb JC, IV, Chapin RE. Experimental models of male reproductive toxicology. In: Thomas JA, Korach KS, McLachlan JA, editors. Endocrine toxicology. New York: Raven Press, 1985:85–115.
4. Mallidis C, Volpe V, Ostor A, Lopata A, Baker HWG. Fixation and staining of testicular tissue. J Histotechnol 1994;17:111–14.
5. Holstein AF, Eckmann C. Multinucleated spermatocytes and spermatids in human seminiferous tubules. Andrologia 1986;18:5–16.
6. Gomes WR. Chemical agents affecting testicular function and male fertility. In: Johnson AD, Gomes WR, Van de Mark NL, editors. The testis. III. Influencing factors. New York: Academic Press, 1970:483–545.
7. Craft I, Bennett V, Nicholson N. Fertilising ability of testicular spermatozoa. Lancet 1993;342:864.
8. Silber SJ, Devroey P, Tournaye H, Van Steirteghem AC. Fertilizing capacity of epididymal and testicular sperm using intracytoplasmic sperm injection (ICSI). Reprod Fertil Dev 1995;7:281–93.
9. Schoysman R, Vandezwalmen P, Nijs M, et al. Pregnancy after fertilization with human testicular spermatozoa. Lancet 1993;342:1237.
10. Devroey P, Liu J, Nagy Z, et al. Pregnancies after testicular sperm extraction and cytoplasmic sperm injection in non-obstructive azoospermia. Hum Reprod 1995;10:1457–60.
11. Bourne H, Watkins W, Speirs A, Baker HWG. Pregnancies after intracytoplasmic injection of sperm collected by fine needle biopsy of the testis. Fertil Steril 1995;64:433–36.
12. Jardin A, Izard V, Jouannet P, Benoît G. Fécondation in vitro et infertilité masculine. Aspects techniques. Indications. Treizièmes séminaires d'uro-néphrologie. Paris: Masson, 1987:27–35.
13. Jardin A, Izard V, Benoît G, Testart J, Belaisch-Allart J, Volante M, et al. Fécondance in vivo et in vitro de spermatozoïdes épididymaires humains immatures. Reprod Nutr Dev 1988;28:375–85.
14. Izard V, Vogt B, Jardin A. Epididymal microsurgery. Technique and results. In: Epididymis: role and importance in male infertility treatment, Frontiers in endocrinology, Vol. XI. Rome: Ares-Serono Symposia Series, 1995:245–58.
15. Van De Mark NL, Free MJ. Temperature effects. In: Johnson AD, Gomes WR, Van de Mark NL, editors. The testis. III. Influencing factors. New York: Academic Press, 1970:233–312.

Part VI

Conceptus Quality in ICSI with Testicular Sperm and Ethical Problems of ART

Part VI

Conceptus Quality in ICSI with Testicular Sperm and Ethical Problems of ART

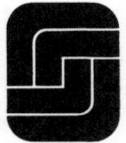

24

Genetic Aspects of Male Sterility

PETER H. VOGT

Introduction

The complex cell differentiation process of the male germ cell, spermatogenesis, is a typical example of a regulative biological network based on the interaction of multiple genes, respectively, the interactions of their expression products (RNAs, proteins). This process starts between days 21 and 26 postconception [i.e., in early embryogenesis (1)], and produces the first wave of motile spermatozoa at puberty. Genetic networks are generally nested one inside the other, building up a complex interactive and open system. Thus, the process of spermatogenesis is nested in the process of development of the male gonad. The process of male gonad development is nested in the process of embryo development. As a consequence, male sterility, as a secondary effect, is also caused by the disruption of genes functioning in the development of the male gonad and by disruption of genes functioning in somatic tissues ("pleiotropic male sterility").

From mutation analysis in Drosophila, genes expressed for male fertility were estimated to range from between 1250 and 1750 (2). In men, it is not known how many genes are essential for the male germ line. Because many genes transcribed in the testis do not have a biological function (3), it is difficult to assign a functional role to a certain gene only by analyzing its transcriptional activity in the testis. In order to identify a functional spermatogenic gene, gene-specific mutations are needed that induce disruption of human spermatogenesis. In human genetics, however, this can become a lengthy and cumbersome task unless the gene to be analyzed has a high mutation rate. Before the patients carrying such mutations are diagnosed, therefore, animal models carrying these mutations, such as "transgenic" or "knock-out" mice, are frequently used and analyzed for their fertility and testis histology. Such studies contribute significantly to our knowledge of the specific spermatogenic defects induced by disruption of the genes expressed in the testis. They also show that the genetic control of human spermatogenesis is a complex regulative network.

This chapter presents a short overview of our current knowledge on the genetic aspects of male sterility. This overview, however, is by no means complete. The current rapid expansion of molecular research in the field of reproduction genetics makes it difficult to present a comprehensive review of the topic; therefore, readers engaged in this field who are interested in more detailed information are advised to study other reviews published on the same subject (e.g., Refs. 4,5). Genetic aspects of male sterility can be studied at two levels: the molecular level, by analyzing gene mutations that disrupt spermatogenesis, and the chromosome level, by analyzing chromosome aneuploidies interfering with meiotic cell divisions. Here, asynaptic chromosome pairing events and/or distortion of the sex vesicle formation are the visible diagnostic indications (6).

The Study of Sex-Specific Gene Expression Patterns

With the exception of postmeiotic germ cells, all human cell nuclei contain two gene copies (two alleles). Genes located on the sex chromosomes (X and Y), however, may have a sex-specific expression pattern because a double dose of the X gene is female specific. Men have only one X chromosome and the male-specific Y chromosome. The genes located in the so-called pseudoautosomal regions (PARs) at the tip of both sex chromosomes may be the exceptions. Due to a high rate of crossing over in these X–Y regions, an identical gene structure is expected on both sex chromosomes (7). A high rate of crossing over, however, is not observed in other parts of the sex chromosomes. As a consequence, in cases where both gene copies on the sex chromosomes are functional, the female-specific sex chromosome constitution (X,X) and the male-specific sex chromosome constitution (X,Y) might display a different functional expression pattern. It is now thought that the Y chromosome provides a sanctuary for spermatogenic genes, both in men, as well as in mice, and in Drosophila (2,8–10). There is no other known human chromosome that contains so many genes expressed solely in the human testis. Genes for male fertility on the autosomes and on the sex chromosomes will therefore be discussed in separate sections.

Genes for Male Fertility on the Autosomes

Genes on autosomes expressed in the male germ line can be divided into two main groups: (A) genes expressed only in the human testis; (B) genes expressed in multiple human tissues but with a specific expression pattern in testis tissue.

Genes that are expressed only during the meiotic cell cycle are examples of genes in group A (11). Mutations in the meiotic genes are expected to cause chromosome aneuploidies in postmeiotic germ cells. Protamines and transition-proteins gradually replace the histones in the DNA of postmeiotic spermatid nuclei, which is a prerequisite for its higher compaction in the developing sperm heads. Protamine and transition-protein encoding genes are expressed only in the spermatids (12); therefore, they are group A genes. They are closely linked in different mammalian genomes (13)—in humans on the short arm of chromosome 6 (6p 13.3). It is interesting to note that the major histone gene cluster also resides on the short arm of chromosome 6 (6p 21.1–22.2; Ref. 14). Testicular isoforms of histones have been described in different mammals (15). The testis-specific H1 histone gene (H1t) transcribed only in spermatocytes seems to be regulated by a specific promoter structure (16).

Other group A genes that are important in spermiogenesis are the preproacrosin gene (mapped to 2q13-qter) encoding acrosin, a germ line-specific protease (17) and the Major mitochondrial Capsule Selenoprotein (MCS) gene (mapped to 1q21; Ref. 18). The selenoprotein is important for the maintenance and stabilization of the crescent structure of sperm mitochondria. Rats on a selenium-deficient diet show a sperm motility disorder and disorganization of sperm mitochondria (19). Genes expressed specifically only in the epididymis were isolated by Kirchhoff and co-workers (20).

Group B genes are the cyclin genes that are generally involved in the regulation of the cell cycle. According to Wolgemuth and co-workers they are also functional in spermatogenesis (21). They have been subdivided into different groups (A, B, C, D, E, F, G, H) depending on their time of function. A cyclins are expressed in G2, B cyclins are expressed during mitosis, D cyclins are expressed at G1, and E cyclins are expressed during DNA synthesis. As a result in spermatogenesis, these genes are predominantly expressed during the proliferation and differentiation of spermatogonia and spermatocytes (21).

Other autosomal B genes encode the cAMP response element binding protein (CREB) and the cAMP responsive element modulator (CREM). They are expressed in germ cells and Sertoli cells in a circadian fashion dependent on cAMP signaling induced by the pituitary gonadotropic hormones FSH and LH (22). These hormones are important during sexual maturation of the testis and spermatogenesis; thus, they link the genetic network of male gonad development to that of spermatogenesis. By alternative promoter usage and exon splicing events, different protein products are translated that function as transcription activators or repressors for specific target genes. The complex CREB/CREM expression patterns in the testis suggest that the functional adaptation of their multiple target genes is critical for the proper development of the male germ cell along its whole pathway. The CREM knock-out mouse shows a severe disruption of postmeiotic spermiogenesis. Late spermatids are completely absent (23,24). In men, CREM was mapped to the short arm of chromosome 10 (10p12.1-p11.2; Ref. 25).

Spermatogenic disruptions by mutations in the autosomal genes of group A (i.e., functioning only in the germ line) are difficult to detect because the genotypical haploid spermatids seem to be phenotypically diploid (26). This means only dominant gene mutations can be recognized phenotypically.

Autosomal germline genes of group B also function in somatic tissues, where disruption of spermatogenesis occurs as a pleiotropic effect (e.g., the immotile cilia syndome, also called Kartagener syndrome) (27). Spermatozoa of men with Kartagener syndrome (KS patients) are usually immobile like the cilia in their respiratory tract ("motility disorder"). The complete absence of dynein arms could be demonstrated as a causative agent. The arms form temporary cross-links between adjacent ciliary filaments and are believed to be responsible for generating movement in cilia and sperm tails. These ultrastructural defects in KS patients are variable (28), however, and there are known patients with the phenotype of Kartagener syndrome in their somatic cells whose sperm motility is not affected (29). Pedigree analysis suggests an autosomal recessive inheritance pattern for KS, but X-linked and autosomal dominant inheritance patterns exist as well (30). This points to the possibility that Kartagener syndrome can be induced by mutations in multiple genes.

An autosomal gene with a distinct dominant inheritance pattern in its pathology is the Dystrophica Myotonica (DM) gene on the short arm of chromosome 17 (31); however, the phenotypical penetrance of this pathology and its influence on male fertility is variable. A high mutation rate in Caucasian populations (1:25; i.e. 4%) and a distinct influence on male fertility have been observed for the Cystic Fibrosis Transmembrane conductance regulator (CFTR) gene on the long arm of chromosome 7 (32). The CFTR gene encodes a protein that functions as a transmembrane channel for chloride ions (33). CFTR mutations manifest as a dysfunction of the pancreas and result in the individual being more prone to infections of the respiratory tract, frequently inducing cystic fibrosis (CF) in somatic cells and congenital bilateral aplasia of the vas deferens (CBAVD) in the male gonads (34). CBAVD is diagnosed in 1.5% of all cases of male sterility. In addition, men with idiopathic obstructive azoospermia and no CF phenotype have an increased rate of CFTR mutations (35). Most frequent is the 5T allele in the 3′splicing region of CFTR intron 8 (36). Three T alleles (5T, 7T, 9T) were found in this region. The reduction in the number of Ts results in reduction of the efficiency of splicing exon 9 in CFTR mRNA. In the presence of the 5T allele, only 10–40% of CFTR mRNA contains exon 9. Men with CBAVD have the 5T allele with a high frequency (84%). Compound heterozygotes of CBAVD (patients with a 5T allele in one gene copy and an R117H mutation in exon 4 of the second gene copy) also have a severe CF phenotype. The severity of the somatic disease is variable and depends on the specific CFTR genotype (Fig. 24.1). This points to cell-type specific quantitative levels for CFTR mRNA and protein in different tissues that are essential for tissue-specific CFTR function.

Gene loci with a specific expression pattern during male gonad development which causes sterility as a secondary effect are listed in Table 24.1. Intersexual phenotypes, in addition to the complete female and male phenotypes with a large variation of expression, are best known from the androgen resistance syndromes; however, all of them are sterile. Their pathology is based on mutations in the androgen receptor gene (AR). Most point mutations causing these syndromes are clustered in the hormone-binding domain (37). AR mutations specifically found

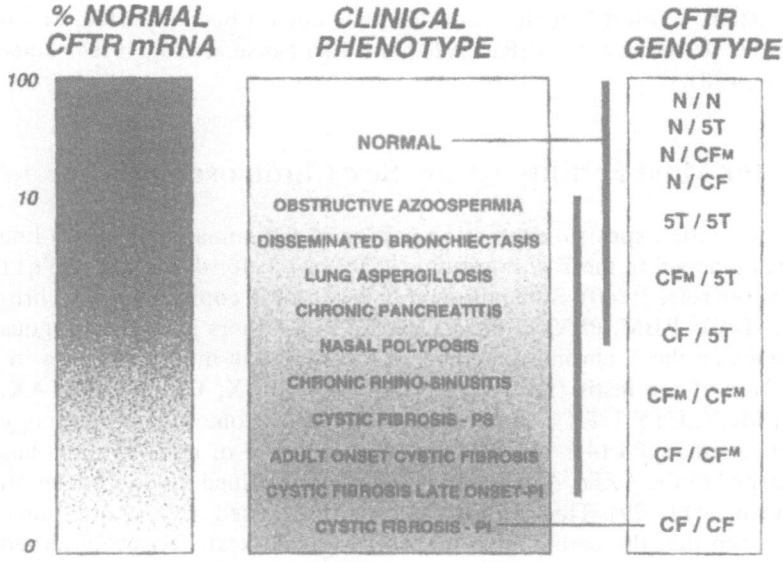

FIGURE 24.1. Different levels of CFTR mRNA produce a wide range of clinical phenotypes, depending on the CFTR genotype. As an example, the 5T allele is presented combined in different mutant genotypes (CF/5T; CF^M/5T; 5T/5T; N/5T). Only the most severe mutations (CF/CF) give rise to the classic cystic fibrosis (CF) phenotype (CF^M: different CF mutations; N: normal CFTR gene; reproduced with permission from Ref 66).

TABLE 24.1. Gene loci involved in male gonad development.

Gene locus	Chromosomal position	Clinical syndrome	MIM reference number
AMH	19p13.3-p13.2	AMH-resistance I (PMDS I)	261550
AMHR	12q13	AMH-resistance II (PMDS II)	261550
AR	Xq12	Androgen resistance (Testicular Feminization, Reifenstein, Infertile Male)	300068
CYP19	15q21.1	Aromatase deficiency	107910
DAX1	Xp21	DSS (Dosage Sensitive Sex)	300200
FGDY	Xp11.21	Aarskog-Scott Syndrome	305400
KAL-1	Xp22.3	Kallmann Syndrome 1	308700
NS1	12q22-qter	Noonan Syndrome	163950
SF1	9q33	Corticol steroid deficiency	184757
SOX9	17q24.3-q25.1	Campomelic dysplasia	211970
SRD5A2	2p23	Male pseudohermaphroditism	264600
WT1	11p	Wilms tumor Denys-Drash Syndrome	194080
XH2	Xq13	Alpha-Thalassemia, (ATRX) Mental-Retardation (X-linked)	301040

*See MIM: Mendelian Inheritance in Man (http://www3.ucbi.ulm.nih.gov/Omim/) for detailed description.

in Reifenstein or infertile male syndrome have not yet been reported. Mutations in the 5α-reductase 2 (SRD5A2) gene also cause androgen resistance syndromes (38).

Genes for Male Fertility on the Sex Chromosomes

Most genes with a specific expression pattern in the human male germ line have been mapped to the Y chromosome (Table 24.2; for definition of Yq11 intervals, see refs. 39,40). Some of them have multiple copies on the Y chromosome (DAZ, RBM, PRY, TSPY, TTY1, TTY2). Others have homologous gene copies on the X chromosome and are expressed in multiple tissues including that of the testis (DBY/DBX; DFFRY/DFFRX; EIF1AY/EIF1AX; SMCY/SMCX; UTY/UTX). One of them (DAZ) has a homologous gene copy on chromosome 3p24 (41–44). The genomic structure of most of them has been mapped to the AZFa, AZFb, and AZFc region defined by microdeletion mapping in Yq11 (39). This is intriguing and has raised several questions. Does it mean that the pathological phenotype in the testis tissue observed after deletion of one of the AZF regions will be created only after deletion of all Y genes mapped to this AZF region? Can the same phenotype be induced by mutation of one or more Y genes in this AZF region, and, if it is induced by more than one Y gene, are they expressed independently or in a functional interaction?

It is safe to assume that at least one functional Y spermatogenic gene must be present in each AZF region. However, this functional Y gene still has to be identified. Any of the Y genes mapped to them and listed in Table 24.2, therefore, are only spermatogenic "candidate genes." One possibility for approving a candidate gene as a functional spermatogenic gene is to identify gene-specific mutations in patients with a specific spermatogenic disorder diagnosed as "idiopathic" by the infertility clinic. This disorder need not necessarily be the same as that observed after deletion of the whole corresponding AZF region. A second possibility is to isolate the homologous mouse gene and, by experimentally inducing its deletion in embryonic stem cells ('knock-out' mouse), cross mice strains with these knockout genes in the heterozygous and homozygous state to study their fertility.

The Y-specific genes in AZFb (RBM/TSPY) and in AZFc (BPY2/DAZ/PRY/TTY2) have been described as multicopy genes (10,40). This makes it difficult to perform an exon-specific mutation analysis using, for example, the SSCP method because each exon is repetitive and single exon mutations can be hidden behind an apparently "normal SSCP pattern." Functional analyses of the TSPY, RBM and DAZ gene families were therefore recently transposed to the protein level (45–47). RBM and DAZ genes encode testis-specific RNA binding proteins. RBM proteins are mostly present in the nuclei of premeiotic germ cells (46), which suggests their involvement in the nuclear metabolism of newly synthesized testis RNA at this phase of human sper-

TABLE 24.2. Human Y candidate spermatogenesis genes.

Gene symbol	Gene name	Protein homolog to	Tissue expression	Yp interv.	Yq11 interv.	X chrom. homol.	Autosome homolog
BPY1	Basic protein Y, pl 9	Novel	Only testis	No	D8	No	
BPY2	Basic protein Y, pl 10	Novel	Only tesis	No	AZFc	No	
CDY	Chromo domain Y	Chromatin package protein	Only testis	No	D10–11; 23–24	No	
DAZ	Deleted in azoospermia	RNA binding RRM proteins	Only testis	No	AZFc	No	3p24; DAZL1
DBY	DEAD box Y	RNA helicases	Multiple	No	AZFa	Yes; DBX	
DFFRY	Drosophila fat facets related Y	Ubiquitin-specific proteases	Multiple	No	AZFa	Yes; DFFRX	
EIF1AY	Essential initiation-translation factor 1AY	Translation initiation factor	Multiple	No	AZFb	Yes; EIF1AX	
PRY	PTP-BL related Y	Protein tyrosin phosphatase	Only testis	Prox. Yp11	AZFc	No	
RBM	RNA binding motif	RNA binding RRM-proteins	Only testis	Prox. Yp11	AZFb; AZFc	No	
SMCY	Selected mouse C DNA Y	H–Y antigen HLA B7	Multiple	No	AZFb	Yes; SMCX	
TSPY	Testis-specific protein Y encoded	SET/NAP-1 regul. cell proliferation	Only testis	Prox. Yp11	AZFb	No	
TTY1	Testis transcript Y1	No-protein encod. RNA	Only testis	Prox. Yp11	AZFc	No	
TTY2	Testis transcript Y2	No-protein encod. RNA	Only testis	Prox. Yp11	AZFc	No	
UTY	Ubiquitous transcribed Y	H–Y antigen HYD[b]	Multiple	No	AFZa	Yes; UTK	
XKRY	XK related Y	Putative membrane transport protein	Only testis	No	D10–11	No	

matogenesis. After deletion of AZFb, these proteins are absent. Most functional RBM gene copies, therefore, must be located in the Y region designated as AZFb. It is not known how many RBM gene copies are functional in AZFb because deletion of one RBM gene in AZFb has not yet been diagnosed. In mice, deletion of all RBM genes, apart from one or two copies on the proximal part of the short Y arm, does not seem to reduce their fertility, although an increase in the number of dysmorphic sperms is observed (48). If the same is true for men, then partial RBM gene deletions will not be found in our azoospermic patient collective.

DAZ proteins seem to be predominantly present in the cytoplasm of late spermatids and in sperm tails (47). They might be functional, therefore, in the translational control of mRNAs in these germ cells. Another possibility may be a structural role in the formation of the complex tail structure. In patients with deletion of AZFc, DAZ proteins are absent from the sperm tails, which suggests that most functional DAZ gene copies are clustered in AZFc. AZFc deletions, however, do not have a distinct pathological phenotype, as do AZFa and AZFb deletions (39). The testis histology of this patient class does not show spermatid arrest as expected, assuming that DAZ proteins function as translational control proteins in late spermatids. Moreover, DAZ deletions do not interfere with the production of mature spermatozoa, although there is a reduction in numbers. This suggests that DAZ proteins are not essential for the terminal differentiation of the human germ cell but are required for optimal function. A similar mutation effect has been described for the POU protein sperm-1 in mouse spermatogenesis (49). AZFc deletions therefore cause subfertility but not azoospermia as their primary mutation effect.

The DAZ homologue on chromosome 3 is highly conserved from Drosophila to man and is now designated as DAZL1 (44). In contrast to this, DAZ genes on the Y chromosome were created first during primate evolution (40, 42). In mice, it has been shown that Dazl1 proteins are predominantly present in spermatogonia and spermatocytes (50). Homozygous deletion of the Dazl1 gene results in a premeiotic disruption of spermatogenesis. There is no reason to assume that the homologous human DAZL1 protein has a different function in human spermatogenesis (89% identity of both proteins along their total lengths). If this holds true, then it is expected that the DAZ genes on the Y chromosome, although homologous to DAZL1, have changed their functional expression pattern because their deletion can be inherited. Further arguments for this are the differences between DAZ and DAZL1 proteins in their C-termini (47). Exon 8 in the DAZ gene is reduced in comparison with the homologous DAZL1 exon 8 by 11 nucleotides and DAZL1 exon 9 is integrated in DAZ intron 8 by deletion of its splicing signals. Different C-terminal peptides (encoded from exon 8 on downstream) in length and sequence are the result.

DAZL1 Peptide

MPPQWPVGEQRSYVVPPAYSAVNYHCNEVDPGAEVVPNECSVHEAT
PPSGNGPQKKSVDRSIQTVVSCLFNPENRLRNSVVTQDDYFKDKRVHHF
RRSRAMLKSV

DAZ Peptide
MPPQCPVGEQRRNLWTEAYKWWYLVCLIQRRD

RBM and TSPY gene copies seem to be interspersed in AZFb and on the short arm of the Y chromosome, although most TSPY genes are in Yp and most RBM genes in AZFb (51). TSPY proteins have been found to be expressed mainly in spermatogonia (45), and it cannot be excluded that their deletion in AZFb contributes to the pathological AZFb phenotype. Like the RBM gene family, however, the TSPY gene family also contains pseudogenes. It is not yet known how many functional TSPY genes are present in Yp and AZFb, respectively.

The dispersed pattern of gene copies of the three other Y-specific genes (PRY, TTY1, TTY2) in Yp and in Yq11 (Table 24.2) resembles that of the RBM and TSPY genes. This suggests a common evolutionary origin. All of them have been found to be expressed exclusively in testis tissue; however, their functional state in human spermatogenesis is not yet known.

Most intriguing is the presence of Y genes in AZFa and AZFb with homologous gene copies on the X chromosome (Table 24.2). RNA blot analysis suggests a multiple tissue expression of all of them (10). Additional testis-specific RNA populations could only be detected for the DBY and EIF1AY genes. Some X–Y genes encode proteins presumed to be involved in the production of male-specific antigens of the H–Y class (UTY in AZFa, SMCY in AZFb). The expression of H–Y antigens in mouse preimplantation embryos (52) suggests that these proteins are early embryonic male cell markers leading, perhaps, to the higher proliferation rate of male cells or to the induction of the male germ line, and/or repression of the female germ line, respectively (53).

To date, there is no pathological phenotype known for the Y genes transcribed in testis tissue but located outside the AZFa,b,c regions (BPY1, CDY, XKRY in Yq11; TTY1, TSPY, ZFY in Yp). This might suggest that their mutation rate is low or that their transcriptional activity is not essential in human spermatogenesis, as discussed earlier for the DAZ genes and perhaps all other AZFc genes (BPY2, PRY, TTY2) in distal Yq11.

Chromosome Constitution in the Male Germ Line Interfering with Male Fertility

The first association of a spermatogenic disorder (azoospermia) with a specific chromosome aneuploidy was recognized in men with the syndrome of Klinefelter (47,XXY). Among sterile men with chromosome aberrations, the karyotype 47,XXY is now known to be the most frequent (54), but it is still not known why this chromosome constitution induces the observed sterile phenotypes. For male gonad development, the balance of sex chromosomes (X and Y) seems to be crucial. Men with increasing numbers of X chromosomes in their karyotype (48,XXXY; 49,XXXXY) shift their sexual phenotype to the female site. Penis development is reduced and cryptorchidism is

found in many cases. Men with Klinefelter syndrome also have disproportionate growth of their legs and achieve consistently low scores in their verbal IQ (55). This suggests that sex chromosome aneuploidies also influence
male gonad and male brain development in early embryogenesis. Men with
azoospermia and a 46,XX karyotype are found less frequently (1:20,000 newborns). In most cases, part of the short arm of the Y chromosome including the
sex-determining SRY (Sex Region Y) gene is translocated to the short arm tip
of one of their X chromosomes. In most cases, therefore, their sex and gonad
development seems to be normal. Cryptorchidism, micropenis, and hypospa-
dia are only observed if the Y breakpoint is in the neighborhood of the SRY
gene in distal Yp (20% of all cases; Ref. 56). This breakpoint, however, is
mostly in proximal Yp in the gene structure of the PRKY (Protein Kinase Y)
gene (57). Despite the location of the PRKY gene outside the PAR region, its
gene structure is highly homologous to its X chromosomal gene copy PRKX
in Xp22.3.

Men with azoospermia and the karyotype 45,X are also known, but this
occurs only rarely. They have an unbalanced karyotype because the distal
part of the long Y arm is lost. The other part of the Y chromosome including
the SRY gene locus is translocated to an autosome (most frequently to the
short arm of one of the acrocentric chromosomes 13, 15, or 22). The Y
breakpoint is in the proximal part of the long Y arm (for review, see Ref. 9).

Autosome aneuploidies, like trisomies of chromosome 21 (Down's syndrome), seem to have individual effects on male fertility. Both infertile and
fertile men have been found with this chromosome constitution (58,59). It is
assumed that the extra chromosome 21 interferes with a normal pairing structure of this autosome during formation of its synaptonemal complex before
meiosis. Partial trisomies or monosomies of the short arm of chromosomes 3
and 9 (60,61) and of the long arm of chromosomes 13 and 10 (62,63) have
been found to be associated with sex reversal and gonad dysgenesis and, as a
result, a distortion of spermatogenesis. In 60% of all cases, a Robertsonian
translocation was found between two acrocentric chromosomes: 13 and 14;
however, (13,14)-translocations are found in fertile couples as well and sometimes in the same pedigree (64).

Even now there are only hypotheses to explain the variable expression of
chromosomally based male sterility factors. It can be assumed that such chromosome mutations are counterselected in a manner specifically oriented to
the individual by the meiotic segregation mechanisms. As a result, men with
autosomal chromosome anomalies in diploid lymphocytes (usually analyzed)
are expected to have variable karyotypes in their postmeiotic germ cells
(germ-cell mosaics). In sterile men with a diagnosed chromosome anomaly in
lymphocytes, the frequency of chromosomally unbalanced sperms seems
to be generally increased (65). To evaluate which chromosome constitutions
in man are essential for spermatogenesis, therefore, routine analyses of
meiotic chromosomes in their testis biopsies should perhaps be an essential
prerequisite.

References

1. Witschi E. Migration of the germ cells of human embryos from the yolk sac to the primitive gonadal folds. Contrib Embryol 1948;209:67–80.
2. Lindsley DL, Tokuyasu KT. Spermatogenesis. In: Ashburner M, Wright TRF, editors. The genetics and biology of drosophila, Vol. 2. London: Academic Press, 1980:225–94.
3. Willison K, Ashworth A. Mammalian spermatogenic gene expression. Trends Genet 1987;3:351–55.
4. Fauser BCJM, Hsueh AJ. Genetic basis of human reproductive endocrine disorders. Hum Reprod 1995;10:826–46.
5. Mak V, Jarvi KA. The genetics of male infertility. J Urol 1996;156:1245–57.
6. Chaganti RS, Jhanwar SC, Ehrenbard LT, Kourides IA, Williams JJ. Genetically determined asynapsis, spermatogenic degeneration and infertility in men. Am J Hum Genet 1980;32:833–48.
7. Rappold GA. Pseudoautosomal regions at the tip of the short and long arms of the human sex chromosomes. Adv Genome Biol 1996;4:205–28.
8. Burgoyne PS. Y chromosome function in mammalian development. Adv Dev Biol 1991;1:1–29.
9. Vogt PH. Human Y chromosome function in male germ cell development. Adv Dev Biol 1996;4:191–257.
10. Lahn BT, Page DC. Functional coherence of the human Y chromosome. Science 1997;278:675–79.
11. Page AW, Orr-Weaver TL. Stopping and starting the meiotic cell cycle. Genet Dev 1997;7:23–31.
12. Hecht NB. Regulation of "haploid expressed genes" in male germ cells. J Reprod Fertil 1990;88:679–93.
13. Engel W, Keime S, Kremling H, Hameister H, Schluter G. The genes for protamine 1 and 2 (PRM1 and PRM2) and transition protein 2 (TNP2) are closely linked in the mammalian genome. Cytogenet Cell Genet 1992;61:158–59.
14. Albig W, Darbent B, Kunz J, Kalff-Suske M, Grzeschik KH, Doenecke D. All known human H1 histone genes except the H1(0) gene are clustered on chromosome 6. Genomics 1993;16:649–54.
15. Doenecke D, Albig W, Bode C, et al. Histones: genetic diversity and tissue-specific gene expression. Histochem Cell Biol 1997;107:1–10.
16. Grimes SR, Jr, van Wert J, Wolfe SA. Regulation of transcription of the testis-specific histone H1t gene by multiple promoter elements. Mol Biol Reprod 1997;24:175–84.
17. Adham IM, Grzeschik KH, Guerts van Kessel AH, Engel W. The gene encoding the human preproacrosin (ACR) maps to the q13-qter region on chromosome 22. Hum Genet 1989;84:59–62.
18. Aho H, Schwemmer M, Tessman D, et al. Isolation, expression, and chromosomal localization of the human mitochondrial capsule selenoprotein gene (MCSP). Genomics 1996;32:184–90.
19. Wu AS, Oldfield J, Shull LR, Cheeke PR. Specific effect of selenium deficiency on rat sperm. Biol Reprod 1979;20:793–98.
20. Krull N, Ivell R, Osterhoff C, Kirchhoff C. Region-specific variation of gene expression in the human epididymis as revealed by in situ hybridization with tissue-specific cDNAs. Mol Reprod Dev 1993;34:16–24.
21. Wolgemuth DJ, Rhee K, Wu S, Ravnik SE. Genetic control of mitosis, meiosis and

cellular differentiation during mammalian spermatogenesis. Reprod Fertil Dev 1995;7:669–83.

22. Walker WH, Habener JF. Role of transcription factors CREB and CREM in cAMP-regulated transcription during spermatogenesis. Trends Endocrinol Metab 1996;7:133–38.

23. Nantel F, Monaco L, Foulkes NS, et al. Spermiogenesis deficiency and germ-cell apoptosis in CREM-mutant mice. Nature 1996;380:159–62.

24. Blendy JA, Kaestner KH, Weinbauer GF, Nieschlag E, Schütz G. Severe impairment of spermatogenesis in mice lacking the CREM gene. Nature 1996;380: 162–65.

25. Masquilier D, Foulkes NS, Mattei MG, Sassone-Corsi P. Human CREM gene: evolutionary conservation, chromosomal localization, and inducibility of the transcript. Cell Growth Differ 1993;4:931–37.

26. Braun RE, Behringer RR, Peschon JJ, Brinster RL, Palmiter RD. Genotypically haploid spermatids are phenotypically diploid. Nature 1989;337:373–76.

27. Rott HD. Kartagener's syndrome and the syndrome of immotile cilia. Hum Genet 1979;46:249–61.

28. Afzelius BA, Mossberg B. Immotile-cilia syndrome (primary ciliary dyskinesia), including Kartagener syndrome. In: Scriver CR, Beaudet AL, Sly WS, Valle D, editors. The metabolic and molecular bases of inherited disease. New York: McGraw-Hill, 1995:3943–54.

29. Samuel I. Kartagener's syndrome with normal spermatozoa (letter). J Am Med Assoc 1987;258:1329–30.

30. Narayan D, Krishnan SN, Upender M, et al. Unusual inheritance of primary ciliary dyskinesia (Kartagener's syndrome). J Med Genet 1994;31:493–96.

31. Harper PS. Myotoic dystrophy and other autosomal muscular dystrophies. In: Scriver CR, Beaudet AL, Sly WS, et al., editors. The metabolic and molecular bases of inherited disease. New York: McGraw-Hill, 1995:4227–51.

32. Welsh MJ, Tsui LC, Boat TF, Beaudet AL. Cystic fibrosis. In: Scriver CR, Beaudet AL, Sly WS, et al., editors. The metabolic and molecular bases of inherited disease. New York: McGraw-Hill, 1995:3799–873.

33. Riordan JR, Rommens JM, Kerem B, et al. Identification of the cystic fibrosis gene: cloning and characterization of complementary DNA. Science 1989;245:1066–73.

34. Oates RD, Amos JA. The genetic basis of congenital bilateral absence of the vas deferens and cystic fibrosis. J Androl 1994;15:1–8.

35. Jarvi K, Zielenski J, Wilschanski M, et al. Cystic fibrosis: transmembrane conductance regulator and obstructive azoospermia. Lancet 1995;345:1578.

36. Zielenski J, Patrizio P, Corey M, et al. CFTR gene variant for patients with congenital absence of vas deferens. Am J Hum Genet 1995;57:958–60.

37. Quigley CA, De Bellis A, Marschke KB, el-Awady MK, Wilson EM, French FS. Androgen receptor defects: historical, clinical, and molecular perspectives. Endocr Rev 1995;16:271–321.

38. Griffin JE, McPhaul MJ, Russel DW, Wilson JD. The androgen resistance syndromes: steroid 5a-reductase 2 deficiency, testicular feminization, and related disorders. In: Scriver CR, Beaudet AL, Sly WS, et al., editors. The metabolic and molecular bases of inherited disease. New York: McGraw-Hill, 1995:2967–98.

39. Vogt PH, Edelmann A, Kirsch S, et al. Human Y chromosome azoospermia factors (AZF) mapped to different subregions in Yq11. Hum Mol Genet 1996;5:933–43.

40. Vogt PH, Affara N, Davey P, et al. Report of the third international workshop on Y chromosome mapping 1997. Cytogenet Cell Genet (in press).

41. Saxena R, Brown LG, Hawkins T, et al. The DAZ gene cluster on the human Y chromosome arose from an autosomal gene that was transposed, repeatedly amplified and pruned. Nat Genet 1996;14:292–9.
42. Shan Z, Hirschmann P, Seebacher T, et al. A SPGY copy homologous to the mouse gene Dazla and the Drosophila gene boule is autosomal and expressed only in the human male gonad. Hum Mol Genet 1996;5:2005–11.
43. Yen PH, Chai NN, Salido EC. The human autosomal gene DAZLA: testis specificity and a candidate for male infertility. Hum Mol Genet 1996;12:2012–17.
44. Seboun E, Barbaux S, Bourgeron T, et al. Gene sequence, localization, and evolutionary conservation of DAZLA, a candidate male sterility gene. Genomics 1997;41:227–35.
45. Schnieders F, Dörk T, Arnemann J, Vogel T, Werner M, Schmidtke J. Testis-specific protein, Y-encoded (TSPY) expression in testicular tissues. Hum Mol Genet 1996;5:1801–7.
46. Elliott DJ, Millar MR, Oghene K, et al. Expression of RBM in the nuclei of human germ cells is dependent on a critical region of the Y chromosome long arm. Proc Natl Acad Sci USA 1997;94:3848–53.
47. Habermann B, Mi HF, Edelmann A, Bohring C. DAZ (Deleted in AZoospermia) genes encode proteins located in human late spermatids and in sperm tails. Hum Reprod 1998;13:363.
48. Mahadeviah SK, Odorisio T, Szot M, Laval SH, Cattanach BM, Burgoyne PS. Deletion of the majority of copies of the mouse Rbm gene family is associated with abnormal sperm development. In: Vogt PH, et al., editors. Report of the Third International Workshop on Y Chromosome Mapping, Heidelberg, 1997. Cytogenet Cell Genet (in press).
49. Pearse RV, II, Drolet DW, Kalla KA, Hooshmand F, Bermingham JR, Jr, Rosenfeld MG. Reduced fertility in mice deficient for the POU protein sperm-1. Proc Natl Acad Sci USA 1997;94:7555–60.
50. Ruggiu M, Speed R, Taggart M, et al. The mouse Dazla gene encodes a cytoplasmic protein essential for gametogenesis. Nature 1997;389:73–77.
51. Gläser B, Hierl T, Taylor K, et al. High-resolution fluorescence in situ hybridization of human Y-linked genes on released chromatin. Chromosome Res 1997;5:23–30.
52. Krco C, Goldberg EH. H-Y (male) antigen: detection on eight-cell mouse embryos. Science 1976;193:1134–35.
53. Mittwoch U. Sex differentiation in mammals and tempo of growth: probabilities vs. switches. J Theor Biol 1989;137:445–55.
54. Paulsen CA, Plymate SR. Klinefelter's syndrome. In: King RA, Rotter JI, Motulsky AG, editors. The genetic basis of common diseases. Oxford monographs on medical genetics, No. 20. New York: Oxford University Press, 1992:876–94.
55. Rovet J, Netley C, Bailey J, Keenan M, Stewart D. Intelligence and achievement in children with extra X aneuploidy: a longitudinal perspective. Am J Med Genet 1995;60:356–63.
56. Boucekkine C, Toublanc JE, Abbas N, et al. Clinical and anatomical spectrum in XX sex reversed patients. Relationship to the presence of Y specific DNA-sequences. Clin Endocrinol 1994;40:733–42.
57. Schiebel K, Winkelmann M, Mertz A, et al. Abnormal XY interchange between a novel isolated protein kinase gene, PRKY, and its homologue, PRKX, accounts for one third of all (Y+)XX males and (Y-)XY females. Hum Mol Genet 1997;6:1985–89.
58. Sheridan R, Llerena J, Jr, Matkins S, Debenham P, Cawood A, Bobrow M. Fertility in a male with trisomy 21. J Med Genet 1989;26:294–98.
59. Zühlke C, Thies U, Braulke I, Reis A, Schirren C. Down syndrome and male

fertility: PCR-derived fingerprinting, serological and andrological investigations. Clin Genet 1994;46:324–26.

60. Fryns JP, Kleczkowksa A, Casaer P, van den Berghe H. Double autosomal chromosomal aberration (3p trisomy/9p monosomy) and sex reversal. Ann Genet 1986;29:49–52.

61. Magenis RE, Allen LJ, Brown MG. 9p monosomy associated with XY gonadal dysgenesis: a contiguous gene syndrome. Am J Hum Genet 1990;47:A33.

62. Jotterand M, Juillard EA. A new case of trisomy for the distal part of 3q due to maternal translocation t(9;13)(p21;q21). Hum Genet 1976;33:213–22.

63. Wilkie AO, Campbell FM, Daubeney P, et al. Complete and partial XY sex reversal associated with terminal deletion of 10q: report of 2 cases and literature review. Am J Med Genet 1993;46:597–600.

64. Koskull VH, Aula P. Inherited (13;14) translocation and reproduction. Hum Genet 1974;24:85–91.

65. Martin RH, Hulten M. Chromosome complements in 695 sperm from three men heterozygous for reciprocal translocations and a review of the literature. Hereditas 1993;118:165–76.

66. Estivill X. Complexity in a monogenic disease. Nat Genet 1996;12:348–50.

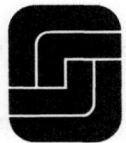

25

Conceptus Quality from ICSI with Testicular Sperm

ANDRE HAZOUT, MARTINE DUMONT-HASSAN, AND PAUL COHEN-BACRIE

Introduction

Since the conception of in vitro fertilization (IVF), it has been gradually accepted that artificial reproductive technology does not imply a higher risk of congenital malformation.

The outcome of intracytoplasmic sperm injection (ICSI) with ejaculate sperm, a more invasive assisted reproductive procedure, has been carefully analysed in a number of prospective and retrospective studies (1–3) which concluded, albeit from a limited number of births, that ICSI does not lead to additional risks when compared with regular IVF.

Concerns have been raised about the risks associated with ICSI using sperm from azoospermic men (4). ICSI was used initially to treat obstructive azoospermia where there was a congenital absence of the vas deferens (CAVD) and sperm were retrieved by microsurgical epididymal sperm aspiration (MESA). It has subsequently been demonstrated that sperm can be obtained from the testis, when none were otherwise available from the epididymis, by testicular sperm aspiration (TESA) and used in successful ICSI (4).

This chapter presents details of 23 pregnancies obtained following ICSI with testicular sperm taken from 15 men with nonobstructive azoospermia and eight men with obstructive azoospermia. In one instance, cryopreserved sperm previously extracted from a patient with obstructive azoospermia were used.

Materials and Methods

Between January 1996 and December 1997, 65 patients were recruited to our ICSI program for azoospermia. All patients underwent detailed physical, biological, and sonographical screening (5).

Testicular sperm samples were successfully retrieved from 72% of our patients, and 11 testicular biopsies were cryopreserved. The mean age of the men investigated was 37 ± 7 years in the obstructive azoospermia group and 36 ± 8 years in the nonobstructive group. Cytological analysis revealed normal karyotypes in all patients. Several ejaculates from each patient were studied before surgical sperm retrieval. In six patients with obstructive azoospermia, previous histologic examination of testicular tissue was performed, whereas only 8 of the 12 patients with nonobstructive azoospemia underwent such an examination. In other patients, the decision to procede with sperm retrieval was determined by the existence of normal anatomy, volume, and consistency of the testis, as well as each patient's hormone profile. Patients with small, soft testes and high levels of FSH were rejected from the study.

Surgical sperm retrieval and preparation was performed as described by Silber and colleagues (4). Any remaining testicular tissue extract was cryopreserved using our standard freezing protocol.

Oocyte Preparation

The mean age of the women was 33 ± 6 years (range, 23–39). Evaluation of follicle stimulating hormone (FSH), leutinizing hormone (LH), oestradiol (E2), and prolactin levels at day 3 of a previous menstrual cycle, was normal in all women recruits.

Ovulation induction and oocyte retrieval were performed using a protocol that included GnRH agonist supression (Decapeptyl 0,1 mg daily by subcutaneous way; Ipsen Biotech Laboratory, France) with urinary or recombinant FSH (Metrodin®, Gonal® F; Serono Laboratories, France) for ovarian stimulation.

ICSI using metaphase II oocytes was performed as described by Nagy et al. (6). Fertilization was assessed 16–18 hours after sperm injection. If two distinct pronuclei were observed, then fertilization was considered to have occurred. Embryos were scored according to the regularity of the blastomeres and the number of anucleate fragments. Cleaved embryos with less than 50% of their volume filled with anucleate fragments were eligible for transfer. Embryo replacement was usually performed approximately 48 hours after the microinjection procedure.

Pregnancy was confirmed by detection of increasing serum levels of hCG 14 days after retrieval of the oocytes. Clinical pregnancy was detected by the observation of a gestational sac by sonography at 7 weeks of pregnancy.

Results

Obstructive Azoospermia

Eight ongoing and achieved pregnancies were obtained: five using testicular sperm gathered from patients with post infectious obstruction of the vas

TABLE 25.1. Results of pregnancies in the obstructive azoospermia group.

	CAVD	Post inf. obstruction
No. of oocytes	19	48
No. of 2 PN	11	27
No. of cleaved embryos	10	25
No. of clinical pregnancies	3 (5)	6 (14)
		(5 with fresh embryos, 1 with cryopreserved embryos, 1 twin pregnancy)
No. of abortions	1	1 (trisomy 18)

deferens and three from patients with congenital absence of the vas deferens with negative cystic fibrosis transmembrane regulation (CFTR) (Table 25.1). Sperm retrieval was straightforward and all surplus spermatozoa were cryopreserved.

The high pregnancy rate (47%) obtained using sperm from three patients with CAVD was due to the excellent ovarian function of their partners, despite the relatively low number of oocytes retrieved (14, 3, and 2 oocytes, respectively). The fertilization and cleavage rates were, respectively, 57% and 52%. Pregnancies resulted from transfer of 3, 2, and 1 embryo, respectively. Twelve weeks after transfer of two embryos to one patient, one abortion occured.

In the group of patients with postinfectious obstructions, fertilization and cleavage rates were 56% and 52%, respectively. One pregnancy was aborted following detection of Trisomy 18 (the same patient became pregnant with two cryopreserved embryos in a subsequent cycle). In both groups of patients, prenatal dignosis was not systematically performed and occurred in three of the nine pregnancies. There were no abnormalities apparent at birth in any of the children.

Nonobstructive Azoospermia

Fifteen ongoing and achieved pregnancies were obtained. Sperm retrieval was straightforward except in one instance where it became necessary to extract 12 pieces of the extruding testicular tissue. Assessment of normal ovarian function and the stimulation protocol for oocyte retrieval were the same as described for obstructive azoospermia.

The results obtained when ICSI was performed in patients with nonobstructive azoospermia are given in Table 25.2. Of the eight pregnancies resulting following intervention in men with so-called normal spermatogenesis, one abortion, one mild abnormality, and one Down syndrome occured. In pregnancies resulting from ICSI with sperm from men with hypospermatogenesis or maturation

TABLE 25.2. Pregnancy characteristics in the nonobstructive azoospermia group.

Characteristics	Normal spermatogenesis	Hypo spermatogenesis	Maturation arrest
Pregnancies	8 (1 twin)	4	3 (1 twin)
Abortions	1 (12 weeks)	0	0
Abnormalities	2 (Down syndrome) (KartagenerΣ)	1 (anencephalia)	1 (anenceph) 1 minor cardiac abnormality
Pathology of pregnancy	0	3 (fetal growth delay: 1 dead)	1 (fetal growth delay: 1 dead)
Normal babies born	6	2	2

arrest, two incidences of anencephaly, one mild cardiac abnormality, and four fetal growth delays, including two deaths, occurred.

For the majority of patients whose fresh sperm was used, two pregnancies were twin pregnancies and the remainder were singleton. Of the twin pregnancies, one terminated in spontaneous delivery at 37 weeks and the other at 36 weeks. One ongoing pregnancy was obtained from cryopreserved embryos, and another pregnancy was obtained with cryopreserved spermatozoa and reached term without any problem.

Details of each stage of ICSI in nonobstructive azoospermia are shown in Table 25.3. Fertilization rates and pregnancy rates were comparable in the three groups (58% and 36%, respectively). The implantation rates were 44%, 36%, and 50%, respectively, in women whose occytes were impregnated with sperm taken from men with "normal" sperm, hypospermatogenesis, and maturation arrest.

Comparisons of embryo quality in obstructive and nonobstructive azoospermia were made, the results of which are shown in Table 25.4. Good quality was defined as four regular blastomeres without granulations and vacuoles and a maximum of 20% of fragmentation; fair embryo was defined

TABLE 25.3. Characteristics and implantation rate in the nonobstructive azoospermia group.

	Normal spermatogenesis	Hypo spermatogenesis	Maturation arrest
No. of metaphase II oocytes	62	30	14
No. of 2 PN	36	15	11
No. of cleaved embryo	34	17	10
No. embryo transferred	24	11	8
Ongoing pregnancies	8	4	3
No. of fetal sacs	10	4	4

TABLE 25.4. Embryo quality in the obstructive and nonobstructive azoospermia groups.

Embryo quality	Obstructive azoospermia	Nonobstructive azoospermia
Good quality	17	18
Fair	15	12
Poor	3	4

as less than 50% of fragments and an odd number of regular blastomere; poor embryos signified more than 50% of fragmentation with irregular and dark blastomeres.

Discussion

When obstructive azoospermia cannot be treated successfully with microsurgery, such as in cases of CAVD, it is clear that ICSI using sperm retrieved from the testes is effective. Patients such as these are considered the best candidates for ICSI because of their theoretically good quality of spermatogenesis. Nevertheless, we must be aware of potential sperm damage occurring in the testes.

In certain of our patients we noted an alteration of spermatic maturation. In these patients it appears that the only obstacle to successful pregnancy is the age and ovarian reserve of the female partner.

If we compare the results from this short series of interventions with those obtained from ICSI using sperm retrieved from spermatozoa obtained from the epididymis or ejaculate, we observed the same fertilization and cleavage rates and similar pregnancy rates (65.6% and 62.2% with fresh and frozen epididymal sperm; 62% with ejaculate sperm, and a pregnancy rate of 35% per transfer; Table 25.5).

The results of our 1996 general program suggest that the use of frozen testicular spermatozoa for ICSI is equally as efficient as fresh spermatozoa, producing a fertilization rate of 56% and six pregnancies from 17 embryos transferred, and one miscarriage and one therapeutic abortion for anencephaly.

Our experience of nonobstructive azoospermia, although limited, is sufficient to conclude that an anatomical exploration of the testis (volume consistency, and endocrinological activity, FSH, Testosterone and Inhibine B levels) should take place before deciding to proceed with surgery and sperm retrieval. Following this approach, and according to the female evaluation, we have found spermatozoa to microinject in more than 60% of our patients.

After sperm recovery, we can conclude, as have others (4), that azoospermia associated with "normal spermatogenesis," hypospermatogenesis, and maturation arrest each produces similar results in terms of fertilization, cleavage, and pregnancy rate.

TABLE 25.5. Overall results of ICSI in our center.

| Overall results of ICSI | Ejaculate sperm | Epididymal sperm | |
		Fresh	Frozen
Cycles	2277	127	86
Injected oocytes	15406	920	630
Fertilization rate	62%	65.6%	62.2%
Transfers	2058	119	82
% clin.preg./transfer	33.4	39.5	36.6

In addition, cryopreservation of testicular sperm is effective. Nevertheless, at 34%, our rate of abortion, even if not statistically significant, is concerning.

ICSI with fresh and cryopreserved testicular spermatozoa in patients with nonobstructive azoospermia gave a pregnancy rate of more than 37%. These patients represent the most extreme cases of male infertility, producing the lowest number of testicular spermatozoa. It was sometimes necessary to search for spermatozoa in testicular tissue for 2 or 3 hours before finding even a few spermatozoa. The success of such a program, also therefore depends upon the patience and the experience of the biologist.

As others have also reported (4), we observed that even in azoospermic men with apparently absent spermatogenesis (diagnosed as "Sertoli cell only syndrome") a tiny focus of sperm production could very frequently still be found somewhere in the testis. An extremely diminished quantity of sperm production in the testes will result in absolute azoospermia in the ejaculate, even though some sperm is being produced.

In this carefully selected group of men suffering from nonobstructive azoospermia, testicular sperm could be cryopreserved, irrespective to the number and the motility of the spermatozoa or the histology of the testicular tissue.

Our data also indicate that freezing of any surplus testicular spermatozoa has to be considered mandatory. Even though Romero and colleagues (7) did not mention any clinical pregnancy when using frozen testicular spermatozoa, Friedler et al. (8) reported 27% clinical pregnancies by transfer.

Are our results in cases of nonobstructive azoospermia alarmist? The relatively high fertilization rates achieved using sperm from men with maturation arrest were rather surprising. This condition appears to be one of a problem affecting meiosis, and carries with it a higher risk of subsequent genetic problems.

Among fifteen pregnancies we observed one Down syndrome, two anencephalia, one minor cardiac abnormality, one Kartagener Σ, one abortion, and four instances of fetal growth delay that ended in two fetal deaths.

Although we cannot come to any definite conclusions due to the limited size of this short series of patients, the children resulting form these pregnancies need to be followed closely. In particular, we noted a high rate of fetal growth delay even in one twin pregnancy; even though our first impressions are pessimistic, we strongly advocate that a further study be performed on a larger cohort of children to confirm or invalidate our findings.

The growing assumption that spermatogenesis is affected by defects in the Y chromosome suggest that it is likely that any male offspring will have the same spermatogenetic defect as their father. Although this condition will be as readily treatable in the offspring as it has been in their fathers, caution is again recommended as we are still largely ignorant of all the genetic and epigenetic problems generated by testicular sperm with maturation arrest or from "sertoli cell only" syndrome.

Acknowledgment. We thank D. Delafontaine for his help and collaboration.

References

1. Palermo G, Joris H, Devroey P, Van Steirteghem AC. Pregnancies after intracytoplasmic injection of single spermatozooan into an oocyte. Lancet 1992;340:17–18.
2. Van Steirteghem AC, Liu J, Joris H, et al. Higher success rate by ICSI than by subzonal insemination. Report of a second series of 300 consecutive treatment cycles. Human Reprod 1993;8:1055–64.
3. Bonduelle M, Legein J, Buysse A, et al. Prospective follow up study of 423 children born after ICSI. Human Reprod 1996;11:1558–64.
4. Silber SJ, Van Steirteghem AC, Nagy Z, Liu J, Tournaye H, Devroey P. Normal pregnancies resulting from testicular sperm extraction and intracytoplasmic sperm injection for azoospermia for maturation arrest. Fertil Steril 1996;66:110–17.
5. Craft I, Tzirigotis M. Simplified recovery, preparation and cryopreservation of testicular spermatozoa. Human Reprod. 1995;10:1623–27.
6. Nagy Z, Liu J, Janssenwillen C, Silber S, Devroey P, Van Steirteghem AC. Using ejaculated, fresh and frozen-thawed epididymal and testicular spermatozoa gives rise to comparable results after intracytoplasmic sperm injection. Fertil Steril 1995,63:808–15.
7. Romero J, Remohi J, Minguez Y, Rubio C, Pellicer A, Gil Salom M. Fertilization after intracytoplasmic sperm injection with cryopreserved testicular spermatozoa. Fertil Steril 1996;65:877–79.
8. Friedler S, Raziel A, Soffer Y, Strassburger D, Komarovsky D, Ron-El R. Intracytoplasmc injection of fresh and cryopreserved testicular spermatozoa in patients with nonobstructive azoospermia—a comparative study. Fertil Steril 1997;68:892–95.

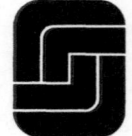

26

Genetic Problems and Congenital Malformations in 1987 ICSI Children

MARYSE BONDUELLE, AYSE AYTOZ, ANN WILIKENS,
ANDREA BUYSSE, ELVIRE VAN ASSCHE, PAUL DEVROEY,
ANDRE VAN STEIRTEGHEM, AND INGE LIEBAERS

Introduction

When assisted fertilization and intracytoplasmic sperm injection (ICSI) were introduced, there was major concern about the safety of the newly introduced technique. Intracytoplasmic sperm injection is indeed a more invasive procedure than routine IVF because one spermatozoon is injected through the oocyte membrane and because fertilization can be obtained from sperm that could never have been used before in fertility treatment. Even more questions arose and concern was again expressed when ICSI with nonejaculated spermatozoa, either epidididymal or testicular, was introduced. Emphasis was put on the fact that because more chromosomal aberrations are found in azoospermic males and more in particular in case of nonobstructive azoospermia, the risk for chromosomal aberrations in the offspring might even be higher. Other heritable genetic causes might also be involved. On the other hand, it was suspected that imprinting may be less complete at the time of fertilization if testicular sperm is used. If this were so, then it would be unlikely to impair fertilization and early development, but anomalies might become manifest at birth or only later in life.

The safety of this novel procedure of assisted fertilization had therefore to be assessed carefully (1–4). In previous publications, we (and other groups) failed to find any increased risk of major congenital malformations as compared with the general population, but we did find an increased risk of chromosomal aberrations, mostly sex-chromosomal aneuploidies (5–11).

In this chapter we will evaluate the safety of the ICSI procedure further by studying data on karyotypes, congenital malformations, growth parameters, and developmental milestones in a larger cohort of 1987 children born after

ICSI. Children born after SUZI or SUZI together with ICSI are no longer included in this series, although they were included in our first study of 55 children (5).

Materials and Methods

From April 1991 onward, 2375 pregnancies, leading to the birth of 1987 children before September 1997, were studied. The follow up of this cohort of children was carried out by the Centre for Medical Genetics in collaboration with the Centre for Reproductive Medicine. Part of this cohort has already been described in previous articles (5–10).

Before starting ICSI, couples were asked to agree to the follow-up conditions of our study. These conditions include genetic counseling and agreement to prenatal karyotype analysis as well as participation in a prospective clinical follow-up study of the children. This includes completing a standardized questionnaire as described in the article by Wisanto et al. (12), returning it to the research nurse, and, where possible, visiting the Centre for Medical Genetics with the child after birth.

All couples referred for assisted fertilization were evaluated for possible genetic problems, either before starting in cases of maternal age above 35 years, positive family history or a chromosomal aberration carried by a parent, or at 6–8 weeks of pregnancy. A history, including a pedigree, was obtained in order to identify genetic risks or possible causes of congenital malformations. This history included details of medication, alcohol abuse, and environmental or occupational risk factors and socioeconomic status. A karyotype was routinely performed for the couple. In view of possible risk factors due to the new techniques of assisted fertilization and taking into account the results of prenatal diagnosis obtained in our ICSI patients, couples during the first year of our program were counseled to have a prenatal test (8,9). Patients were gradually able to be informed more precisely about the different types of risk factor and were left free to opt for a prenatal test procedure or not. Pros and cons of the different types of prenatal diagnosis were discussed in detail at approximately 6–8 weeks of gestation; amniocentesis was suggested for singleton pregnancies, and chorionic villus sampling was proposed for multiple pregnancies (13). If indicated, prenatal tests or preimplantation diagnosis for other genetic diseases were planned.

The follow-up study of the expected child was further explained: It was to consist of a visit to the geneticist-pediatrician at 2 and at 12 months of age, and then once a year. For all pregnancies, written data concerning pregnancy outcome with regard to the babies were obtained from the gynecologists in charge. Perinatal data, including gestational age, mode of delivery, birthweight, Apgar scores, presence or absence of malformations, and neonatal problems were registered. If any problem was mentioned, detailed information was also requested from the pediatrician in charge. For babies born in our university hospital, a detailed physical examination was done at birth, looking for major and minor malformations and including evaluation of neurological and psychomotor development. For babies born elsewhere, written reports were obtained from gynecologists as well as from pediatricians, and a detailed morphological examination by a geneticist-pediatrician from our center was carried out at 2 months whenever possible. Additional investigations were carried out if the anamnestic data or the physical examination suggested them.

At follow-up examination at 12 months and 2 years, the physical, neurological, and psychomotor examinations were repeated by the same team of geneticist-pediatricians. At approximately 2 years or more, a Bailey test was performed in order to quantify the psychomotor evolution of the children. Further psychomotor evaluation and social functioning will be evaluated at the age of 4–6 years. If parents did not come spontaneously to the follow-up consultations, they were reminded by phone to make an appointment.

A widely accepted definition of major malformations was used (i.e., malformations that generally cause functional impairment or require surgical correction). The remaining malformations were considered minor. A minor malformation was distinguished from normal variation by the fact that it occurs in 4% or fewer of the infants of the same ethnic group. Malformations or anomalies were considered synonymous with structural abnormality (14,15).

Results

In the group of 1987 children studied, 1072 were singletons, 816 were from twin pregnancies, and 99 were from triplet pregnancies. Of the 1987 children, 1699 were born after a cycle using fresh embryos obtained by ICSI with ejaculated sperm, 91 after ICSI using epididymal spermatozoa obtained after microsurgical epididymal sperm aspiration (including 58 with fresh spermatozoa and 33 with frozen spermatozoa), 118 after ICSI using testicular sperm, and 79 after replacement of cryopreserved embryos obtained after ICSI with ejaculated spermatozoa (Table 26.1). Of the 1987 children born, 1966 were livebirths and 21 were stillbirths (defined as fetal death $\geq$ 20 weeks or $\geq$ 400g). The stillbirth rate was 1.06% varying from 0.83% in the singletons to 1.34% in the twins. For 1951 of the 1987 children (98.2%) we had complete information at birth: For 36 children, data remained incomplete, even after several attempts to obtain the information. During the follow-up at 2 months, 1652 of the 1966 liveborn children (84.02%) were examined by one of the geneticists; 868 of the 1409 children (61.60%) who reached 1 year have so far been examined a second time at 1 year.

Overall, the mean maternal age as regards the children born was 32.4 years (range, 19.9–45.1); the mean maternal age was 32.6 years for the singleton pregnancies, 31.9 years for multiple pregnancies. The overall mean paternal age was 35.0 years (range, 25.5–64.7).

TABLE 26.1. Number of children born after replacement of embryos using intracytoplasmic sperm injection (ICSI).

	Ejaculated spermatozoa	Epididymal spermatozoa		Testicular spermatozoa	Cryopreserved embryos[*]	Total
		Fresh	Frozen			
Singleton	893	31	51 20	65	63	1072
Twin	734	18	10	38	16	816
Triplet	72	9	3	15	—	99
Total	1699	58	33	118	79	1987

[*]Transfer of frozen–thawed supernumerary embryos obtained after ICSI with ejaculated spermatozoa.

We obtained data from the physical examination at birth for 98.2% of the children. We compiled this information from the medical records as well as from careful questioning of the parents during follow-up consultations. For the children living further away, or where the parents were no longer willing to come to the clinic, detailed histories (except for one major malformation where we were given only the name of the malformation) were obtained from the pediatrician if any problem was mentioned in response to the questionnaire.

Genetic Counseling

At the genetic counseling session, we saw 1304 of the 1513 couples (86%) and concluded that there was an increased genetic risk for 557 children. This increased risk was due to maternal age (404); paternal age (9); chromosomal aberrations (27); monogenic disease (79); multifactorial disease (32), and consanguinity (7). We found 20 out of 415 (4.8%) abnormal karyotypes in the tested men and 7 out of 480 (1.5%) in the tested women. Within the monogenic diseases, CF-related problems were encountered in 61 couples, seven of whom were carriers of CF detected on routine CF screening offered for ICSI couples. Two of the couples had a 1 in 4 risk for CF, for which a preimplantation diagnosis could be offered. Half of the 18 other monogenic diseases were found in couples who came to the Centre with the request for preimplantation diagnosis for the disease at risk for the couple (Table 26.2).

Prenatal Diagnosis

Abnormal fetal karyotypes were found in 28 cases out of 1082 tested fetuses: 690 amniocenteses (AC) (15 of which were abnormal), 392 chorionvillus biopsies (CVS) (13 of which were abnormal), and seven cord blood punctures that were control samples of previous amniopunctures and were normal. No result was obtained for two amniocenteses.

Overall, the mean maternal age of the mothers undergoing a prenatal test procedure was 33.3 years (21.4–45.1); the mean maternal age was 33.5 years

TABLE 26.2. Follow-up rate of the cohort of 1987 children born.

	Ejaculated spermatozoa	Epididymal spermatozoa	Testicular spermatozoa	Cryopreserved embryos	Total
Children born	1699	91	118	79	1987
Liveborn	1680	90	118	78	1966
Stillbirth	19	1	—	1	21
Complete information at birth	1674/1699 (98.52%)	87/91 (95.60%)	117/118 (99.15%)	77/79 (97.46%)	1951/1987 (98.18%)
Follow-up at 2 months	1432/1680 (85.23%)	64/90 (71.11%)	90/118 (76.27%)	66/78 (84.61%)	1652/1966 (84.02%)
Follow-up at 1 year					868/1409 (61.60%)

for mothers undergoing AC (standard deviation 4.06) and 32.9 years for mothers undergoing CVS (standard deviation 4.08). In these 1082 tests we observed 18, or 1.66%, de-novo chromosomal aberrations: Nine of these, or 0.83%, were sex-chromosomal aberrations and nine, or 0.83%, were autosomal (trisomies and structural aberrations) (Table 26.3). Table 26.4 gives more details of the type of abnormal results, maternal age, and the outcome of the pregnancies after an abnormal result. In all, nine pregnancy interruptions were carried out after an abnormal karyotype result (5 trisomies and 4 sex-chromosomal aberrations) and one after a DNA diagnosis for fragile X, where the fetus was affected.

The Figures in Table 26.5 show that there is a statistically significant increase in sex-chromosomal aberrations (0.83%) because the 95% confidence limit of this percentage (0.4–1.7%) does not contain the percentage of aberrations (0.19–0.23%) described in the literature in a neonatal population (16,17). The increase in autosomal aberrations is partly due to the increase in trisomies, linked with higher maternal ages. On the other hand there is also an increase in structural de novo aberrations (0.46% compared with 0.07% in the literature), which is significanty higher. The number of inherited aberrations, one of which was nonbalanced, is of course higher than it is in the general population, but it was predictable for the individual couples in all but one of whom the father was carrying the structural anomaly.

It is interesting to observe that all de novo sex-chromosomal aberrations were found in cases using spermatozoa from men with extreme oligoasthenoteratospermia (concentration 0.1–4, 600,000/ml; normal morphology 0–40%; A progressive motility 0–18%) (18, unpublished observations). So far, however, there is no statistical correlation between standard semen parameters (concentration, motility, % normal morphology), and de novo chromosomal aberrations.

In a study group of 460 consecutive ICSI singleton pregnancies with AC and 360 consecutive ICSI singleton pregnancies without AC there is no statistical

TABLE 26.3. Genetic and environmental problems encountered in the genetic counseling sessions in early pregnancy for 1304 couples.

Number of couples seen at the genetic counseling session	Ejaculated spermatozoa	Epididymal spermatozoa	Testicular spermatozoa	Cryopreserved embryos	Total
No. couples	1284	69	89	71	1513
Not seen	180	10	25	6	221
Seen	1104	59	64	77	1304
(%)	(86)	(86)	(72)	(92)	(86)
Parental age at birth					
Mat. age ≥ 35 y	347	14	27	16	404
Pat.age ≥ 50 y	7	—	2	—	9
Total	354	14	29	16	413
Karyotype anomalies in parents					
Normal 46,XX	411	9	22	31	473
Abnormal (%)	7 (1.07)	—	—	—	7 (1.5)
Total	418	9	22	31	480
Normal 46,XY	347	8	17	23	395
Abnormal (%)	18 (4.9)	—	1	1	20 (4.8)
Total	365	8	18	24	415
Monogenic disease					
CF related					
CBAVD	1	24	11	1	37
CF patients (+ CBAVD)	—	2	2	—	4
CF 1/4 risk (+ CBAVD)	—	1	1	—	2
CAVD	1	8	1	—	10
epididymal agenesis	—	—	1	—	
CF carrier (− CBAVD)	2 M 5 F	—	—	—	2 M 5 F
Total	9	35	16	1	61
Other					
Adult polycystic kidney d.	3	—	—	—	3
Fra X premutation	3	—	—	—	3
Hemophilia A	3	—	—	—	3
Duchenne's muscular dystrophy	2	—	—	—	2
Huntington 1/4	2	—	—	—	2
X-linked ichtyosis	1	—	—	—	1
Myotonic dystrophy	2	—	—	—	2
X-linked retinitis pigmentosa	1	—	—	—	1
X-linked mental retardation	1	—	—	—	1
Total	18	—	—	—	18

(*Continued*)

TABLE 26.3. (*continued*).

Number of couples seen at the genetic counseling session	Ejaculated spermatozoa	Epididymal spermatozoa	Testicular spermatozoa	Cryopreserved embryos	Total
Multifactorial disease	—	—	—	—	—
Cleft lip & palate	—	—	—	—	—
RR >1%	3	—	—	—	3
RR >1%	—	—	—	1	1
Neural tube defect	—	—	—	—	—
RR >1%	4	—	—	—	4
RR <1%	6	—	—	1	7
Epilepsia	5	—	—	1	6
Diabetes type I	2	—	1	—	3
MODY diabetes	1	—	—	—	1
Bechterew	3	—	—	1	4
Manic depression	2	—	—	—	2
Schizophrenia	1	—	—	—	1
Total	27	—	1	4	32
Consanguinity					
3th	2	—	—	1	3
4th	1	—	—	—	1
5th	3	—	—	—	3
Total	6	—	—	1	7

difference in outcome measured in terms of prematurity, low birthweight, very low birthweight, or loss of pregnancy. The same findings are observed in 109 consecutive ICSI twin pregnancies with chorionic villus sampling and 174 ICSI twin pregnancies without chorionic villus sampling (19).

Neonatal Data

Neonatal measurements for 1966 liveborn children of 20 or more than 20 weeks of gestation are listed in Table 26.6. For the total group, mean birthweight was 2818 g, mean length was 47.9 cm, and mean head circumference was 33.5 cm. Prematurity (birth under or at 37 weeks of pregnancy) was observed in 11.8% of the singletons, 59.% of the twin children, and 96% of the triplet children. Birthweight under 2500 g was observed for 8.2% of the singletons, 51.6% of the twin, and 84.8% of the triplet children. Very low birthweight (under 1500 g) was observed for 1.8% of the singletons, 5.0% of the twin, and 36% of the triplet children.

Sex ratio of male-to-female is 0.98% in the total group and 0.98%, 1.39%, 0.73%, and 1 in the different subgroups of ICSI children born, respectively, after ICSI with ejaculated, epididymal, or testicular sperm or after cryopreservation.

TABLE 26.4. Prenatal diagnosis: Type of abnormal results from 1082 tests.

De novo (18) Sex chromosomes (9)	Maternal age (y)	Outcome	
45,X	37	CVS	→ TOP
46,XX/47,XXX	44	CVS	→ IUD (>40w)
47,XXX	37	AC	→ born
47,XXX	32	CVS (twin)	→ born
47,XXY	32	CVS (twin)	→ TOP/2 affected[*]
47,XXY	28	CVS (twin)	→ born
47,XXY	28	amniop	→ TOP
47,XXY	26	amniop	→ TOP
47,XYY	25	amniop	→ born
Autosomal trisomies (5)			
47,XY + 21	41	AC (twin)	→ selective TOP
47,XY + 21	41	CVS	→ TOP
trisomy 21	37	AC	→ TOP
47,XY + 21	32	CVS (twin)	→ TOP/2 affected[*]
47,XY (+ ?)		AC	→ IUD 37w.
Structural anomalies (4)			
46,XY,t(4;5)	34	CVS (twin)	→ born 28w.
46,XX,t(2;5)	30	AC	→ born
46,XX,t(2;13)	36	AC	→ born
46,XX,inv(1qh)	39	AC	→ ongoing
Inherited structural aberrations (10)			
Balanced (9)			
46,XY,inv(1)(p22p23.1)		AC	/ pat.origin
46,XY,inv(5)(p13q13)		AC	/ pat.origin
46,XX,t(14;15)		AC	/ pat.origin
46,XX,t(13;14)		CVS	/ mat.origin
46,XX, + invdup(15p)		CVS	/ pat.origin
46,XX, + invdup(15p)		CVS	/ pat.origin
45,XY,t(13;14)		CVS	/ pat.origin
45,XX,t(14;15)		AC	/ pat.origin
45,XY,t(13q;14q)		AC	/ pat.origin
Nonbalanced (1)			
46,XY,t(14;21) + 21		CVS → TOP /pat.inherited	

[*]Same pregnancy with two affected fetuses.
CVS:chorionic villus biopsy; AC:amniotic fluid puncture; TOP:termination of pregnancy.

Major Malformations

Major malformations were found in seven interruptions and in four intrauterine deaths in a total of 21 stillbirths after 20 weeks. No other malformations were detected prenatally, apart from one twin child with a holoprosencephaly detected at the age of 15 weeks of pregnancy, where the multiplicity and the

TABLE 26.5. Prenatal diagnosis on 1082 children: Abnormal results.

Type of abnormal results	Number	Percentage	95% confidence interval
De novo	18	1.66%	1.0–2.7%
Autosomal	9	0.83%	0.3–1.6%
Structural	4	0.36%	
Trisomies	5	0.46%	
Sex chromosomal	9	0.83%	0.4–1.7%
Inherited	10	0.92%	3.0–5.7%
Balanced	9	0.83%	
Nonbalanced	1	0.09%	

risk involved in a selective abortion led to the option of continuing the pregnancy. This child died at birth.

Major malformations were found in 22 out of 1063 (2.1%) singleton children, 22 out of 805 (2.7%) twin children, and 2 out of 98 (2.0%) triplet children (Table 26.7). This is 22 out of 1966, or 2.3%, of all babies born alive. If we define the malformation rate as (affected livebirths + affected fetal deaths + induced abortions for malformations) divided by (livebirths + stillbirths) the figures are: $(46 + 4 + 77) / (1966 + 21) = 2.9\%$ (Eurocat, 1993).

During the follow-up consultations of 2 months and 1 year, 10 more major malformations were detected. This gives a total malformation rate after 1 year of 56 out of 1987 or 2.8%, taking into account that not all the children had reached 1 year at the time. Investigations *psychomotor and neurological development* at the age of 1 year revealed problems in 39 children. Neurological problems were encountered in 7.2% of the premature children and in 3% of the children born at term. At the age of approximately 2 years a Bayley test was performed for 145 ICSI children, where the mean test age is above the

TABLE 26.6. Neonatal measurements in children born after the replacement of embryos using ICSI.

	Weight		Length		Head circumference	
Singleton	3220.1	±583.6	49.6	±3.1	34.3	±1.8
	(610–4970)		(31–59)		(21.5–43)	
Twin	2421.8	±518.1	46.2	±3.1	32.6	±2.1
	(520–4080)		(30–54)		(22–44)	
Triplet	1724.1	±565.7	41.4	±4.4	29.6	±3.0
	(610–3100)		(31–49.5)		(22–34)	
Total	2818.5	±720.1	47.9	±3.8	33.5	±2.3
	(520–4970)		(30–59)		(21.5–44)	

chronological age in the group of singletons, twins, and triplets. For nine children (five singletons, three twins, and one triplet) chronological age was 3 or more months more than the test age. These data will be compared with the test results in the IVF group.

Discussion and Conclusion

Although all pregnancy outcomes were registered, the data were not analyzed in this chapter. In a previous article by Wisanto, the incidence of pregnancy loss (i.e. subclinical pregnancies), clinical abortions, and ectopic pregnancies was 21.9% in the group with ejaculated sperm, 37.8% in the group with epididymal sperm, 33.3% in the group with testicular sperm, and 61.4% in the pregnancies from frozen–thawed embryos; perinatal mortality was 1.71% (20). The stillbirth rate of 1.06% observed in this study is not higher than the number reported in the literature for IVF pregnancies (21–23).

From the beginning of our ICSI treatments, nearly all patients have been seen at the Centre for Medical Genetics either before starting or at 6–8 weeks of pregnancy. Because many of our patients are living abroad, they tend to leave the country early and not to attend the *genetic counseling session*. We have still seen 86% of the couples and have concluded an increased risk (of 1/4 to 1/2) for 79 children due to monogenic disorders. As mentioned earlier in this group of the monogenic disorders a number of couples is included in our ICSI patients because they requested a preimplantation genetic diagnosis which is performed in combination with ICSI (in order to reduce the risk for contamination). For 27 children there was an increased risk due to the karyotype anomalies in their parents, most often the fathers with either sex-chromosomal aberrations or structural anomalies (4.8%). This percentage is much higher than the expected figure of 0.5% in the general population (17) and is associated with the severe male-factor infertility often present in the patient population for ICSI (24–26). The different possibilities for the offspring were explained to all the parents carrying a structural aberration, in terms of the specific chromosomal aberration and the sex of the parent: A normal karyotype is of course possible, but so is a higher

TABLE 26.7. Major congenital malformations at birth in liveborn children.

	Total	Ejaculated spermatozoa	Epididymal spermatozoa	Testicular spermatozoa	Cryopreserved embryos
Singletons (n = 1063)	22	17	3	1	1
Twins (n = 805)	22	22	—	—	—
Triplets (n = 98)	2	1	—	1	—
Total (n = 1966)	46	40	3/90	2/118	1/78
Percentage	2.3%	2.4%	3.3%	1.7%	1.3%

miscarriage rate and perhaps a lower implantation rate, which both lead to a lower success rate for the ICSI procedure, a risk of nonbalanced offspring that can be detected by a prenatal diagnosis, and a risk of transmitting exactly the same structural aberration as present in the parent. As well as being told about the risk of transmitting the same chromosomal abnormality to the offspring, which leads to greater genetic risks for the latter, parents were also informed about the possible higher risk of infertility, mainly for their male children. When indicated, a preimplantation diagnosis for sex chromosomal aneuploidy was discussed or a specific diagnosis for translocation carriers was evaluated and further discussed if technically feasible.

We think it is necessary to continue to perform parental karyotypes because for the couples with a structural aberration the general chance of success of the treatment procedure shoud be explained, as well as the strict indications for a prenatal test and the risks for the offspring. It would be of help for future counseling if chromosome analysis of spermatozoa cells was possible on a routine basis because some studies have described a higher percentage of gonosomal aneuploidy present in male with severe oligo-asthenoteratozoospermia (27), which could lead to a more differentiated way of counseling for a prenatal diagnosis. For the first 2 years, 85% of the counseled pregnant patients participated in the *prenatal diagnosis* program. At that time we were still in an experimental stage of our ICSI program and no data on prenatal karyotypes in ICSI were available beside our own. Patients had to agree to a prenatal diagnostic procedure as an entry criterion for the treatment. Now, however, we discuss our actual risk figures and can offer a free choice for testing. Under these conditions only 54.5% of the couples accept either CVS or AC. Patients also take into consideration that the increased risk of, mainly, sex-chromosomal aberrations is more acceptable because children with sex-chromosomal aneuploidies usually have a normal physical appearance and are likely to have IQs within the normal range of the population, because mental retardation, defined as an IQ less than 70, is not typically associated with sex chromosome aneuploidy. There is, however, a moderate risk of developmental problems in the areas of speech, motor skills, and learning abilities. Infertility is often present (28).

More singletons than twins were tested because parents of a multiple pregnancy were afraid of the test procedure as we counseled them to have a CVS rather than AC and attributed a higher risk (of 1%) of miscarriage to the latter during the counseling. Because a study of our group has demonstrated that there is no difference in outcome either with or without a prenatal test procedure, we shall also discuss these data with our patients in the future (19).

Abnormal fetal karyotypes were found in 28 cases out of 1082 tested fetuses, 18 of which (1.66%) were de novo chromosomal aberrations The mean maternal age of the mothers who conceived was 32.5 years, which does not explain the higher rate of chromosomal aberrations found. For a mean maternal age of 32 years we would expect a figure of approximately 0.3% chromosomal aberrations at the time of prenatal diagnosis (29,30) rather than 1.66%, including the 0.83% of sex-chromosomal aberrations. The incidence of these sex-chromosomal aberrations at the time of prenatal diagnosis is comparable with the incidence at birth (because these aberrations are not critical to survival) (16,17). The figure of 0.83% of sex-chromosomal aberrations can thus be compared with the total newborn population and is approximately four times higher than the figures of 0.19% (16), 0.2% (30), and 0.23% (17) found in an unselected newborn population. These figures are also statistically significant. The hypothesis for the higher incidence of chromosomal aberrations (i.e., that sperm from men with a fertility problem contains a higher number of gametes with chromosomal abnormalities) is now increasingly well supported (24,27,31,32). Even if data from the literature are somewhat contradictory, we may take our own observations as going in the same direction and conclude that the higher frequency of chromosomal aberrations in sperm from men with OAT is a risk factor in ICSI treatment, which in itself is the origin of the higher percentage of chromosomal aberrations observed. This might also be the explanation for the observation of a six-fold increase in de novo structural aberrations, but insufficient data on structural aberrations in sperm are available.

Ten out of a total of 1082 results (0.92%) were familial structural aberrations. These were certainly not induced by the microinjection technique because they were all detected in the infertile males (or partners) before the treatment. It was seen statistically that familial structural aberrations can lead to normal karyotypes, to exactly the same structural aberration as in the parent, or to a percentage from 0% to 50% of nonbalanced karyotypes. In this group of parents carrying a structural aberration, however, only one unbalanced fetus was found: A child with a trisomy 21 due to a paternal translocation 14.21.

Neonatal data indicate that prematurity, low birthweight, and very low birthweight are mainly due to multiple pregnancies. For singletons, the rates of low birthweight (8.2%) and very low birthweight (1.8%) are comparable to or lower than the percentages described in the IVF population in the literature (21–23), but they are still higher than in cases of natural conception. The figure of 2.3% *major malformation* rate is similar to that found in most of the *general population* national registries (33,34) and the assisted reproduction surveys (22,35–37). We have here taken the livebirth malformation rate as this is the most frequenly used, rather than a more precise calculation of the ratio, taking fetal deaths and interruptions of affected fetuses into account, which is used in only a very few malformation surveys. National registries most often register anomalies at birth or during the first week of life, whereas in this study the follow-up is carried through to 2 years; therefore, and the higher figure at the age of 1 year (2.8%) should be likened to comparable data. Belgium is one of the countries were registration for Eurocat (38) is done. In the Province of Antwerp, registered by the "Provinciaal Instituut voor Hygiene, 1997," major anomalies up to the age of 1 year were 2.28% from 1989 to 1996. This seems lower than what we found, but risk figures in the national statistics will probably also be somewhat lower because it is unlikely that malformations generally should be looked for as carefully as in this survey.

Assisted reproduction surveys have their limitations, too: Data were obtained through standard data collection forms, most often completed at birth. The children born after assisted procreation were not examined in a systematic manner and no follow-up was provided to detect congenital malformations or developmental problems, which become manifest only later. There is no system in place to check the reported results and the missing data. This explains why we expect to find malformation rates to be lower in the reported surveys after IVF than in this detailed prospective follow-up study of children after ICSI.

A few smaller studies were done to compare outcomes of IVF to natural conception, as in the study by Morin et al. (39) of 83 IVF children and 93 matched controls, where a systematic examination for 130 major and minor malformations showed no difference between IVF and the control group. In a U.S. retrospective study by Schattman et al. (40) 3.6% (11 out of 303 children) had major anomalies after regular IVF within the first year of life, attested by questionnaires (with a 68% response). These rates were considered comparable to those observed in the New York population (41). Even if only a small number of good studies on malformation rates after ART are available, it is generally accepted that there are no more malformations than there are in the general population.

We have already published a few articles on the basis of our ICSI population: A first article on 55 children born after subzonal insemination and ICSI (5) reported one child with multiple congenital anomalies. We were unable to find any difference in malformation rates between children born after ICSI in a larger but still limited group of 130 children, compared with a group of 130 children born after IVF. This observation of *2.6 % major malformations* in 1995 is comparable to the figures found in IVF surveys and some reported ICSI surveys (6,7).

In an article Kurinczuk et al. (42) provided a less reassuring interpretation of our data. Using the classification scheme from the Western Australia birth defects registry they note that many (mostly cardiac) major defects in the Belgian series had been incorrectly classified as minor. In the commentary to this article we replied that most of the minor heart defects were found by routine heart ultrasonography, and that the disproportionate numbers of cardiac malformations who all resolved spontaneously at 1 year of age and are thus minor malformations, are due to overreporting rather than to the ICSI technique itself (10). Low percentages of major malformations were observed in the different subgroups: 3.3 % (3 out of 90) in cases of ICSI with epididymal spermatozoa, 1.6% (2 out of 118) in the testicular spermatozoa group, and 1.26% (1 out of 78) in the children born after replacement of frozen–thawed supernumerary ICSI embryos. As the totals in the subgroups are still low, it is too early to conclude on any difference due to the origins of the sperm or to additional techniques, but there seems to be no particular reason for concern.

These observations should be completed by others and by collaborative efforts. In the meanwhile and before any treatment is started, patients should be informed of the available data: The risk of transmitting chromosomal aberrations, the risk of de novo, mainly sex chromosomal as well as structural, aberrations, and the risk of transmitting fertility problems to the offspring. Patients should also be reassured that there seems to be no higher incidence of congenital malformations in children born after ICSI.

Acknowledgments. We are indebted to many colleagues: The clinical, scientific, nursing, and technical staff of the Centre for Medical Genetics and the Centre for Reproductive Medicine, Hubert Joris, for his efforts in computing these data, and M.-Paule Derde for statistical calculations. Research grants from the Belgian Fund for Medical Research and an unconditional educational grant from Organon International are kindly acknowledged.

References

1. Palermo G, Camus M, Joris H, et al. Sperm characteristics and outcome of human assited fertilization by subzonal insemination and intracytoplasmic sperm injection. Fertil Steril 1993;59:826–35.
2. Van Steirteghem AC, Liu J, Joris H, et al. Higher success rate by intracytoplasmic sperm injection than by subzonal insemination. Report of a 11second series of 300 consecutive treatment cycles. Hum Reprod 1993a;8:1055–60.
3. Van Steirteghem AC, Nagy Z, Joris H, et al. High fertilization and implantation rates after intra-cytoplasmic sperm injection. Hum Reprod 1993b;8:1061–66.
4. Van Steirteghem A, Nagy Z, Liu J, Joris H, Janssenswillen C, Tournaye H, Smitz J, Bonduelle M, Devroey P. Intracytoplasmic sperm injection. Assisted Reprod Rev 1993c;3:160–63.
5. Bonduelle M, Desmyttere S, Buysse A, et al. Prospective follow-up study of 55 children born after subzonal insemination and intracytoplasmic sperm injection. Hum Reprod 1994;9:1765–69.
6. Bonduelle M, Legein J, Derde MP, et al. Comparative follow-up study of 130 children born after ICSI and 130 children born after IVF. Hum Reprod 1995a;10:3327–31.
7. Bonduelle M, Hamberger L, Joris H. Assisted reproduction by ICSI: an ESHRE survey of clinical experiences until 3 December 1993. (ICSI Task Force) Hum Reprod Update 1995b;1: May, CD ROM.
8. Bonduelle M, Legein J, Buysse A, et al. Prospective follow-up study of 423 children born after intracytoplasmic sperm injection. Hum Reprod 1996a;11:1558–64.
9. Bonduelle M, Wilikens A, Buysse A, et al. Prospective study of 877 children born after intracytoplasmic sperm injection, with ejaculated epididymal and testicular spermatozoa and after replacement of cryopreserved embryos obtained after ICSI. Hum Reprod 1996b;11:131–59.
10. Bonduelle M, Devroey P, Liebaers I, Van Steirteghem A. Commentary: major defects are overestimated. BMJ 1997;7118:1265–66.

11. Palermo G, Colombero L, Schattman G, et al. Evolution of pregnancies and initial follow-up of newborns delivered after intracytoplasmic sperm injection. JAMA 1996;276:1893–97.
12. Wisanto A, Magnus M, Bonduelle M, et al. Obstetric outcome of 424 pregnancies after intracytoplasmic sperm injection (ICSI). Hum. Reprod. 1995;10:2713–18.
13. De Catte L, Liebaers I, Foulon W, et al. First trimester chorion villus sampling in twin gestations. Am J Perinat 1996;13:413–17.
14. Smith DW. Classification, nomenclature, and naming of morphologic defects. J Pediatr 1975;87:162–64.
15. Holmes LB. Congenital malformations. N Engl J Med 1976;295:204–7.
16. Jacobs P, Browne C, Gregson N, Joyce C, White H. Estimates of the frequency of chromosome abnormalities detectable in unselected newborns using moderate levels of banding. J Med Genet 1992;29:103–6.
17. Nielsen J, Wohlert M. Chromosome abnormalities found among 34910 newborn children: results from a 13-year study in Arhus, Denmark. Hum Genet 1991;87:81–83.
18. Devroey P. Clinical application of new technologies to treat the male. Hum Reprod (Suppl) (in press).
19. Aytoz A, De Catte L, Bonduelle M, et al. Obstetrical outcome after prenatal diagnosis in intracytoplasmic sperm injection pregnancies (submitted).
20. Wisanto A, Bonduelle M, Camus M, Tournaye H, Magnus M, Liebaers I, et al. Obstetric outcome of 904 pregnancies after intracytoplasmic sperm injection. Hum Reprod 1996;11(suppl) 4:121–29.
21. Rizk B, Doyle P, Tan SL, et al. Perinatal outcome and congenital malformations in in-vitro fertilization babies from the Bourn-Hallam group. Hum Reprod 1991;6:1259–64.
22. Bachelot A, Thepot F, Deffontaines D, et al. Bilan FIVNAT 1994. Contracept Fert Sex 1995;23:490–93.
23. Lancaster P, Shafir E, Hurst T, Huang J. Assisted Conception Australia and New-Zealand 1994 and 1995. AIHW National Perinatal Statistics Unit sydney. 1997.
24. Moosani N, Pattinson HA, Carter MD, et al. Chromosomal analysis of sperm from men with idiopathic infertility using sperm karyotyping and fluorescence in situ hybridisation. Fertil Steril 1995;64:811–17.
25. Van Assche E, Bonduelle M, Tournaye H, Joris H, Verheyen G, Devroey P, Van Steierteghem A, Liebaers I. Cytogenetics of infertile men. Hum Reprod 1996;11:25–26. In: Van Steirteghem A, Devroey P, Liebaers I, editors. Genetics and assisted human conception. Oxford, U.K.: Oxford University Press.
26. Vogt P. Genetic aspects of artificial fertilization. Hum Reprod 1995;10(Suppl 1):128–37.
27. Bernardini L, Martini E, Geraedts J, et al. Comparison of gonosomal aneuploidy in spermatozoa of normal fertile men and those with severe male factor detected by in-situ hybridisation. Mol Hum Reprod 1997;3:431–38.
28. Linden MG, Bender BG, Robinson A. Intrauterine diagnosis of sex chromosome aneuploidy. Obstet Gynecol 1997;87:468–75.
29. Ferguson-Smith M. Prenatal chromosomal analysis and its impact on the birth incidence of chromosomal disorders. Br Med Bull 1983;3:355–64.
30. Hook E, Hamerton J (eds). Population cytogenetics: studies in humans. New York: Academic Press, 1977:63–79.
31. Hoegerman S, Pang MG, Kearns W. Sex chromosome abnormalities after intracytoplasmic sperm injection Letter to the editor. Lancet 1995;346:1095.

32. Pang M, Zackowski J, et al. Detection by fluorescence in situ hybridisation of chromosome 7, 11, 12, 18, X and Y sperm abnormalities in of an in vitro fertilization program. J Assist Reprod Gen 1995;12:OC 105, 1995.
33. Office of Population Censuses and Surveys. Mortality statistics: perinatal and infant (social and biological factors) Nos 18 and 20, 1985 and 1986 London: HMSO (OPC series DH3), 1987–88.
34. National Perinatal Statistics Unit and The Fertility Society of Australia (1992) IVF and GIFT pregnancies, Australia and New Zealand. Sydney National Perinatal Statistics Unit (NPSU) 1990.
35. Beral V, Doyle P. Report of the MRC Working Party on children conceived by in vitro fertilization. Births in Great Britain resulting from assisted conception, 1978–87. Br Med J 1990;300:1229–33.
36. Lancaster P, Shafir E, Huang J. Assisted conception Australia and New Zealand 1992 and 1993. AIHW National Perinatal Statistics Unit Sydney. 1995;1–71.
37. Medical Research International, Society for Assisted Reproductive Technology (SART) and The American Fertility Society. Assisted reproductive technology in the United States and Canada: results generated from the American Society for Reproductive Medicine/Society for Assisted Reproductive Technology Registry. Fertil Steril 1992;64:13–21.
38. Lechat MF, Dolk H. Registers of congenital anomalies: Eurocat environ heath persect 1993;101:153–57.
39. Morin NC, Wirth FH, Johnson DH, et al. Congenital malformations and psychosocial development in children conceived by in vitro fertilization. J Pediatr 1989;115:222–27.
40. Cohen J, Schattman G, Suzman M, Adler A, Alikani A, Rosenwaks Z. Micromanipulating human gametes. Reprod Fertil Dev 1994;6:69–83.
41. New York State Department of Health. Congenital malformations registry annual report. Statistical summary of children born in 1986 and diagnosed through 1988. 1990.
42. Kurinczuk J, Bower C. Birth defects conceived by intracytoplasmic injection: an alternative interpretation. Bonduelle M, Devroey P, Liebaers IA, Van Steirteghem A. Commentary: major defects are overestimated. BMJ 1997;7118:1260–66.

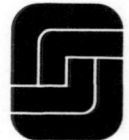

27

Ethical Dilemmas in Assisted Reproduction

Francoise Shenfield

Introduction

There are a plethora of ethical dilemmas in assisted reproduction: There is no doubt that the status of the embryo, the subject of 3 days of debate at the Council of Europe in December 1996 (1), is at the core of most concerns because of what it represents symbolically—life itself from syngamy (for Catholics for instance), or the potential for a person (2,3). In either case it is an entity worthy of respect (4), even though terminology appeared to have been used in order to defuse the strong emotions raised by related issues to assisted reproductive techniques, in particular research and the fate of spare embryos, when the term preembryo was coined (5).

Nevertheless, as a practitioner, the duty of care both toward the patients and the future child (with the responsibility involved and possible conflicts) is often our first consideration because we have a duty to respect the patients (often a couple), and the respect of their autonomy, which could be in conflict with our duty to their potential offspring. Finally, we do not practice in a vacuum, but at societal level, and the interface between ethics and law is a symbol of what any society, preferably democratically, at any point in time, has deemed is the appropriate compromise between often clashing principles.

As it is impossible to cover all ethical dilemmas in the field even in books dedicated to the subject (6), selected topics in the context of andrology and the treatment of motility disorders will be discussed. Because intracytoplasmic sperm injection (ICSI) has already replaced several indications for (gamete) sperm donation, the new issues raised by the technique should be discussed, while alluding to the already well-thrashed-out issues in sperm donation. I shall also discuss preimplantation diagnosis as it represents both a new technique and a challenge in ethical terms, taking us back to the status of the embryo, which has led to so many debates at the core of assisted reproduction issues. It is indeed one of newest the tools available in prenatal diagnosis, a subject that must be discussed in the context of the genetic anomalies described in ICSI, without forgetting.

Finally, in the wake of the publication in *Nature* of the Dolly (7) experiment, which has led to so much debate worldwide in relation to the field of reproduction, the arguments involved will be laid out for further scrutiny of the relevance to the ethical core of our arguments.

The Specific Example of New Techniques in Andrology: ICSI and a Few Words about DI

In 1992 the Brussels Free University Center for Reproductive Medicine reported the first pregnancies and births after a novel procedure of assisted fertilization [i.e., intracytoplasmic sperm injection (8), which is the direct injection of a single spermatozoon into the cytoplasm of the oocyte by means of micromanipulation procedure]. This has transformed the outlook for many cases of male infertility, but it also raises new ethical questions in that there is at least a theoretical possibility of transmitting a risk of infertility to a male child (9,10) as well as association in some cases of bilateral vas agenesis with cystic fibrosis mutations. Counseling of the candidate couples, screening of candidate-fathers, and longitudinal follow-up of the babies born have become key issues in the treatment. With regard to informing and counseling the future parents, the general ethical dilemmas concerning genetic screening and information have been well rehearsed (11). The debate has also been revived (12). More concerns follow the actual birth of the child from new techniques in that both (responsible) parents and practitioners face the arduous decision whether to observe and follow up those born of the new techniques. This epitomizes the difficulty of singularizing without discriminating. This close follow up is the result of the concern to avoid a higher prevalence of anomalies than what exists in natural conceptions. The whole debate about eugenics then raises its ugly head because of the historical connotations of the word. I shall only briefly mention the debate here, because it is worthy of a whole book itself.

Several problems arise as far as the children are concerned: The length of time the follow up may be necessary entails an invasion of the privacy of the family concerned. Furthermore, the more mature the children, the more inappropriate it becomes to perform any test or observation with the consent (or dissent) given by their parents, and not by themselves. The psychological aspects are intricate and they demand sensitive handling, which legislation may not always portray, although the opportunity for counseling is mandatory in English law (13).

Before the introduction of ICSI, male factors of extreme severity were palliated by DI. There are still instances where there is no alternative, but severe OAT can certainly be treated with ICSI, where the only obstacle is sometimes a financial one. This, of course, is a fundamental question of justice and access to health care (14), and it would be interesting to know the hard facts and figures of how finances influence the choice that couples have to access appropriate treatment, which we can only surmise for the time being in the United Kingdom. In France, where both treatments are encompassed within the national health care system, the number of DI cycles per year has been decreasing, and that of IVF/ICSI cycles has been increasing. The other ethical dilemmas, particularly in the sphere of payment of donors, anonymity, selection of donors, and recipients have been well rehearsed and subject to many debates that revolve around respect of the person symbolized in the noncommercial profit from donation (15) and actually enshrined in the European Convention for Bioethics (16). Secrecy of the procedure and the consequence to the future family, as well as anonymity of the donors with the possible effects for the child and family relationship, have also led to several debates, with different attitudes enshrined for instance in Swedish legislation (17) which requires sperm donors willing to reveal their identity to the mature child, and the French legislation, which makes anonymity compulsory. There is little hard evidence concerning the consequences of these opposed attitudes for the children for now, and it seems reasonable to leave the parents to decide in privacy how they will fulfill their responsibility to their DI child while awaiting any evidence that may be published later (18).

Techniques at the Cutting Edge of Assisted Reproduction, from the Actual to the Fantastic

In this section we will discuss a current practice—preimplantation diagnosis—even though it is seldom used (to date, less than 100 healthy children born at the latest report, 19); and one that has made perhaps more headlines than any other in reproduction before—cloning.

Preimplantation Diagnosis

If one accepts the premise that it is ethical to perform embryo research (20), and study the embryo in vitro, then the most complex ethical question is what might be the consequences of its evolving techniques, not so much the current practice. There is no forceable upper limit to the number of genes that will be accessible to evaluation on one or two blastomeres.

The serious dilemma in the carer–patient relationship concerns the reluctance most practitioners would feel when faced with a parental request to sort out, at the time of preimplantation diagnosis for severe genetic disease, embryos also carrying genes associated with diseases that although serious, are amenable to treatment, like diabetes or cardiovascular disease. The problem is different if the request concerns the BCRA1 gene or Huntington's chorea, which are conditions for which no efficient therapy exists. The same concerns have long burdened all those involved in the decision of performing therapeutic terminations of pregnancy. There has not been an established list of "proper reasons" for which a practitioner may in his or her conscience accept the request of a patient to terminate a pregnancy within the legal grounds of the national legislation. The terms of the 1967 English abortion Act, as modified by the HFE Act 1990, offer a good example of this (21).

The semantic problem regarding the definition of a "serious" (potential) handicap, even though it is different from extreme conditions at birth that entail such suffering as to make then "unbearably so awful," which is a jurisprudential term used in court (22) in cases of selective nontreatment, leads us to question further the gray area between prevention of handicap, avoidance, and eradication. For the time being, the majority of preimplantation diagnosis has been performed for embryos at risk of cystic fibrosis.

Will couples demand, after preimplantation diagnosis, the assurance of a "perfect" baby? This fear was stigmatized by Testard and Sele (23), who discuss the "production of survivors of this choice, escapees and obligatory servants of an ideology of performance and exclusion" with the danger of exclusion of handicapped people, and "a more and more restrictive definition of normality and humanity."

Eugenics is defined by its focus on population, however, and not on an individual couple's choice to reproduce or not when faced with a high chance of having a child with a serious anomaly. Indeed the spirit of the French legislation that forbids "practices" (24) reflects this postulate.

Indeed, this accusation of "eugenics," with the emotionally laden connotations that relate to the European history, alluded to in the U.S. report on cloning ["a path which humanity has treaded before for its everlasting shame," (25)] is a topic that has also been an argument in the condemnation of human cloning by the European GAIEB report on cloning, and to which we shall return.

Cloning

The application, either theoretical or fantastic, of the somatic cloning that resulted in the birth of (*Nature*) Dolly the sheep to the human has arguably been the most eventful mediatic event at an international scale, even in one which has been replete with headlines in the last few years (26,27).

All over the world powerful political figures like the French and U.S. presidents asked national ethical committees to address the issue (25,28); parliaments, both national (like the British Parliament, where questions were answered) and international (like the European Parliament), convened special meetings and asked august bodies to reflect or to pronounce on the implications of this experiment, which was only successful to the tune of 1 in 277.

The questions raised by this successful somatic nucleus transfer into an enucleated oocyte cytoplasm are ethically numerous. Charged words like *human dignity* and *respect* have been the matter of arguments in the pages of *Nature* (29), and it has been a renewed pretext to condemn assisted treatments in general and the debasement of the embryo for the prolife lobby (30). Scientists are aware that the achievements of this experiment may be a model for learning more about somatic cell differentiation, the possibility of targeted cell types of value in transplantation (skin, blood, perhaps neuronal tissue), the development of transgenic animals, and the preservation of endangered species (31), but we will only comment here on the ethical implications of the possible application to the human.

Various responses show an array of concerns. For instance, in the United Kingdom, the physics Nobel prize winner, Joseph Rotblat, voiced his fears in the Guardian, of the incipient "danger of a mass destruction of humankind" by eugenic selection (32). The chair of the Human Fertilization and Embryology Authority (HFEA) stressed to the parliamentary commission on science and technology that cloning of human embryos is illegal, and that all embryo research is submitted to the HFEA because it has to fall within five allowed categories. Another legal interpretation is that while the intention of Parliament was to ban human cloning, the Act only applies to techniques known in 1990 (33). Technical precision may also be harmful to the application of the law, and it may be more useful to stay in the general principle, rather than to forbid a specific technique soon to be scientifically modified and not within its remit any more. This is precisely why current argument is about the wording of the UNESCO Declaration on the Human genome, and the insertion of Article 11 (34).

The democratic British machine started rapidly, with a report of the Parliamentary Commission for Science and Technology. Even though it found the notion of creation of identical human beings shocking, the summary of the debates of the commission distributed to the press March 20 (31) stresses that the real or imagined dangers of the method described by Wilmut et al. occulted the meaning of this exceptional achievement, but the commission nevertheless suggests an amendment of the law specifically to forbid the creation of experimental human beings and of cloning in general. It also stressed that the HGAC was created in December 1996 in order to study the scientific developments in genetics—their ethical, social, and economical consequences—and it is starting to reflect on somatic cloning. Ethical aspects were specifically covered in the several reports published by autumn 1997. The distaste of the majority for the creation of organs reservoirs by cloning is an example of the infraction of the Kantien precept that insists that a person is treated as an end and not as a mere means. The several reports, however, differed in the emphasis of the argument used. The CCNE (28) report to the French president starts with the caveat that personal (including psychological) identity and genetic identity are not to be confused; however, it also stresses that the technique would totally disrupt the relation (or balance) between genetic and personal identity. The argument of dignity is underlined, in relationship to the unicity of the individual. It also criticizes the importance of the genetic as determinant of the person at the end of the century while highlighting the fact that a clone would not be totally identical to the adult donor of the nucleus because of the recipient cytoplasm bearing the maternal mitochondriae. Thus, the notion of unicity, even though it is necessary, is not sufficient to justify the quasiuniversal rejection of the planned replication of human beings. This is why we must add the consideration of the social dimension of the individual, and where we return to the notion of responsibility, both as interpersonal as described by Levinas (35) ("la responsabilite est initialement pour autrui"), and in a social and universal dimension, as understood by Hans Jonas.

The U.S. Nat Bioethics Commission (25) stated the potential for physical harm, the threat to individuality, and the effect of cloning on the family, with the undesirable attitude to children, as well as, finally, the eugenic concerns. In conclusion it is deemed to be the matter of public policy—this report is only the beginning of the public process.

At the European level (36) GAIEB (group of advisers to the EU on the ethical implications of biotechnology) states logically that as there is no discrimination against twins per se, so it follows that there is no per se objections to genetically identical human beings; human reproductive cloning is unacceptable on the grounds of risks (*responsibility* is underlined), instrumentalization, and eugenics. One would have to be wary of the danger of lowering genetic diversity. As far as the human applications are concerned, it distinguishes between reproductive and nonreproductive (research), as well as nuclear and replacement and embryo splitting. It is limited at the in vitro phase (i.e., as a research tool), as in the possible development of stem cells cultures for repairing organs. As all research, the objectives are essential in analyzing the ethical quality.

Finally, a resolution of Council of Europe (37) is similar to that of the GAEIB, but it is much stricter concerning human cloning, which is also forbidden as a research activity. Article 13-b of the Convention on Human rights and biomedicine proposes the following addendum: Any intervention seeking to produce genetically identical human individuals in the sense of individuals sharing the same nuclear gene set.

Conclusion

When society feels strongly about a matter with moral implications, it may be translated into law. The danger, beautifully expressed by Dickens, is that "the urge to use law to enforce moral conclusions may be pursued at too heavy a cost to the health of the moral sensitivity and judgment the law was intended to promote" (38).

On a hopeful note, however, there is an observable trend to widen the debate at societal level. UNESCO, the Council of Europe, and groups in the United Kingdom, have all declared their will to inform society at all levels, and they have enshrined this in declarations that show a powerful amount of good will.

It is in this spirit that this chapter, despite being addressed to an enlightened audience, has been written. Our common responsibility goes beyond our personal duties to patients: It is also one of responsible citizens to broaden the debate of this essential ethical issues to all.

References

1. Shenfield F, Sureau C. Report on the status of the embryo conference at the Council of Europe, December 1996, Focus in reproduction (European Society for Human Reproduction and Embryology newsletter, Tarlatzis B, editor) May 1997.
2. Comite Consultatif National d'Ethique pour les Sciences de la vie et de la Sante (1984–1991), Avis concernant l'embryon, 1986 and 1990, Avis relatif aux recherches sur les embryons humains in vitro, et sur les recherches soumises a un moratoire depuis 1986, Centre de documentation et d'information d'ethique, 101 rue de Tolbiac, 75 654 Paris Cedex 13.
3. Davis v Davis (1992) 842 S.W. 2d 605, Supreme Court of Tennessee: Reid CJ, Anderson, Daughtrey, Drowota and O'Brien JJ. In: Kennedy I, Grubb A, editors. Frozen embryos: legal status, disposition and control, Davis v Davis. Med Law Rev 1993;1:273–78
4. Great Britain Department of Health and Social Security, Warnock M. Report of the Committee of Inquiry into Human Fertilisation and Embryology. London: HMSO, 1984: Cmnd 9314.
5. Jones HW, Schrader C. And just what is a pre-embryo? Fertil Steril 1989;52: 189–91.
6. Shenfield F, Sureau C, editors. Ethical dilemmas in assisted reproduction. London: Parthenon, 1997.
7. Wilmut I, Schnieke E, McWhir J, Kind A.J, Campbell, KHS. Viable offspring derived from fetal and adult mammalian cells. Nature 1997;385:810–13.
8. Palermo G, Joris H, Devroey P, Van Steirteghem AG. Pregnancies after intracytoplasmic injection of a single spermatozoon into an oocyte. Lancet 1992;340:17–18.
9. Patrizio P. Intracytoplasmic sperm injection (ICSI): potential genetic concerns (1995);10:2520–22.
10. Meschede D, De Geyter C, Nieschlag E, Horst J. Genetic risk in micromanipulated assisted reproduction. Hum Reprod 1995;10:2880–86.
11. Nuffield Council on Bioethics, Genetic Screening, Ethical Issues, December 1993, 23 Bedford Square, London WCI 3EG.
12. Pauer HU, Hinney B, Michelmann HW, Krasemann EW, Zoll B, Engel W. Relevance of genetic counselling in couples prior to intracytoplasmic sperm injection. Hum Reprod 1997;12:1909–12.
13. Human Fertilisation and Embryology Act 1990. London, HMSO.
14. Shenfield F. Justice and access to fertility treatments. In: Shenfield F, Sureau C, editors. Ethical dilemmas in assisted reproduction. London: Parthenon, 1997:7–14.
15. Shenfield F, Steele SJ. A gift is a gift is a gift, or why gametes donors should not be paid. Hum Reprod 1995;10:253–55.
16. Convention for the Protection of Human Rights and Dignity of the Human Being with Regard to the Application of Biology and Medicine: Convention on Human Rights and Biomedicine, 1996. Directorate of Legal Affairs, DIR/JUR (96) 14, Council of Europe, Strasbourg.

17. Daniels K, Lalos O. The Swedish insemination act and the availability of donors. Hum Reprod 1995;10:1871–74.
18. Shenfield F, Steele SJ. Information to the children of assisted reproduction. Hum Reprod 1997;12:393–95.
19. Harper JC. Preimplantation diagnosis of inherited disease by embryo biopsy: an update of the world figures. J Assist Reprod Genet 1996;13:90–95.
20. Shenfield F, Sureau C. Ethics of embryo research. In: Shenfield F, Sureau C, editors. Ethical dilemmas in assisted reproduction. London: Parthenon, 1997:15–22.
21. Abortion Act 1967, as modified by the Human Fertilisation and Embryology Act 1990. London: HMSO.
22. Templeman LJ. re B. In Kennedy, Grubb. Medical law, text and materials. London: Butterworth, 1989:951.
23. Testard J, Sele B. Towards an efficient medical eugenics: is the desirable always the feasible? Hum Reprod 1995;11:3086–90.
24. Lois nos 94-653 and 94-654, Journal officiel, 29-7-94, relative au respect du corps humain et relative au don, Assistance Medicale a la Procreation et diagnostic prenatal.
25. National Bioethics Advisory Committee. Report on cloning to President Clinton, Washington, USA, 1997.
26. "Double trouble" but cloning does not herald the end of humanity. *The Times*, February 1997.
27. Winston R. The promise of cloning for human reproduction. Br Med J 1997;314:913–14.
28. Shenfield F. Quelques reflexions d' Outre Manche concernant le clonage. Les cahiers du Comite Consultatif National d'Ethique no 13, October 1997:16–17.
29. Harris J, Kahn A. Is cloning an attack on human dignity and cloning, dignity and ethical revisionism (letters). Nature 1997;387:320.
30. Shenfield F, Lord Alton of Liverpool. Interview on BBC World service, 13 November 1997.
31. Fifth Report of the Parliamentary Committee for Science and Technology on Cloning, HC 373-II, session 1996–1997. London: The Stationary Office, 1997.
32. Scientists 'able to create human clones.' *The Guardian* 26 February 1997:6.
33. Grubb A, Walsh P. I want to be alone, Letter from the Centre for Medical Law and Ethics, Kings College, the Strand, London. Dispatches spring 1997;7:1–6.
34. UNESCO. Human genome declaration. Paris, November 1997.
35. Levinas E. In: Fondements philosophiques de l'ethique medicale. Paris: Suzanne Rameix, Ellipses, editions marketing sa, 132–33.
36. GAIEB Report to the EU on cloning, May 1997, DG12, rue de la Loi, Bruxelles.
37. Comite Directeur pour la Bioethique (CBDI), Council of Europe, November 1997.
38. Dickens B. Interfaces of assisted reproduction, ethics and law. In: Shenfield F, Sureau C, editors. Ethical dilemmas in assisted reproduction. London: Parthenon, 1997.

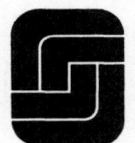

Author Index

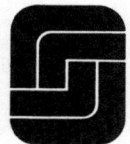

Subject Index

PROCEEDINGS IN THE SERONO SYMPOSIA USA SERIES

Continued from page ii

PROCEEDINGS IN THE SERONO SYMPOSIA USA SERIES

Continued